OVERCOMERS OUTREACH

OVERCOMERS OUTREACH
A Bridge to Recovery

BOB & PAULINE BARTOSCH

© 1994, 2009, 2014 by Overcomers Outreach, Inc. and Bob and Pauline Bartosch. All rights reserved.

© 2004 by Bob and Pauline Bartosch, Founders, Overcomers Outreach

No part of this publication may be reproduced, stored in a retrieval system, or transmitted in any way by any means—electronic, mechanical, photocopy, recording, or otherwise—without the prior permission of the copyright holder, except as provided by USA copyright law.

All rights reserved. Written permission must be secured from Pauline Bartosch to use or reproduce any part of this book, except for brief quotations in critical reviews or articles, in any form or by any means—whether electronic, mechanical, photocopy, recording, or any other means.

The Twelve Steps and other quotes from A. A. literature (as noted) are reprinted with permission of Alcoholics Anonymous World Services, Inc. Permission to reprint this material does not mean that AA has reviewed or approved the contents of this publicaton, nor that AA agrees with the views expressed herein. Nor is AA in any way affiliated with Overcomers Outreach. AA is a program of recovery from alcoholism only—use of the 12 Steps and excerpts that appear throughout this publication in connection with programs and activities that are patterned after AA, but that address other problems, does not imply otherwise.

Requests for permission to use portions, or for purchase of this book, may be directed to the author:

> Pauline Bartosch c/o Overcomers Outreach
> 6528 Greenleaf Ave., Ste. 223
> Whittier, California 90601
> Overcomersoutreach.org

Unless otherwise noted, all Scripture passages quoted are from *The Living Bible*, © 1971 Tyndale House Publishers Inc., Wheaton, IL 60189. All rights reserved. Used by permission.

Scripture references marked KJV are taken from the *King James Version* of the Bible.

Library of Congress Cataloging-in-Publication Data

Bartosch, Bob and Pauline Overcomers outreach: a bridge to recovery / Bob and Pauline Bartosch

p. cm. Includes bibliographical references. ISBN 1-929753-18-7 1. 12-step groups—history of 2. Recovery movement—history of 3. Christian recovery organization—Overcomers Outreach—history of 4. Addictions and compulsions—recovery from, religious teachings 5. Alcoholics Anonymous—unaffiliated adjunct groups I. Title

Printed in the United States of America

ISBN 13: 978-0-578-14133-6
Library of Congress Catalog Card Number: 2009903973

The book is dedicated in loving memory to four of God's most dynamic Overcomers who helped pioneer the Christian Recovery Movement before anyone knew what it was:

>Bob Bartosch
>Wally Starr
>Jess Maples
>Al Southern

These four shining beacons are now celebrating their salvation and sobriety in the presence of our Highest Power, Jesus Christ. The completion of the third edition of this book would definitely put a smile on their faces.

Robert H. Bartosch
12/31/27–12/26/06

Bob Bartosch, perpetually jolly and larger than life, is now with the Lord! How he loved Jesus and welcomed each day with gusto! Before dawn he would bounce out of bed, make coffee, and prepare to dash off to his first stop, the local 6:30 A.M. meeting of Alcoholics Anonymous. For the last thirty-three years of his life he was embracing sobriety and "getting high" on life, thanks be to God and this incredible twelve-step program.

Although Bob was originally a ministerial student, he had no conception of the specialized work God eventually had in mind for him. After working in the life insurance business for decades, Bob became known as a pioneer in the Christian recovery field, touching many with his own testimony of God's power. Ultimately, the ministry of Overcomers Outreach became the vehicle that multiplied successful recovery in literally thousands of lives around the world.

Each and every day Bob would spend time in personal prayer, especially for his family and multitude of friends. How he loved his church. His rich baritone voice would resonate as he sang praises to God. He took great pleasure in making the world laugh, and was best known for his vast repertoire of jokes, usually delivered at a moment's notice. Tagged the "king of huggers" by his three sons and nine grandchildren, he would invariably reach out to anyone who might need a quick embrace or a joke!

After a delightfully busy December playing Santa Claus, Bob went to be with Jesus the day after Christmas 2006. He is with our Savior today, and has probably organized the first Overcomers Outreach Celebration Meeting for the many program people who preceded him through the Pearly Gates. Someday we will join him, singing praises to God for His mercy and grace on life's amazingly wild ride while here on planet earth.

—Pauline Bartosch

CONTENTS

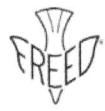

Biblical Description of an Alcoholic xi
Acknowledgments xiii
Foreword: *By Stephen F. Arterburn* xv

Preface: The Power of Pain xix

PART I: BEGINNINGS
1. Beyond Recovery into Discovery 1
2. An Incredible Journey of Hope 5
3. The Founders: Bob's Story 11
4. The Founders: Pauline's Story 27
5. Bridging the Gap 47
6. Birth of a Ministry 57

PART II: FROM THE PROFESSIONALS
7. From the Pastor: Heart—Mending as the Church's Task 79
   By Anthony L. Jordan, D. Min.
8. From the Physician: Healing Body, Mind, and Spirit 87
   By Willard E. Hawkins, M.D.

9. From the Psychologist: 12-Step Programs
   Make My Job Easier 95
   By Earl R. Henslin, Psy.D.

PART III: CHANGED LIVES: OVERCOMERS SHARE THEIR EXPERIENCE, STRENGTH, AND HOPE

10. Fatal Attraction: My Love Affair with Ethyl 107
    By Jack J.
11. Don't Quit Before the Miracle Happens! 115
    By Debbie K.
12. Food Was My Life 121
    By Doris R.
13. Skeptical Attorney Finds His "Higher Power" 125
    By Mike H.
14. Addicted to Lust, Alcohol, and Drugs 129
    By Bill R.
15. Dealing with My Husband's Sexual Addiction 137
    By Lindsey E.
16. A Preacher's Kid Overcomes Drug Addiction 147
    By Larry W.
17. Her Master Plan 151
    By Ruth W.
18. Drug Addict Set Free to Serve Jesus 155
    By Robin S.
19. From Black Magic to the Power of Christ 161
    By Bernard M.
20. Jesus, My Leaning Post in Recovery 169
    By Philip B.
21. Such an Addict! 173
    By Jeff M.

22. A Biker Freed from Bondage 179
    By Jerry C.
23. Our Son's Addiction Led to Our Recovery 183
    By Pat M.
24. New Life Without Alcohol 191
    By Vern A.
25. Only by His Grace—Only for His Glory 195
    By Rolf P., Germany
26. Antics of an Escape Artist 201
    By Peggy M.
27. Freedom from Fear 205
    By Al A.
28. There Are No Coincidences 211
    By Christa B.
29. Stuffed Feelings Added Pounds 217
    By Loraine W.
30. A Workaholic Gets a New Heart 223
    By Kim G.
31. Addict Encounters "Amazing Grace" 229
    By Don T.
32. Riding High with the Hell's Angels 235
    By Jay S.
33. Gambling Away My Dreams 239
    By Wayne D.
34. The Relapse Roller Coaster 243
    By Mike F.
35. My Daily Bread Almost Killed Me! 249
    By Lynn B.
36. Workaholism Is a Lonely Business 253
    By Duke V.

37. The Patchwork of My Life 261
    By Frances H.
38. Nightmare to Miracle 267
    By Mary Jean B.
39. Spending It All 271
    By Jim S.
40. Christian Nurse Needed Her "Fix" 275
    By Phyllis H.
41. From the Heart of an ACA 281
    By Bob Noonan
42. Those Other Meetings 287
    By Bill D.
43. Lucky 291
    By Jess Maples

PART IV: OVERCOMERS OUTREACH SUPPORT GROUPS: A CHRIST-CENTERED PROGRAM OF DISCOVERY

44. The Heart of Overcomers Outreach 295
    The 12 Steps, 12 Traditions and View of our Higher Power
45. The 12 Steps Come A-L-I-V-E in the Scriptures 309

APPENDICES:

Appendix A: Overcomers Outreach Publications 331
Appendix B: International Ministry 333
Appendix C: Referrals for Recovery 335

Endnotes 339

BIBLICAL DESCRIPTION OF AN ALCOHOLIC

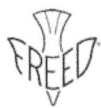

"Whose heart is filled with anguish and sorrow?
Who is always fighting and quarreling?
Who is the man with bloodshot eyes and many wounds?

It is the one who spends long hours in the taverns, trying out new mixtures.

Don't let the sparkle and the smooth taste of strong wine deceive you.

For in the end it bites like a poisonous serpent; it stings like an adder.

You will see hallucinations and have delirium tremens, and you will say foolish, silly things that would embarrass you no end when sober.

You will stagger like a sailor tossed at sea, clinging to a swaying mast.

And afterwards you will say, 'I didn't even know it when they beat me up....

Let's go and have another drink!' "

—Proverbs 23:29–35 (TLB)

ACKNOWLEDGMENTS

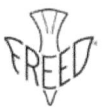

This book was originally compiled by:
Bob and Pauline Bartosch, Founders,
Overcomers Outreach
with the assistance of:
R. Duncan Jaenicke, Editor and Publisher, First Edition
Elfie Neber
Stephen F. Arterburn
and especially all the Overcomers
who put their remarkable stories into writing.
This third edition of OO's big book has become a reality
due to the professional assistance of
Jeffrey MacLeod, OO's executive director and
Julie Martin, the third edition's preliminary editor.
With heartfelt gratitude to Robert D. Winter and other donors
who provided generous gifts toward the
Bob Bartosch Memorial Fund, making this project possible.

"Cheer up, for I have OVERCOME the world!"
—John 16:33b

Thanks be to God!

FOREWORD

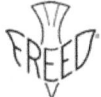

I first heard of Overcomers Outreach on a beautiful day while traveling, ironically enough, through the wine country of Northern California. *How significant,* I thought as I traveled through the vineyards on my way to one of the alcohol and drug treatment centers I managed, *that today of all days I would hear two rare and clear voices who expressed my own frustrations about recovery and the church.* Listening to the *Focus On The Family* radio program as its host, Dr. James Dobson, interviewed Bob and Pauline Bartosch, I realized that they could be part of God's plan to build a bridge from the church to the recovery world.

Over the past fifty-plus years, recovery had become so secularized that the Person of Jesus Christ was rarely a topic of conversation or object of devotion—even though He, we firmly believe, is the "Higher Power" who enables so much change in millions of lives around the world. Unfortunately, by delivering a message of condemnation rather than a message of hope and healing, the church had alienated many who needed to recover. Sadly, most of those in the church who are recovering are seldom open about it, fearing that they will be judged and rejected by their fellow believers because of their moral weakness. It occurred to me that there needed to be a bridge that could bring Christ into recovery and, conversely, bring recovery back into the church. Through the radio airwaves that day, I heard the first sounds of hope that this bridge could be built.

OVERCOMERS OUTREACH

Since that first chance encounter, I have come to know the Bartosches and the foundations upon which Overcomers Outreach (OO) has been built. Today I know that no two people have done more to build that biblically-sound bridge between the recovery movement and the church than Bob and Pauline Bartosch. The strength of that bridge grows greater with each day that a new Overcomers group is started in a church or community center.

This bridge is sorely needed because of a gross misuse of 12-step recovery programs and a deep fear of many in the church of any program that talks of recovery and the 12 Steps. Ironically, these steps and the recovery process itself began with alcoholics helping each other stay sober. They are based on biblically-based principles like acceptance, confession, honesty, accountability, and service. According to Dr. Bob S. and Bill W., founders of Alcoholics Anonymous, these principles were gleaned from the Sermon on the Mount, 1 Corinthians 13, and the book of James, among other passages. The principles were developed into 12 Steps that have helped and offered hope to more addicted and abused people than any other program.

Although Christ was at the center of the 12 Steps' development, He was not overtly mentioned in them, so as not to alienate either agnostics or those of other faiths. In an effort to attract more people into sober living, what was done was to genericize the reference to deity, referring to God instead as the "Higher Power." Sadly, this became a dilutive factor, as many abandoned the search for the God of the Bible and instead sought to construct gods to their own liking. Although there were many who already were Christians recovering in AA and many unbelievers moving beyond AA to find Christ, some church leaders unfortunately backed away from 12-step support groups, seeing them as competition to the church, offering good feelings on earth rather than eternal life in heaven.

The way church leaders saw it, the church had a simple solution for the eradication of alcoholism: their commands to "not drink" seemed to make sense and be obviously sufficient. Their motives were good—wanting to follow God in the path that seemed to them to be right—but their actions unfortunately were not very helpful. The mistake they made was in only understanding the beverage alcohol and not the condition of alcoholism. They did not realize there was, in addition to the spiritual battle for the soul of the alcoholic, a physical battle that leads to an addiction so powerful that all the power and money in the world cannot counter its grip.

FOREWORD

What was needed was God Himself, revealed in flesh and blood through caring arms wrapped around those in despair, helping them break free from the addiction trap. Alcoholics didn't need more guilt (which only increased the need to drink); they didn't need more sermons (the ones they silently preached to themselves out-shamed any sermon from a church pulpit). What they did need were people who cared enough to spend time with them, cared enough to hold them accountable, and cared enough to be there when the individual finally decided it was time to get well. As the church's lack of concern and understanding alienated alcoholics, thankfully AA groups were there for them—literally saving their lives in many cases. Millions found the answer outside of church while the church refused to look at their attitudes and actions toward addicts.

Others, who were not alcoholics, but struggled with codependency, sexual abuse, depression, and eating disorders, came to discover the hope found in working the 12 Steps and began attending recovery groups. They saw the Steps as a 12-point sermon that could be successfully applied every day.

As more people were finding hope from secular recovery groups outside the church, there were Christians in recovery inside the church who were starting to be heard. Their voices were crying out for a new understanding of the 12 Steps and of those who could benefit from them. Finally, in the late '70s and early '80s, churches began to open new doors to hurting people. These doors opened to the basements and annexes of churches where people could find support and hope from recovery groups with Christ at the center. Some church leaders—those with wisdom—came to see 12-step groups as a way to attract people to the church, rather than as a force eradicating the need for salvation through Jesus Christ.

Overcomers Outreach has done more than any other group to assist with the construction of the bridge (and in its subsequent maintenance and repair) between recovery programs and the church. Its groups have been established in communities around the world, bringing recovery from past hurts to people and discovery of a loving God so full of grace that He sent His Son to save each person, no matter how difficult or horrible his/her past. While encouraging ongoing attendance at meetings outside the church, where honesty continues to be of great value, Overcomers Outreach groups offer the greatest hope for Christ-centered recovery that is healthy and balanced.

OVERCOMERS OUTREACH

The book you hold in your hands is a true miracle, one I have prayed for for some time. It reflects the handiwork of God as He has moved through the OO program to change myriad lives. I heartily recommend it to you.

If you have been in a recovery group where Christ was either never mentioned or was brought up inappropriately by someone with toxic faith, you will be delighted at the healthy way in which Christ is incorporated into Overcomers Outreach groups. Within this book you will find the biblical principles that form the foundation of the group meetings, and the powerful testimonies of recovery from those who attend. While no one can recover for you, this book can assist you in finding strength and hope once you have made the decision to change. If you want to know if God is real and relevant to your recovery, you will find the answers right here, within this large and expanding connection that extends from the reality of our world to our hope for eternity.

—Stephen F. Arterburn
Founder and Chairman, New Life Clinics
Laguna Beach, California

PREFACE: THE POWER OF PAIN

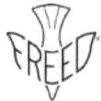

Life wasn't meant to be easy, yet we human beings continuously attempt to use our ingenuity to try to disprove this simple truth. In an age of designer drugs and pharmaceutical fixes, many of us refuse to endure even the slightest hint of pain, whether it be physical or emotional. In fact, the media has brainwashed us with the delusion that pain should not be even a small part of lives. We view pain as the enemy—one that must be quickly subdued and anesthetized with drugs, alcohol, pills, food, work, religiosity, sex, gambling, television, the internet, computer games, shopping-'til-we-drop, or merely by attempting to take care of other people's problems so that we don't have to look at our own.

One of our dilemmas is we have come to expect that all of our desires must be fulfilled immediately. This myth can totally sabotage our serenity; we can get tangled in a web of perpetual unrest, almost accepting this anxiety as a normal state, as long as we can get a quick fix from our favorite mood-altering chemical or compulsion. Life in the fast lane does not allow for delayed gratification. We find ourselves looking for ways to soothe away life's inevitable disappointments, and especially the hurts of the past that haunt us from time to time.

Often, we continue to escape life's realities in this way until we lose touch with the truth about ourselves and become totally immersed in denial. As a general rule of thumb, we have found that about ten percent of the U.S. population who drink alcohol will eventually become alcoholics. In a church population (due to the guilt factor, mainly), more like 25% of people who drink will eventually cross over an invisible line into addiction. Usually, our compulsions sneak up on us when we least expect it. Our love affair with alcohol, drugs, or other substances or compulsions, which may have comforted us so effectively in the past, can literally turn on us and bite like a snake!

Even though we find it hard to believe (and would never admit it because of denial), at that point we have become powerless. The door of addiction slams shut with a resounding "clang." We are caught in a disease of body, mind, emotion, and soul. As depressive thoughts start to close in on our minds in such a dependent state, we may come to believe that we will be in bondage for the rest of our lives, because we have unsuccessfully tried so many times to stop. The good news is that this downward progression is not necessarily our guaranteed fate—the stories in this book are proof of that.

Yet along the route to recovery, we may mask our pain with an accumulation of things in a controlled effort to look good to our friends, both inside the church and outside. Some of us schedule constant activity or entertainment so that we won't have to face our reality, but the trouble is we eventually run out of things to do. Finally, some of us who got tired of running away from ourselves turn to the Bible for a fresh look at the truth. Jesus said, "I have told you all this so that you *will* have peace of heart and mind. Here on earth you will have many trials and sorrows; but cheer up, for *I have overcome the world*" (John 16:33, emphasis added).

Those of us who overcame life-threatening addictions will be the first to say that it was pain that finally brought us to our knees. Though we had medicated it many ways, pain eventually proved to be God's gift to us—indicating that something was very wrong and that we needed help from outside ourselves. Many of us who finally surrendered to that pain and need in our lives found hope and healing through the discovery of the 12-step programs of recovery: e.g., Alcoholics Anonymous (AA), Al-Anon, etc. And no wonder—it wasn't long before we realized that those 12 Steps originated in the Scriptures!

The encouraging news is that we can not only overcome through the power of Christ and the 12 Steps, but we can also live abundant lives of joyful celebration if we're willing to give up our anesthetizers and rely upon Him. Jesus also said, "...you will know the truth, and the truth will set you *free*" (John 8:32, emphasis added).

The truth is we are greatly loved by our "Higher Power."

PREFACE: THE POWER OF PAIN

As Christians who have found hope, we invite you to forsake denial and go ahead and walk through the pain with God by your side, taking advantage of the other sources of help He has provided. God works in a thousand different ways, so it is wise to keep an open mind regarding His methods of healing. We really don't have to figure it all out; He knows much better than we do what is best for us. We're the ones who have messed up our lives with our own methods of fixing them. Our methods haven't worked! We need to become honest, open, and willing to follow His direction.

Why did we compile this book? Its primary purpose is to serve as a strong scriptural support base and positive network for thousands of Overcomers all over the world who can identify with and profit from the miraculous stories recorded by other Overcomers.

It is also intended to keep building bridges between people in 12-step programs and those in the church. Many people from both perspectives find it difficult or even impossible to talk about their recovery program and their personal faith all in the same breath. Somehow, a wide gap still exists in their minds. Recovering people in traditional groups, though sometimes skeptical, are still looking for the link between their religion and their 12-step program. Out of fear of judgment or lack of understanding from their peers, some have given up on their church altogether and cling to their recovery group for their only spiritual sustenance. In addition, some Christians in recovery still hesitate to make the traditional 12-step support group an integral part of their lives, fearing that these groups may compromise their faith, or not be spiritual enough, because they don't overtly name Jesus as Lord. They find themselves straining to hear about their own personal struggle with addiction in their Bible study or Sunday school group at church, sometimes feeling very lonely, isolated, or simply different from their friends.

Our message to people who have never found Christ as their "Higher Power," or have been hurt by the church (and are therefore running in the opposite direction), or who have resisted the available help offered by traditional 12-step groups in the community, is that the program of Overcomers Outreach helps marry your faith with your recovery program. The vital link is in the person of our "Higher Power," Jesus Christ. It has been demonstrated time and time again that recovery enhances one's Christian faith, making it come alive. By the same token, a personal faith in Christ adds a whole new powerful dimension to one's recovery. Those who discover this "marriage" become double winners, both in this life and in the life to come.

OVERCOMERS OUTREACH

The most important thought at this point is that there is hope after all—no matter how bad it's been. It really is possible to emerge from the other side of this dark tunnel of the unknown into a brand new life of celebration and discovery, taking life one day at a time.

Jesus stands quietly, waiting to heal us, if we will only let go of our lives and let Him do it.

—**Bob and Pauline Bartosch**
Founders, Overcomers Outreach

PART I
BEGINNINGS

1

BEYOND RECOVERY INTO DISCOVERY

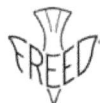

Webster's dictionary tells us that *recovery* is "the act of getting something back, restoration to any lost state, as health."[1] Yet the definition of recovery does not even begin to describe the awesome new life that God has provided for those of us who had once utterly given up in the pit of our despair. After surrendering to His will we were granted a whole new life we never could have imagined!

In contrast, we as Overcomers feel the word *discovery* more adequately describes what is happening to us. Webster's says that discovery is "the act of discovering, or that which is brought to light or knowledge."[2] That sounds more like what our Savior, Jesus Christ, is causing to happen in our recovery.

It is exciting to watch countless individuals and families not only get into recovery, but move one step further into a "discovery mode," discovering who God is in the person of His Son, experiencing His great love for us, and encountering an entirely new dimension of living. We are among all people most blessed because we have found that it is OK to be powerless, as long as Christ becomes our "Higher Power."

Overcomers come from all walks of life but share a certain camaraderie, a unique common bond that is difficult to describe to those who cannot identify with the crushing crises we have weathered and survived. In nearly every instance, we knew what it was like to come crashing to the bottom in our lives and completely give up hope. When God intervened and gave us the fresh, new beginning we never expected, no one was more surprised than we!

Those of us whose lives have been miraculously turned around and freed from addictions or compulsions as a direct result of Overcomers Outreach and a 12-step program are very grateful to God. Psalm 116:6–12 reads: "...I was facing death and then He saved me. Now I can relax. For the Lord has done this wonderful miracle for me. He has saved me from death, my eyes from tears, my feet from stumbling. I shall live! Yes, in His presence—here on earth! In my discouragement I thought, 'They are lying when they say I will recover.' But now what can I offer Jehovah for all He has done for me?"

In our overwhelming gratitude, we found that we dared not be quiet about what God had done. Just as AA's founders discovered healing in the giving away of their stories, Christians in recovery no longer desire to hide or cover up as they had before. We quit being people pleasers and began to experience new dimensions of healing by being honest with ourselves and with others. We are learning to celebrate each new day and to carry the message to those who are still suffering. We no longer wage our battles alone, but are surrounded by the loving support of our new recovery family who truly understands because they've been there too. God has put a remarkable support system in place.

Today, our journey of discovery comes in manageable one-day-at-a-time segments and what an adventure life now is! As humans, of course we fail, but now when we do, we know that it isn't the end of the world. An entire new set of attitudes and goals characterizes our lives. No longer are we filled with the remorse of yesterday or dominated by fears about tomorrow. Just for today we make the positive choice to live in serenity, sober and abstinent, with God's help. We no longer need to blame someone else for our condition, but we are learning to take responsibility for our own actions. It is not our desire to control anyone else but to turn them over to God and set our own focus on the Lord. We no longer feel compelled to react to those around us, but instead we can choose to release them to their own choices with love. We don't have to retaliate when others hurt us. In fact, we've found that holding a grudge can threaten the very sobriety or serenity we treasure. Today, we don't have to be perfect, because life is all about progress rather than perfection.

Discovery is all about making our journey with our best friend and "Higher Power," Jesus Christ, by our side. It's about facing each day with anticipation instead of dread, and making a point of being good

BEYOND RECOVERY INTO DISCOVERY

to ourselves even in small ways. It's about giving ourselves choices in every circumstance: Plan A, Plan B, etc. We learn to live our own lives, with our eyes focused on Christ, and we turn other people over to His almighty care.

God changes our hearts so that it becomes possible to forgive others and ourselves, just as He has forgiven us. We begin to set healthy boundaries. We begin to live without guilt because Christ has forgiven our sins on the cross. We let go of shame because He's paid the price and has granted us a new life, whether we deserved it or not.

Living in discovery means putting first things first and keeping it simple. It's about admitting when we are wrong. It's about taking life step by step and doing the next indicated thing, instead of getting all riled up about trying to solve our whole life's problems at once. It's letting go of anger, expressing it when we need to, in healthy ways, but refusing to harbor it within our souls. It's forsaking the shroud of fear that has engulfed us and living in the light of His loving presence. We find that the more we give away of ourselves, the more we receive.

At first, this new way of processing our thoughts may seem utterly impossible. How can we change so radically after all we've been through? What if we don't really want to change, but just wish to stop our addiction or compulsion? Those of us who have experienced the miracle of recovery cannot totally explain how it works. All we know is that God can do for us what we are powerless to do for ourselves.

Discovery is experiencing God's joy and having it spill over to those around us. It's celebrating the fact that we're still alive and feeling more alive than ever before! Though we were once chained to our problems, addictions, or compulsions, or could have easily been locked up in a real prison, today we are happy, joyous, and free!

How can we get well? By becoming Honest, Open and Willing to surrender to God's will for us. This means giving up our wills and trusting God. This means going to 12-step meetings and more meetings! And this means becoming accountable to a sponsor and others traveling the discovery road with us.

What we thought was the end of our world—that crushing pain that brought us to our knees—turned out to be only the beginning of a new world for each of us. God can take our wreckage and put the pieces back together again, only this time, the pieces fit much better than they did before! He arranges them into a beautiful picture that reflects both His love and a lifetime of discovery if we'll only trust Him.

2

AN INCREDIBLE JOURNEY OF HOPE

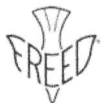

When Jesus Christ was here on earth, He was particularly compassionate toward people who were suffering from physical ailments. He healed people around Him using many different methods. He seemed to take special joy in healing those who were blind. In some cases it took merely a touch or even just a word from Him to produce instant healing or deliverance.

One of the stories in the New Testament describes a man who had been blind since birth (John 9). In this instance, Jesus used a very strange method to bring healing: He spat on the ground, made a lump of mud from the mixture of dirt and spit, and smoothed it over the man's blind eyes. Then He told the man to take the next step toward his healing, instructing him to go wash in the Pool of Siloam. As soon as he took this step of faith, the man could see!

Curiously, following this particular blind man's healing, the Pharisees (the church leaders of the day) did everything they could to cast doubt upon this miracle. They contended that not only was Jesus an impostor, but He had broken the law by working (healing) on the Sabbath Day. So how could this healing possibly be valid?

The healed man avoided any entanglement with such legalistic questions, and simply responded to the Pharisees: "...I know this: I was blind, and now I see!" (John. 9:25). When Jesus spoke with the healed man afterwards, He said, "I have come into the world to give sight to those who are spiritually blind and to show those who think they see that they are blind" (John 6:39). Obviously, our Higher Power, Jesus Christ, works in a million different ways to heal us, too. How could we possibly presume to impose our puny limits on the Creator of the Universe? As Scripture tells us, "There are many ways in which God works in our lives..." (1 Cor. 12:6).

Paths to recovery from addictions and compulsions are no exception. If anyone wishes to take issue with the particular method He uses to bring healing to those of us in Overcomers Outreach, we, like the blind man, should only have one reply: "Once I was powerless over (insert your addiction or compulsion here) and my life was unmanageable. Today, God has restored my spiritual eyesight, and I am in recovery! Once I was blind, but now I see!"

Overcomers are Christian men and women whose eyes have been opened, defying all odds. Many of us were at one time in secret bondage to our emotional wounds, which we attempted to medicate in a variety of ways. We had lost all hope, because no matter how hard we tried to deny it, we were still held captive by those recurring problems and could not get free in our own strength.

Some of us were strangled by alcoholism or drug dependency. Others of us were held tightly in bondage to eating disorders, gambling, or sexual addiction. Some of us were raised in alcoholic or dysfunctional homes, causing painful memories to surface and our whole world to be distorted.

Those of us who are spouses or family members of the addicted or compulsive persons began to center our lives around the erratic behavior of our addict or alcoholic, and in valiant but vain attempts to fix them, we became codependent. We were obsessed with our loved ones, and tried our best to control or change them. In our own denial, we tried hard to excuse, cover up, or rationalize their behavior. In our countless attempts to calm the troubled sea of our lives and gain control, we bailed them out, time and time again. These methods seemed to work for a while, but when we failed repeatedly and our loved one just got worse, we felt it was our fault.

Perhaps we had come from fine, upstanding Christian families and never dreamed these types of problems would—could—ever occur in our lives. Yet we found that as Christians we were not immune from addictions, compulsions, and shameful family problems. When they did occur, we found ourselves making an extra effort to hide them. We disguised our pain and secret despair behind plastic smiles, which turned out to be dark cloaks of denial. We valiantly tried to be lone rangers and to manage our chaotic lives using our own remedies——vitamins, exercise, more Bible reading, and especially agonized prayers for deliverance.

Every time we looked into a mirror, we despised the dismal eyes that gazed back at us, abhorring the stranger we had become. We really didn't want to reveal our true identity to anyone else because we were so ashamed. Yet, even though we were full of self-loathing, our pride always seemed to come first, and we felt it necessary to protect our image. Sometimes we found ourselves protecting the very bottle or substance that kept us sick. If someone threatened to take our magic potion away, we panicked, subconsciously picturing our minds and bodies disintegrating on the spot.

In one sense we seemed to have a problem we couldn't solve and wished to hide, yet on the other hand, it was our firm belief that our substance or compulsion seemed to temporarily keep our heads together. How could we exist in our crazy world comfortably without our stabilizers? How would we be able to cope?

This was the delusion that ruled our minds: we were convinced that our chemicals or compulsions were actually our best friends. If our loved ones became suspicious of our bad habits or deteriorating condition, we always assured them that we could stop anytime we wanted to. We tried hard to believe this ourselves, but inwardly we had doubts, because we had tried too many times to stay clean, sober, or abstinent, and it hadn't worked for long. We were secretly terrified and filled with guilt, but were not about to let anyone know it.

So before we could get well, each of us had to come crashing down until we hit bottom, usually in the midst of a painful crisis. Frequently, our crisis occurred after we tried every single method we could think of to stop on our own and get our lives under control. Just like switching brands of liquor to one we could supposedly handle, we traded one obsession for another. We were afraid that our friends or family would discover the private nightmare in which we were existing. Or perhaps we were quite alone, and everyone of significance had abandoned us in utter disgust because of our bizarre behavior or repetitious problems. Even then, it was still too difficult to admit defeat until we were morally and spiritually bankrupt.

Whether we were one of the afflicted (i.e., the addicted person) or the affected, (i.e., the loved one of the addicted person), we concealed our hurting inner selves in an effort to live victorious Christian lives. Many of us attended church regularly, perhaps even sang in the choir or taught a Sunday school class. Outwardly, we displayed a cheery composure, giving the impression that we had it all together. In the midst of our facade, however, we somehow lost track of the basic truth about ourselves. Frightened at our own loss of control, we manufactured excuses and covered up our pain as best we could.

As addicted, born–again Christians, at one time we made a decision to accept Jesus Christ as our Savior. With thankful hearts we believed that His death and resurrection assured us of the cleansing of our sins and the promise of eternal life. At that point in time, some of us seemed to be instantly delivered from our addictions or compulsions. Many of us remained free the rest of our lives; others felt quite strong for a while, but after weeks or months, we found ourselves hanging on for dear life. White–knuckling it became our normal condition. We could always be found gritting our teeth and clenching our fists in an effort to stay sober.

In such a state, we battled fear that we might slip and fall back into those dreaded addictions and compulsions that had gotten us into so much trouble in the first place. Sometimes we even forgot how much trouble they had caused. Many of us relapsed over and over again. Other times, we didn't actually take up our old habits but substituted other addictions. Even worse, we often tried to use willpower to cure our ills, and we only ended up with rigid irritation, stark hypersensitivity, and a jittery sense of unrest. In this state of mind, peace was nowhere to be found and we felt terribly alone.

We were baffled. If Christ had redeemed us, why weren't we experiencing a sense of victory? Our continuing bondage to alcohol, drugs, or other crippling compulsions ravaged us with crushing guilt and shame, yet we felt certain that we, of all people, should know better. In our shame, we went about building more walls of denial, thus keeping ourselves in a state of self-perpetuating turmoil and defeat.

Whatever we did, we could never seem to get it right; our faith seemed inferior to others', only confirming our feelings of despair and inferiority. As much as we tried, we couldn't sweep the cobwebs out of our souls or find the strength to put a stop to those sins that "so easily beset us" (Heb. 12:1, KJV). Instead, our lives were lived contrary to our belief systems, causing an inner conflict that never ceased.

In one breath, we clung to our Christian faith, uttering thousands of prayers asking God to remove our pain while wondering why He didn't seem to answer our agonized pleas, and in the other, we felt that because of our sin, we probably deserved to be abandoned by Him. Sometimes we were angry at God, since He had seemingly deserted us.

Somehow, we didn't fit in anymore with our church friends. We were ashamed to share our true condition with them, feeling sure they would never understand. They might reject us, judge us, offer us their well–meaning advice, or even worse, express pity for us (the ultimate put-down). There was always that gnawing sense of never measuring up, no matter how controlled or serene we tried to appear. We felt imprisoned by our secrets as they loomed large and ugly within our souls. Even if we did get honest, we got the feeling that the church had become a kind of country club for saints, and that the club members would just as soon have people like ourselves either become invisible or find another place to worship. Though our search was largely unsuccessful, we were desperately looking for a hospital for sinners like ourselves.

12-STEP GROUPS

In a last desperate attempt to get help, we tried attending traditional 12-step groups and found to our astonishment that we were totally accepted there without having to make any explanations. In fact, the people there displayed a genuine love and caring that we had seldom experienced before, even in church. We found that quite a number of the recovering people we met had something we didn't have—serenity. Not only that, they were winning over their addictions! (This was very embarrassing for us as Christians, who were supposed to have it all together.) Was this the "hospital for sinners" we had been searching for?

Twelve-step group meetings were comprised of all sorts of people. As Christians, most of us had been clinging to our faith throughout our ordeal of defeat, carrying an extra load of guilt because of our own failures. Others had a faith in God at one time, but had fallen away. Also present in these meetings were agnostics, people who questioned the existence of God or the possibility of knowing Him.

Our common problem was that we needed help and were not able to generate it on our own. Many of us began to form honest, healthy relationships for the first time. These new 12-step friends talked about a "Higher Power" and "God as we understood Him."

We began to witness what an almighty God could do when an individual would turn his or her life and will over to His care, no matter whether it was a church 12-step group or a so-called "secular" support group! The miracles that were happening in people's lives in these traditional 12-step groups were too powerful not to notice.

We were profoundly affected by witnessing these miracles, not only in ourselves, but in the lives of some of the most unlikely people around us. We started to understand that these miracles became possible because these people had literally been brought to their knees in brokenness, resulting in total surrender to "God as they understood Him." We began to question: Was it because these people gave up their control with complete abandon that God was willing to step in and take control? We pondered these things in our hearts, reflecting back with deepest gratitude upon how God stepped into our lives once we finally "let go."

As we considered these thoughts, seeds were being planted in our hearts that eventually led to our founding Overcomers Outreach.

3

THE FOUNDERS: BOB'S STORY

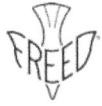

BY BOB BARTOSCH
1927–2006

Even though my story is related to alcoholism, the struggle, pain, and eventual healing are all similar to the experience of anyone caught in addictive/compulsive bondage.

I had my first experience with alcoholism as a young boy growing up in the Baptist church. It was a church of several hundred members and served as the evangelistic center for our community. I'll never forget my impression of a man in our congregation who would come to church drunk. We could count on him to go forward whenever an invitation to accept Christ was given. Each time he did, we would get our hopes up that he would change for good, only to be disappointed when he went back to drinking. Little did I dream that some years down the road I would find myself in this same predicament. Alcoholism is indeed "cunning, baffling, and powerful."[1]

I had been raised in a wonderful Christian home. My mother had been a missionary to Cuba in her younger days, before marrying my father. Both my parents were in their forties when I was born and as an only child, I was spoiled rotten. My mom and dad would do just about anything within reason to fulfill my wishes. We didn't have a lot of material things, but that has never been important in my life. I can remember little things, like my dad driving several miles out of his way so I could go on a pony ride. I really believe their whole life centered around their little son. I only mention this because I know many people do not have such fond memories of their childhood. Some had alcoholic parents or were abused in one way or another. It's easy to blame the past for the trouble we get into later on. A sentence from the AA "Big Book" says it best, "So our troubles, we think, are basically of our own making."[2] I couldn't agree more; even with an ideal childhood, we can lose control of our lives as adults.

Even though I was raised in the church, my parents never tried to force their belief system on me. At the age of twelve, I made up my own mind about which religious path I wanted to follow. After hearing a gospel message about how Jesus died for my sins, I made a personal commitment to Jesus Christ, accepting Him as my Lord and Savior. I'm sure it was childlike faith, but after all, that is what God wants from us. To this day God has never left me, although I have certainly wandered from Him on many occasions. I guess that's why the biblical story of the prodigal son is so meaningful to me. No matter what we do, God is always waiting with open arms to welcome us back home.

As a young person, I became very involved in church activities. On a typical Sunday I could be found in Sunday school, the morning worship service, the young peoples' meeting, and the evening service. I loved church and wanted to learn all I could about God and about His Son, Jesus Christ. It's not surprising that at the age of fifteen I jumped at the opportunity to go away to a Christian high school. I can remember my father crying as I left to travel across the country to attend school. I was so self-centered that I had no understanding of his feelings. My father was a very hard-working man, but my mother was the spiritual leader of our family, and I sensed I was carrying out her wishes in my decision about schooling. I'm certain my parents had no idea of the dysfunctional situation into which their son was heading.

For many people, high school days were filled with laughter, football games, proms, etc. Some got into trouble as they began sowing their oats in adolescence. I too remember a few fun times, but in looking back, what stands out is the list of crazy rules I was forced to accept. I'm not talking about the clear guidelines for living that God has specified in the Bible; I'm talking about man-made rules. Breaking one of the school's rules would result in demerits that could lead to being expelled. We were not allowed to attend movies, listen to certain types of music, or play cards. Any physical sensation stronger than an itch was considered a sin. We

THE FOUNDERS: BOB'S STORY

were instructed not to pray for Billy Graham, because his theological position was not exactly the same as that of the founder of the school. The rules about dating mandated that fellows could only take a girl to a school lounge, (resembling a furniture store filled with couches and armchairs), and could only talk to her with a chaperon seated close by. Holding hands was considered almost as bad as premarital sex!

I bought into this system hook, line, and sinker. The underlying message was that I didn't need to think—I could let the leaders of the school do that for me. I decided that feelings must be bad, so if a feeling or emotion came up I just repressed it. Since you shouldn't speak about any subject in a way that differed from the official party line, I simply went along with this insanity.

Looking back, the thing that I am the saddest about is my own lack of discernment. I didn't realize how these experiences would affect me later in life.

I graduated from high school in 1945 in the midst of World War II and joined the Navy. I don't have any interesting "war stories" because I wasn't assigned to a ship. The war was winding down, and after boot camp I was sent to one of the separation centers to help with the typing and clerical work in discharging sailors. One of the reasons I even mention my brief Navy career is that this was the first time I had been away from home and in a non-Christian setting. I had many opportunities to drink and get into the partying scene, but I didn't. My home was only a few miles from the base, so when I was given a pass, I always associated with my church friends.

You can probably guess what happened after I got out of the Navy. I returned to the same Christian school and enrolled in their college. I majored in Bible and minored in history. In spite of the legalistic rules, I seemed to thrive in that sheltered atmosphere. I didn't have to make any decisions because they were all made for me.

While in college I had my first exposure to jail, but not in the way you may think. On Saturdays a bunch of guys and I would pile into someone's car and head for a small town that had a jail. Loaded down with gospel tracts (short evangelistic booklets), we set out to save all the drunks in the world. If there weren't any drunks in the jail, we would head for the nearest pool hall, where we would try and preach to anyone who would listen. We usually got kicked out of the pool hall, so then we would set up a meeting on the street corner. Although some people were reached for Christ in this manner, we probably turned more people off than on

OVERCOMERS OUTREACH

to God. Since I had not had my first drink at this point, I had absolutely no concept of what alcoholism was all about. As far as I was concerned, it was just a matter of willpower, and all that those tavern and pool hall people needed to do was shape up and stop drinking. As I found out later, it's not quite that easy.

The year 1950 was a big one for me. Not only did I graduate from college, but the most important event of the year happened on September 22: Pauline and I got married. God gave me an absolutely wonderful wife, even though some of our friends said our marriage wouldn't last six months (since I had dated most of Pauline's friends and couldn't seem to settle down in a serious relationship). Little did we know what God had planned for us.

We soon settled into a tiny apartment in the Los Angeles area, and I continued my education at Fuller Theological Seminary in Pasadena. During the second year of graduate school, our eldest son Bobby was born, and when he was just five months old I began to have trouble feeling comfortable in my school program. Although Fuller is a fine school, at that time in my life I don't think I was ready for the degree of intellectual and spiritual freedom they offered; I was too accustomed to being spoon-fed at the legalistic school where I had done high school and undergraduate work. That seemed to be my only security. I was convinced that it was the only place in the world that had a handle on the truth. So, with a 28-foot travel trailer hitched behind our little Plymouth Club Coupe, we casually waved goodbye to our bewildered parents and headed cross-country again.

During our first few weeks back at my heaven on earth, I had an unfortunate series of legalistic experiences that caused me to want to leave there, too. Certain concerned faculty members and alumni questioned the integrity and practices of some of the school's leadership. When a fellow alumnus asked me for my opinion, I had to admit that I agreed with a few of their concerns. In so doing, I took a tremendous risk, because we had been taught to report anyone to the administration who disagreed with the party line. Sure enough, someone felt compelled to report my rebellion, and I soon received a letter in the mail informing me that I was no longer welcome on campus. I had spent six years of my life (two in high school and four in college) at this institution, and now I was informed that I had been blacklisted. I was deeply hurt by this unjustified action, but following my usual pattern, I tried to stuff these feelings, and as a result, I became bitter and vindictive towards the institution.

THE FOUNDERS: BOB'S STORY

So, once again, we decided to move and headed for my new job as manager with Fuller Brush Co. in Charlotte, North Carolina.

I want to emphasize that the disillusionment with my alma mater is not the reason I became an alcoholic, but it helped set the stage in my rebellion toward God and the values I had been taught as a youth. I said to myself, *If this is what Christianity is all about, who needs it?*

So on a particularly warm, sunny afternoon when I was twenty-four years of age, in a spirit of rebellion, I made the choice to pull into a drive–in restaurant and order my first bottle of beer. Talk about guilt! I was doing something against the teachings of my parents, my church, and the (albeit dysfunctional) school I had so faithfully attended. As I drank that beer, I began to relax, and my problems didn't seem nearly as big. I didn't particularly like the taste, but the effect was wonderful. A couple of drinks did something for me that a whole case of soda pop just couldn't do.

During the next ten years, Pauline was busy giving birth to and raising our three sons, while I was busy becoming a social drinker. I could take it or leave it. I didn't drink on a daily basis, but in times of stress I always knew that I could have a couple of drinks and feel better. In those early years it never failed. There were times when I might overshoot the mark and wake up the next morning with a hangover, but even then I would weigh the fun I had the night before with the minor pain of a hangover and it seemed worthwhile.

I well remember that when we moved back to California after the death of Pauline's father, we used to frequent a little bar called Paddy's Pad. It was a rather sleazy hangout with a pool table and sawdust on the floor, where you could buy a pitcher of beer for about a buck. Paddy's had a bulletin board on which we would place announcements for parties we were going to have at our home the following weekend. By this time, I had developed a tremendous tolerance for alcohol. I could drink more than anyone at the party and then drive my inebriated friends home with no problem at all. At the time, I looked on this as a real sign of manliness. Now I realize that my great tolerance for alcohol should have been a warning sign to me that something was very wrong.

I have to honestly say that during those early years I had a lot of fun with alcohol. At the time, I thought booze was the solution to my problems, rather than the *problem*. When I drank I felt more at ease with other people; alcohol worked wonderfully as a social lubricant for me. We had a small ski boat, and I would spend time with my wife and sons water skiing. Alcohol became a big part of those trips and today I realize it's miraculous that I didn't get my family into any serious accidents because of my drinking.

About ten years down the road, the difficulties really began. Many times I would drink more than I had intended and would make a complete fool of myself in front of my family. My behavior became unpredictable; I had wide mood swings and would promise to go somewhere with my family and then at the last moment change my mind. It must have been very confusing for them. On occasion, I promised myself that I would stop drinking entirely. I would keep my promise for a week or two but would gradually start drinking again, telling myself that I would "watch it this time." I made promises that I really wanted to keep but was unable to. Alcohol had me firmly in its grip.

There is one incident that I would rather not write about, but I need to share it in all honesty. Although I was never arrested for D.U.I. (driving under the influence), I should have been many times. I was never in an alcohol-related accident, but on one occasion I came close to wiping out my entire family.

Our whole family had been visiting my cousins. Red Mountain wine flowed liberally that night, and I had been drinking more than my share. Although I was in no shape to drive, I decided that I could make it the few blocks to our home. When I came to the main thoroughfare, I made my left turn onto the wrong side of the divider. Instantly, all three boys jumped onto the floor of the back seat. Pauline grabbed the steering wheel, stepped on the brake and brought the car to a stop, straddling the curb diagonally, barely clearing the rushing cars on either side.

Pauline shouted at me to get out of the car, and then she drove us the rest of the way home. I was furious with her, feeling that she had deliberately humiliated me. To prove my point, I slapped her. I think this was the only time in our marriage that I behaved in such a manner. I'm just thankful that Pauline had the presence of mind to intervene in that nearly fatal situation.

When I finally realized that alcohol had become a big problem in my life, I decided to get help. With my background in the church, I naturally went to that source first. My pastor knew of my theological training, and when I shared my drinking problem with him, he told me to go home, read the Bible, and pray. That sounded good to me. So I did as he suggested. When the withdrawals from alcohol began to manifest themselves, the only logical solution was to have another drink. My

THE FOUNDERS: BOB'S STORY

pastor was well-meaning but saw my problem only from a spiritual point of view, thereby overlooking the physical as well as emotional aspects of the disease of alcoholism. He offered me no practical ways of combating my problem.

Since I still needed help, the next person I approached was my family physician. I was in sales at the time, and when he asked what my problem was I told him the truth, but not the whole truth. I explained that I was under a lot of stress because of my work. The solution he had was a little pill called Valium. For the next several weeks and months I would continue to drink and then take my Valium, never realizing how close I had come to ending my life! Now I know that combining these two drugs increases the effect nine-to-one over the effect of the drugs separately; death is common when they are used together. I don't fault the doctor, because I wasn't totally honest about how much I was drinking. (I'm not even certain that knowing my alcoholic consumption would have changed his prescription, but I'll give him the benefit of the doubt.)

During the time that I was contacting ministers and doctors, my problem continued to get worse. I couldn't understand why I wasn't able to quit of my own accord—after all, I thought I was in control of most other areas of my life.

By then my marriage was breaking up, and I had been kicked out of the house, but in my gross denial I didn't even associate my alcoholism with my marriage problem.

I was devastated when Pauline asked me to leave. I packed a few clothes and rented a room in a cheap motel. Ironically, I ended up in room #13. The cockroaches must have been having a convention while I was living there. It was very unpleasant. I looked for other living quarters and finally rented a small bachelor apartment. I went to the local grocery store and bought some TV dinners, small shrimp cocktails, a couple of cans of peanuts, and bottles of scotch and vodka—all the essentials of good nutrition! When I returned to my apartment, I discovered that there was no oven (this was before we had microwaves) in which to cook the TV dinners, so I promptly took them back to the store and lived off shrimp cocktail, peanuts, scotch, and vodka.

Of course, during this time if you'd asked me if I had an alcohol problem, I would have laughed. Thankfully, though, after several months of this craziness and through a miracle that only God could perform, Pauline and I did get back together. (Pauline tells about this miracle in more detail in the next chapter.)

OVERCOMERS OUTREACH

Even after our reconciliation, though, I continued to drink. My next effort to get help was to go to a counselor. I'll have to admit that I had some nudging from my wife. She was upset and had come to her wit's end because, thanks to me, I wasn't the only one whose life was a mess. Our whole family was affected by my drinking. We picked a highly qualified Ph.D. who was a Christian, but unfortunately he was not very informed about alcoholism. He did help us learn to communicate better, but he never addressed my problems with alcohol.

We changed churches a great deal during my drinking days. We left the Baptist church and became Presbyterians for awhile. They seemed to be a little more tolerant of my drinking practices—at least it appeared that way, because many of our new church friends also used alcohol. Then followed a time in our lives when we didn't go to church at all, rather preferring to stay home and perhaps catch a religious program on television.

When we moved to Whittier, California, in 1963, I had a secretary who invited us to attend her Lutheran church. I had never been in a Lutheran church before and was really blessed with the emphasis they placed on worship. I also thought I had found some answers for my drinking problem because we were now in a church where just about everybody drank alcohol. Drinking was no big deal. Since many Lutherans come from a Scandinavian or German background, having a glass of beer with lunch or dinner is an acceptable practice. This congregation soon found out about my theological training, and I was voted a member of the Church Council. We held our meetings in a local restaurant, and as far as I knew, everyone on the Council usually had a glass of wine with dinner, except me—I usually had two or three!

In keeping with our pattern, we soon changed churches again. This time we started attending what was then called Garden Grove Community Church and is today known as the Crystal Cathedral. Although we attended church, God used a small talk-it-over group comprised of about six or eight couples to bring us the help we so desperately needed. Ironically, I was known as the spiritual leader of our group. I would usually be well fortified with alcohol before going to the meetings, but even if someone asked me a question about the Bible, I would be able to fall back on my three years of New Testament Greek and my general knowledge of the Scriptures.

At the end of each meeting, we would draw names of prayer partners with whom we would pray during the interval until our next gathering.

THE FOUNDERS: BOB'S STORY

One time, Pauline drew the name of a gal named Sandy, and she shared with her the problem I was having with alcohol. This was a little unusual for Pauline, because she normally did a good job at hiding my alcoholism from others. Thank God she told Sandy the truth, because this became a turning point in my life.

Sandy and her husband just happened to work for a large aerospace firm in the area that had an employee assistance counselor on its staff. Although Pauline and I had never worked for this firm, Sandy was able to set up an appointment for us with this counselor. As I recall, I didn't want to go but was given an ultimatum by Pauline to see the counselor—or else. I was tired of having my suitcase on the porch, so I went to the appointment. Seated across the desk from me was an older man who informed me that he had been sober for more than twenty-five years. He gave me a forty-question test, and I lied on every answer. I was in so much denial about my condition that I couldn't see the truth, even if it hit me in the face.

He shared his story with me, and as I remember, I promised once again to quit drinking. This time I stayed away from alcohol for three whole weeks. I was so proud of myself that I thought it would be a good idea to celebrate this new-found sobriety with a drink! I was just going to have one; I wasn't going to get drunk. Surprisingly, I was able to do it. During that next year, I gradually increased my drinking without Pauline even realizing it for several months.

Pauline used to wash her hair on Saturday mornings. She had one of those really noisy hooded hair dryers. I could hardly wait until I heard that sound, because I knew she would be under that hood and unable to hear me in the kitchen. I would race to the refrigerator, grab a soft drink, go to the sink and pour half of the contents down the drain, then top it off with vodka (or whatever else was in the liquor cabinet). I would then plop myself down in front of the TV with this angelic look on my face that only an alcoholic can conjure up. I don't think Pauline caught on to my shenanigans for several months. Needless to say, that year I got a lot worse, and so did Pauline.

In the late summer of 1973, God began working a miracle in our home, and strange as it may seem, it didn't start with me.

Pauline got so fed up with my drinking that she went back to the counselor, took his advice, and started attending a 12-step program for families or friends of alcoholics: Al-Anon. Gradually her codependent, enabling behavior began to change. For years I had been able to ask her to call the office when I had a hangover and tell them that I was sick and she always cooperated. Now when I would ask her to cover for me, she would just smile and say, "Call them yourself." I was stunned. For the first time, Bob was being held responsible for Bob's actions. It sure felt strange.

In the past, Pauline would get mad at my various behaviors and pour my liquor down the drain. When she stopped doing this as a result of things she had learned at her 12-step meetings, I was angry. I believed that I needed her to take care of me, and yet she refused to play my games.

Sometimes I would pick an argument with Pauline when I would come home half inebriated. In the past she would really react to my baiting her, and then I could reply, "Well, if that's the way you feel, I'll just go back out with the guys and drink some more." After she was in her 12-step group, she would just smile and say she would see me later, as she headed out for her meeting. I was baffled.

My moment of clarity came on October 15, 1973. I don't remember all the details, but I do remember coming home drunk, looking in the mirror, and not liking what I saw. I told Pauline that I would like to go back and see the counselor we had seen a year prior. When the day arrived, we both went. My motivation was completely different this time. Previously I tried to stop drinking for my wife, which was not a strong enough incentive. This time I wanted to quit for me. I knew that if I didn't do something about my drinking, I would die—and I was too young to die.

This time I listened as the counselor discussed the disease of alcoholism. He told me that most alcoholics die prematurely from this disease. He said of those who do get help, about 85 percent get their initial help from Alcoholics Anonymous, about 12 percent from a religious experience completely separate from Alcoholics Anonymous, and about 3 percent from all other methods. Armed with that information, I went to my first Alcoholics Anonymous meeting.

I was scared stiff, fearing that someone there would know me. I didn't seem to care who saw me when I was out there drinking, making a complete jerk of myself, but now my self-image was threatened. I'll never forget that first meeting. The people who came didn't fit the image of what I thought an alcoholic should look like. They were clean-shaven, had smiles on their faces, and seemed to laugh a lot as various people told their stories. I felt immediately accepted with a great deal of love and no one was the least bit judgmental toward me.

THE FOUNDERS: BOB'S STORY

I remember them talking about twelve steps to recovery. It took weeks for me to grasp this concept. At first, I pictured a building that had 12 steps leading up to the door. I kept going back to A. A. and gradually the key ideas began to sink into my thick head. Even after I began to understand, I still fought step number one: "We admitted we were powerless over alcohol—that our lives had become unmanageable." It was hard for me to admit that I was powerless over anything, especially alcohol. I had been successful in most other areas of my life, but I finally had to admit that alcohol had me whipped and that my life was indeed unmanageable. That was a tremendous breakthrough.

I have been attending 12-step meetings for more than thirty years, and in many ways my life is still unmanageable, but I don't have to turn to alcohol anymore to try and make it better. I can turn my unmanageability over to God. He is patient with me, and all I can say is that it's been quite a journey. Recovery to me is a process and not an event. Although God may choose to deliver some people instantly from their addiction, I have found that in many cases He chooses a trust-Me-one-day-at-a-time approach.

Sometimes we alcoholics think that all we have to do is quit drinking and then everything in our family will be OK. I can remember coming home from my first 12-step meeting feeling really excited. I had some unrealistic expectations, however. I wanted my wife and three sons to forgive me immediately for all the harm I had done in the family. Although they were happy to see that I was doing something about the problem, they still doubted that the change was really permanent.

Looking back, I don't blame them a bit. It had taken years to do the damage in our family, and I had to accept the fact that it was going to take some time to repair it. Fortunately, my wife was in a 12-step program, so she had some tools that helped her in this area. My sons adopted a wait-and-see attitude.

Each family member is affected differently in an alcoholic home. Our oldest son, Bob, was already out of the house during some of my heaviest drinking. Our youngest son, Steve, was completely baffled by my behavior and threatened to run away from home. Our middle son, Mike, really got the brunt of my alcoholic behavior. I would get angry at him in a fit of drunkenness and tell him to leave the house. He got more than his share of verbal abuse. What's more, Pauline seemed to take out her anger at me on Mike, since I was usually passed out on the living room sofa.

After we had been attending 12-step groups for about two years, Mike asked Pauline and me to show a film on alcoholism and share our stories at California Lutheran University, where he was attending. Mike's apartment on campus was situated so that students going to the dining room had to pass by his room. Mike made a sign and posted it on his door that read, "My father is an alcoholic, but he got help for himself. Come tonight at 7:30 and perhaps you can learn how you can help a friend." When I saw this on his door, I got tears in my eyes because I realized that this was the beginning of the healing process for us. It had taken two years, but Mike was once again beginning to accept his father.

One of the term papers Mike wrote in the spring of 1975 while in college impacted our whole family. It was called "Alcoholism and the Family," with the last three pages entitled "Personal Reflections." A few excerpts from this paper give a son's-eye view of what it was like in our family during the drinking years. I'd like to share selected portions to give you a flavor of our life then.

> My father is an alcoholic. He's now working on his second year of sobriety, through the help of some 12-step programs and God. Because my mother insulated the problem so well, I did not know that my father was an alcoholic until I was eighteen or nineteen. In fact, even now when I picture my father as an alcoholic, the picture doesn't seem to fit all that well. But he is!
>
> He followed a fairly normal pattern on his road to alcoholism. I knew that he drank a lot sometimes, but I thought that that was the normal, male thing to do. I guess the main reason why I didn't really know the truth was that my father's drinking mostly took place away from home while he entertained insurance clients.
>
> The first ten years of my life are vague to me. But when I was ten, we moved to Whittier, California. Moving into a new neighborhood, I began to establish new friendships. At the time, I didn't think about it, but now it's clear to me that I rarely brought friends home because I was afraid that my father might be in one of his "bad moods."

THE FOUNDERS: BOB'S STORY

My father was the perfect example of a "cat-napper." The only time that I would see my dad, he would be sleeping on the couch with a newspaper over his head. In fact, this would start a couple of hours after he got up from a night's sleep. He became part of the furniture in the family room—a part that needed to be "refurnished" before I would bring my friends home.

A few of the times I thought of my father as having an alcohol problem was when he once drove us head-on into oncoming traffic; another time when he blocked the driveway with his car so we couldn't leave for church; and the many times when my mother would cry.

My father's behavior was very unpredictable. There were times when the family had planned a camping trip and he decided at the last minute that we weren't going to go because he didn't want to. So we went from high hopes to great disappointments. I shared this anxiety and confusion with my two brothers, one older and one younger than I.

It was my mother's strength, with the help of God, that held us together emotionally. There was a time when my parents' relationship was at the point of destruction, the conflict was so severe. During those days, divorce seemed the lesser of two evils, as compared to the misery we were experiencing.

My mother tried to restructure the family without my father for a time, and this was fairly successful as things began to run more smoothly; we could identify with her stability and consistency. But she didn't know how to solve the problem permanently; she tried the "home treatment program" for years, not knowing any better. Fortunately, a counselor was in tune to the traditional 12-step programs and got my parents into that philosophy.

It took awhile, though, until my father would accept the fact that he was an alcoholic. My mother began attending 12-step meetings for herself. As she learned how to cope with the situation (hers, his, and ours), he became open to help.

OVERCOMERS OUTREACH

> The happy ending to this story is that my father went "on the wagon." Today he is more than halfway through his second year of sobriety and our family has successfully restructured itself. At first it was difficult for me to reinstate my father into his former roles; the hardest thing for me was to respect him. Once I could do this, by realizing that alcoholism is a disease and not a deficiency in his personality, it was easier to include him again into my process of growing up.
>
> I now view his authority with respect, his comeback with admiration, and the fact that he is my father and I am his son, with LOVE.[3]

It took two years, but at the time of that writing, my relationship with Mike was beginning to be healed. Given our history, you can imagine how honored I was to be asked later to officiate at his wedding ceremony.

Although the excerpt above seems to focus on the relationship between Mike and me, I don't want to leave the impression that our oldest son, Bob, and our youngest son, Steve, were not also affected by my drinking, although perhaps in lesser degrees. The important thing is that all three have benefited enormously from my being in recovery. My three sons are now all married with families and seem to have overcome any damage that might have resulted from living in such a dysfunctional family as ours was then. They are all active in their churches and are doing a wonderful job of parenting, with the help of their terrific wives. How thankful I am that all nine of our grandchildren are being raised in Christian homes!

Many changes have occurred in my life since those early days of sobriety. After I had been sober approximately six months, I began volunteering at the Orange County Alcoholism Council. I answered telephones, emptied wastebaskets, and performed any other tasks they felt I could handle. As a result, I enrolled in a certificate course on Alcohol Studies at UCLA. I wanted so much to carry the message to others like myself.

One of my professors took me under his wing and suggested that since I already had a college degree, I might want to pursue a graduate level degree in alcoholism counseling. Since the only serious studying I had done in more than twenty years was the daily sports page, this was hard to imagine; however, I enrolled in the master's program at LaVerne

THE FOUNDERS: BOB'S STORY

University to see what God was going to do next. Since I was still working, I took the classes that fit into my work schedule.

The first course I took was Psychological Testing and Statistics. I was completely lost as I listened to the lectures. I would get up at four A.M. and study, work all day, and then drive twenty-five miles to my evening class. I don't know why I stuck it out, but I did, successfully completing that course as well as all the others. I earned a master of science degree in counseling with an emphasis in alcohol counseling. I was able to obtain a job as an alcoholism counselor in a small psychiatric hospital. After two years of working at that facility, God opened another door of opportunity, and I became the executive director of the Alcoholism Council of Greater Long Beach.

Most alcoholism councils have target groups that they are trying to reach such as youth, women, senior citizens, etc. Because of my background, in addition to reaching out to those groups, I felt a strong need to approach the religious community. I knew that I wasn't the only drunk in the church; there had to be another one out there someplace! What I found in my search to help the religious community was that the so-called liberal churches seemed interested in helping people with this type of problem and greeted my efforts with open arms. I was invited to speak in churches and not only share my story, but to lecture on alcoholism in general.

At that time I did not receive the same type of response from the more conservative evangelical churches I approached. I was really saddened by this unexpected turn of events, because this was the branch of Christianity in which I had grown up. These churches seemed to be in tremendous denial about alcoholism even existing as a problem. When the problem did arise, they looked on it strictly as being of a spiritual nature rather than one that affects the whole person spiritually, emotionally, physically, and mentally. It was while working in this job that God gave Pauline and me the vision for the first Overcomers group, which we started at Whittier Area Baptist Fellowship in 1977.

It's been thirty years since I went to that first 12-step meeting that saved my life. I still attend meetings several mornings each week and continue to derive a great deal of benefit from them in every area of my life. In fact, sometimes I go to meetings just to see what happens to people who stop going to meetings. I've found that one of the most important ways to prevent relapse is to continue attendance at the meetings. I also need to hear newcomers share their stories. The longer I get away from that last drink, the easier it becomes to forget the devastation alcohol played in my life. I don't want to go back to where I was, that's for sure!

Attending meetings is like an insurance policy for my continuing recovery. Some people don't understand the 12-step movement and ask if 12-steppers aren't addicted to meetings in the same way they were addicted to booze. My reply, especially with regard to OO meetings, is that I'm addicted to miracles! Moreover, I need the fellowship and support these groups provide. Twelve-step involvement should not replace one's church attendance and participation in Christian fellowship, but rather should complement it. And once you understand it, it's a wonderful complement indeed.

Each time I go to a 12-step meeting, I wholeheartedly agree with the AA saying: "Keep coming back—it works!" I'm living proof that it does!

4

THE FOUNDERS: PAULINE'S STORY

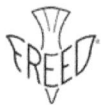

BY PAULINE BARTOSCH

When I first met Bob, I was a painfully shy fourteen-year-old. He would show up at our Baptist church in his Navy uniform and dazzle all the girls. I was busy dating another boy in our youth group at the time and couldn't be bothered. In fact, as each one of my girlfriends fell for this fickle charmer, I would admonish them, "Look out for that guy—he's trouble!" How was I to know that just a couple of years later Bob would turn out to be my knight in shining armor? He didn't have a white horse, but he did have a blue '37 Plymouth with a loud, purring muffler! The very flaws I had warned others about concerning this wild and crazy guy were the very traits that suddenly attracted me the most!

Though my goal was to live happily ever after, I was more than content just to escape my parents' clutches. Bob was a complete renegade, perpetually boisterous and full of spontaneous fun and mischief; his enthusiasm knew no bounds! He always got away with his shenanigans due to that irresistible twinkle in his eye. I had been totally sheltered and restrained as a child, so Bob's unabashed freedom to be himself intrigued me, and I couldn't help but be attracted to this gutsy, free spirit.

My father must have been filled with apprehension as he walked me down the aisle at our wedding. He probably comforted himself with the fact that at least his new son-in-law loved the Lord and was studying for the ministry. Bob was to whisk me off into the sunset at the tender age of 18, allowing me to elude my parents forever (or so I thought). Thus began my great escape.

The "Perils of Pauline" was an accepted way of life for me from the time I was a tiny munchkin with blond Shirley Temple curls. My parents were married in midlife, and I was their little surprise package. Though they thought I was cute and loved to show me off, they weren't quite sure what to do with me most of the time. For many years, I believed I must have been left on their doorstep by mistake!

My father headed up a Christian ministry and authored scores of Bible study books and gospel tracts. He was a quiet, gentle man whose health was always fragile, but he had a quick, dry wit that was guaranteed to tickle my funny bone every time. Even though I never felt very close to him, I loved and admired him greatly. However, there was this other father in him who kept me confused. During his writing times, my dad would completely withdraw—for days at a time—and become an inaccessible stranger. I always felt like I had two fathers, one who considered me the apple of his eye and would make me giggle, and one who occasionally hung out a sign that read "Sorry, we're closed."

My mother was a very strong, take-charge woman who was the picture of health. She fiercely protected my father from noisy distractions—like me. Most of the time I felt it was my job to just be quiet and stay out of their way. The two of them were very close, and though they tried to include me in their displays of affection, I usually viewed my mother as the immovable obstacle between my dad and me. I was entrusted to the care of various housekeepers while both of my parents poured their lives into ministry. My resentment would surface whenever I was called from the neighborhood tree house to wash up and play the piano for their visitors, accompanying my father's masterful performance on our Hammond organ. I learned early to despise these intruders, and took a vow that I would never go into ministry.

I have to say that there were also some warm, wonderful times in my childhood. My father had built a tiny redwood cabin with a pot-bellied stove, nestled in the foothills near Los Angeles, where the three of us would retreat for a day or so. There, I had my parents all to myself and didn't need to play second fiddle to God's work or any strangers. My own special swing hung from a tall oak branch on the hillside and a play corner of smooth blocks, which my daddy had lovingly hewn for me, was my safe haven where I could create a whole fantasy world all my own. My dearest childhood memories were at this small, peaceful hideaway.

THE FOUNDERS: PAULINE'S STORY

Nonetheless, we always had to return home, where I was perpetually ill at ease. While all appearances revealed a smiling little girl with wonderful Christian parents, the silent agreement was that any real feelings were to be kept under wraps. We had to look good, especially to our church friends; therefore, I constantly stuffed shame, anger, and fear, chilling them into a frozen ice cube located in the pit of my stomach. I never felt like I fit anywhere. I was wretchedly lonely and laden with guilt because our regular attendance at the Baptist church gave me the message that I should be happy. The underlying message was that there had to be something dreadfully wrong with me if I didn't truly feel that way.

At the tender age of eight, following a church service, I came home and gave my heart to Christ. I danced up and down the driveway, rejoicing in my decision and feeling a huge burden lifted from my shoulders. When I shared my good news with my parents, they indulgently patted me on the head and sent me off to play. I was not used to being taken seriously anyway, so this reaction was nothing new; however, I was keenly aware that I had a new friend who would never abandon me. His name was Jesus! I vowed to follow Him the rest of my life.

As adolescence overtook me, the Lord provided for many of my needs. A peach of a housekeeper named Blanche came to live with us and became a surrogate mom for the next several years. My parents sensed my intense loneliness and opened their hearts and home at different times to several girls who were in need of a place to stay. God brought these foster sisters—Dolly, Mary, Colleen, and Margaret—to brighten my life, and I cherish their unique contributions to my life to this day. Margaret and I became particularly close, like true sisters in every sense of the word. I loved her dearly. Later in life Colleen proved to be a true confidant.

In high school I was considered a "square" because I hung out with my church friends, and of course was never allowed to go to movies or dances. When I graduated, my parents enrolled me at Biola College, which was then located in Los Angeles. That year, I became more disillusioned. Bob and I were engaged during my freshman year, so I was not allowed to return as a sophomore. Throughout my agonizing year at college, I spent most of my time writing letters to Bob, who was then in South Carolina finishing his undergraduate degree. During the summer, we had a gospel team called the Calvary Crusaders that traveled around to churches. Bob was the preacher, and I accompanied the singing group on the piano. Bob and I fell head-over-heels in love. These two strong-willed, self-centered only children joined together to face the world as a team.

OVERCOMERS OUTREACH

After we got married in 1950, we settled into a one-bedroom apartment in Los Angeles while Bob was attending Fuller Seminary. Every now and then my parents would drop by, unannounced. I was loaded with guilt, because I usually didn't want to see them and would sometimes hide and not answer the door. I vehemently began to resist my mother's control and a battle royal began to rage between us. Bob had become my refuge. I thrived on the fact that he always gave me space to be myself and was rarely critical the way his parents had been toward him.

It wasn't long before I was pregnant with our first son. Bobby's birth was the happiest day I could ever remember. When he was just five months old, we moved into a 28-foot house trailer, hooked it up to our Plymouth club coupe, and cheerfully waved goodbye to our bewildered parents. We headed for South Carolina where Bob continued his seminary training at the same Christian university he had attended for college. Our income consisted of what Bob made selling Fuller brushes part-time, so our diet was comprised of chicken wings and beans most of the time. As Bob told you in his chapter, it took about four months for him to realize that he no longer fit in at the school, and he became extremely disillusioned with Christian leaders who had miserably let him down. I too was ready when Bob suggested we sell the trailer and have him take a job as manager with Fuller Brush Co. in Charlotte, North Carolina.

We started attending a little Presbyterian church near our apartment. One weekend when they held a square dance, Bob, because it was a dance, refused to go, so I went with the minister and his wife—and to my surprise I had a marvelous time! By then, without my knowledge, Bob had started experimenting with a little beer drinking.

Before long, we were expecting our second son. Three weeks following Mike's birth, we received the crushing news that my father had suffered a stroke and was not expected to live. By the time we were on the plane headed for California, my father was dead, and I was numb. Moreover, I despised every fawning person at the funeral. Many of them had robbed me of my father's time and energy during my childhood, with their own so-called Christian agendas. I was devastated and disillusioned. We decided to move cross-country again, back to California. We took an apartment in South Pasadena where Bob continued his employment with the Fuller Brush Co.

We soon purchased a tiny house in Los Angeles. It wasn't long before we were well acquainted with the neighbors in the cul-de-sac. Since most of us didn't have two dimes to rub together, we would sometimes pool our

THE FOUNDERS: PAULINE'S STORY

spaghetti and beans at dinnertime. The normal thing to do after dinner was to play wild music on the hi-fi and dance, an activity I learned to adore. The other activity that seemed to ease all of our troubles and make inhibitions disappear was drinking booze. We were off and running with our new lifestyle!

My first swallow of alcohol initially seared my conscience, burning all the way down. *Surely God will never forgive me*, I thought guiltily. I had committed one of the cardinal sins on my church's list of no-no's. However, the payoff for me was that my intense fear, anger, and guilt all seemed to dissolve with each sip. *How could this be so bad?* I rationalized with relief. After a while, caution was thrown to the wind, my inhibitions were nicely suppressed, and I proclaimed myself free to indulge in all the things I had frowned upon all of my life. Breaking out of the tight little box I'd been raised in took extra effort, so I probably rebelled more strenuously than most people. Our little house would rock with music until the wee hours, while our sons would try to get some sleep in their little bunks. There were painful hangovers the next day, which we always considered hilariously funny. They were all part of the fun of our rebellious new lifestyle.

I began to cool it when Bob and I found we were to be parents again. Steve, our third son, bounced into our world, turning my attention toward home. I began to reassess my life and to think about the Lord again, wondering if there was any hope for me. I was becoming frightened, because Bob's social drinking had taken an ugly turn. At first he could drink everyone under the table and then drive them all home. But after a few years, he began to manifest two distinct personalities, like Dr. Jekyll and Mr. Hyde. He became very unpredictable.

Life became a roller coaster: just as I would begin to worry about Bob's drinking behavior, he would turn into the fun-loving guy whom everybody loved. He always adored his boys and coached Little League for nine years. Our family would head for the river or the mountains with our ski boat for camping trips, and we seemed like any other normal family out on the water (except, of course, that the bow of our boat rode lower in the water because it was loaded down with cases of beer).

There were times when Bob would drink too much, and he would arrive home reeling, reeking, and disgusting us all. His language would be filled with obscenities, and he became less and less capable of taking care of things around the house. *Who is this person?* I asked myself. *Surely he isn't the darling guy I married.* I found myself becoming the manager, controller, referee, and peacemaker all at the same time, taking over all the responsibilities while Bob was out consuming huge amounts of alcohol. However, despite all the evidence to the contrary, I still could not imagine my husband ever being "one of those alcoholics." I would not allow anything like that to happen!

Since by now I was quite adept at living a lie, I accepted the solemn responsibility of inventing excuses for my husband's behavior in an effort to cover up the truth. If someone expressed concern about his actions or the kids questioned me about them, I would just say that he was senile early. At one point I even manufactured a brain tumor for him!

In the depths of my denial, I allowed the situation to get worse through my own dishonesty and by accepting the unacceptable. In my own efforts to cover up what was wrong, I was actually prolonging the disease without even knowing it. I believed that if I thought long enough and prayed hard enough (telling God what He must do) and created just the right sermon for Bob, I could handle it myself. "Letting go and letting God" didn't fit into my agenda at all. Astonishingly, it never crossed my mind that booze had any bearing upon what was happening to my life and our marriage.

At this time Bob took a job in Whittier, California, as a manager with New York Life Insurance Co. We bought the ultimate party house, with vaulted ceilings, huge windows, and a large expanse of yard. The house was on the opposite side of a rippling creek from other homes so that we could make all the noise we wished. It was our job to entertain clients, and entertain we did.

Since all three boys were in school by then, I began to work a string of part-time jobs. The first position I held was as a bookkeeping machine operator at Far East Broadcasting Co., a Christian organization. I was living a double standard at the time, but these wonderful people accepted me. My boss, Evelyn Esselstrom, eventually became my treasured spiritual mentor. The Lord knew exactly what I needed, even though I felt very far from Him.

The whole time we were in this precarious lifestyle, our family continued to go to church. We would usually fight all the way there but would show up in the parking lot with our big plastic smiles firmly in place. Bob would have his big Thompson Chain Reference Bible under his arm and would bellow out the hymns louder than anyone else. We looked like the perfect Christian family. Then we would resume our fighting on

THE FOUNDERS: PAULINE'S STORY

the way home. No one had the least suspicion that anything was awry, and we weren't about to share what was really going on!

After a while, we started feeling a little uncomfortable keeping up appearances at that church and we began to do some church-hopping. Baptists didn't seem to have a sense of humor about partying, so we became Presbyterians for a while. Then we thought we'd found heaven on earth when we were invited to a Lutheran Church where social drinking is a normal, acceptable practice.

I spent much time and energy checking up on Bob. I had been obsessed with my alcoholic's behavior—what he was doing or not doing. I had even kept a calendar of the number of drinks I thought he'd consumed. I made it my business to mark the labels of the bottles in the liquor cabinet at the level he had last left them so I would be able to ascertain if he'd been drinking. Looking back, I'm not quite sure what I planned to do with all this juicy evidence, but my own life was so out of control that I felt I must maintain at least partial control of something somehow. After all, did God have all the facts? He hadn't seemed to be listening, so I felt I should help Him out a little.

But what was happening to me? Sometimes I would catch a glimpse of my contorted face in a mirror and could hardly recognize myself. When caught off-guard, my facial expressions gave me away. That's why I usually worked extra hard to improve my cheery facade.

But it didn't work for long. My anger simmered inside me, and one day it burst loose and I managed to put my dainty fist through the bathroom door! The next day Bob called me from work and demanded that I repair the damage. So I purchased a fish plaque with three little fish and decorated the hole I had made. That was fine until my fist hit the second bathroom door. Then I had to invest in some full-length mirrors to cover the evidence of my wrath.

The next few years were filled with my futile attempts to fix whatever was wrong with Bob. I was thinking, of course, that there was nothing wrong with *me*. I truly believed that it was my job to remedy this situation and that deep down it was probably all my fault. My best-rehearsed sermons were usually delivered at two A.M., when I would raise up in bed on my tired elbow and proceed to outline Bob's problems as I perceived them. I would then quote just the right Scripture verses, with key words enunciated perfectly, thinking each time that this sermon would surely get through his thick skull. His anguished reply was always, "Get off my back and leave me alone!"

OVERCOMERS OUTREACH

Though I was reluctant to share any real problems with my pastor, I was finally driven to do so out of sheer desperation. Strangely enough, I avoided any reference to the drinking and concentrated only on Bob's bizarre behavior. When my pastor's advice to "read the Bible more and pray" didn't produce results, I sought the counsel of other pastors in my area—anyone I could get to listen to my ravings!

One evening as a pastor and I left his office following one of my visits, we passed a door and I noticed a group of people sitting inside in a circle. I asked the pastor what was going on. "Oh, that's Al-Anon," he replied. "It's for family members and friends of alcoholics."

As my ears perked up, I asked, "Does it help?"

"Oh yes—very much so," was his reply. Then we both got into our cars and left. A number of years of agony could have been avoided if I had only had the courage to tell him the whole truth that night.

My Christian physician became concerned about the stress symptoms I was manifesting, so I told him a little more about Bob's drinking. Since he was very concerned, he sat Bob down one day and preached a sermon about his consumption of alcohol and what might happen in the future if he didn't stop drinking or at least cut down. He felt so sorry for me after hearing all my sad tales of woe, that he gave me a prescription for Valium (effectively a martini in pill form) so that I could cope with it all. So instead of one addict in the family, we now had two!

At that point, our marriage seemed to be at its crushing end. Huddled on the bottom step of our front porch one terrible day, I was gripped with fear. I had just insisted that my husband of eighteen years leave our home. I couldn't even have stated what was wrong, I really didn't know. I just knew my life was out of control and it had something to do with him—that guy who used to be so sweet, kind, loving, and cute was turning into a monster. The dull ache in the pit of my stomach seemed to increase with every passing day. I figured that our marriage was over and that there was no hope because I had tried everything to fix it. *This shouldn't be happening to a Christian*, I thought dejectedly. I was terrified of sharing with anyone at my church, because I feared they wouldn't understand. Not only that, I wasn't prepared for their judgment, misguided advice, or the sympathy that might come my way, since I was still more or less proud and hadn't admitted my life was unmanageable yet.

With the assistance of one of the pastors who managed to talk Bob into leaving the house for a trial separation, Bob angrily left and set up housekeeping in a neighborhood motel. Having it all figured out as usual,

THE FOUNDERS: PAULINE'S STORY

I felt that he might see the error of his ways, shape up, and someday return so we could resume our marriage. Instead, during that time, our lives began to go in distinctly opposite directions even involving other people, and our animosity toward each other increased day by day. He began to drink more than ever. This was not the way I had it planned! Before we knew what hit us, we filed for divorce, even though neither one of us really believed in it. We were just swept along in the legal process.

Then began the incredible miracle of God that Bob referred to in his chapter, one of restoring health and sanity to our lives and marriage. One terrible afternoon I paid a visit to one of the pastors on my list because I was feeling so depressed. His words to me were few but potent. "Pauline," he said, "I realize you and Bob will probably never get back together. However, if that should somehow happen, do you think you could ever forgive him?"

I sat dumbfounded. *Forgive him? Why should I, after all he's done?* Suddenly, the Lord's Prayer that we said at our little Lutheran church each Sunday resounded loudly in my ears—something about "forgive us our trespasses, as we forgive others, who trespass against us."

I ventured, "I guess I couldn't say that prayer if I didn't forgive Bob, right?"

Pastor smiled and quietly agreed with me, and in so doing, the first positive seed of hope was gently planted in my heart and mind.

Just as we both had given up on any hopes of reuniting, Bob came over one evening to celebrate Steve's birthday. Bob and I played a fiercely competitive game of pool between verbal snarls at one another. I trounced him for the first time in my life! I was so elated at this accomplishment that I followed him out to his car just to rub it in, and for reasons unknown to me, I found myself sitting in the car with him for several quiet moments without saying a word.

Seemingly from out of the blue, God suddenly popped some words into my brain and they escaped my lips before I could stop them. "I know that we will never get back together again and that our marriage is over. But you know, if we ever did try it again, I think I would be able to forgive you." Tears sprang from Bob's surprised eyes as he reached for me. He had figured that there was far too much water under the bridge to turn back, particularly knowing how unforgiving and spiteful I could normally be. Yet a few words of simple, direct communication had suddenly opened a door of hope for both of us.

Am I ready for this? I fearfully asked myself. I honestly didn't know.

OVERCOMERS OUTREACH

At that point Bob promised to stop drinking, and my joyful response was, "Great—now all our problems are over!" I was still sure he wasn't one of "those alcoholics," but I did know that somehow it would make a tremendous difference in our relationship if he stopped drinking. I was ready to believe anything in order to have our family reunited and to get some sanity back in my life. I was unaware, however, that by then Bob had crossed an invisible line into addiction and that he no longer had that power of choice in the matter.

With the skeptical help of our patient Lutheran pastor (whom we nearly drove to drink), we decided to try this rocky marriage again. We were admonished to get regular counseling; in fact, Pastor Gesch wouldn't leave our home until we made that first appointment. So for the next year, we saw Dr. Bingham, the psychologist, every couple of weeks to work out our differences. Some of the first issues to be dealt with centered not upon our marriage, but upon Bob's unfortunate college experience of rejection and the false heroes who had disappointed him. In digging up these pains of the past, Bob "tapered on" with his drinking again over a three-week interval, this time hiding it from me better than before. I was completely unaware of this, and furthermore, I subconsciously didn't want to know.

Finally I had to acknowledge that it was happening again. Steve, our youngest, was threatening to run away from home. He exclaimed, "Can't you see what's happening, Mom? Dad's acting weird because he's drinking again!" I had been blind to it. All of my excuses and cover-up operations began to collapse and fall upon deaf ears, and I had to look at stark reality. It wasn't a pretty sight.

When our help finally arrived, it came in a most unexpected way. By that time, our family was attending a mega church in Orange County. Bob was the ninth-grade Sunday school teacher and usually arrived at church with a terrible hangover, a green tongue (from breath mints, used to mask his booze breath), and a bottle of breath-freshener in his pocket. Steve had the misfortune of being in the ninth grade at the time, so of course he hated going to church on Sunday.

Bob and I were also involved in a small group of about seven other couples. My prayer partner, Sandy, asked me one Sunday morning how things had gone that week. For the first time, to my great surprise, truthful words popped out of my mouth. "I think Bob might have a drinking problem," I said.

THE FOUNDERS: PAULINE'S STORY

Sandy couldn't believe it. Bob was considered to be the spiritual leader of the group because he knew the Bible inside-out! From that time, Sandy and her husband used a huge amount of tough love on me. They wouldn't take "no" for an answer and literally forced me to the aerospace firm where they both worked to set up an appointment with a counselor who was a recovering alcoholic himself. I finally agreed to go in order to make one more stab at getting my crazy husband fixed. It was there that I encountered the smiling employee assistance counselor who saw right through me and my games.

At that point, in my opinion, I was quite sure that there was nothing wrong with *me*. After all, I had done everything within my power to keep the family together. I made sure the bills were paid, and above all, I kept up a look-good appearance on the outside. Nothing had worked. I felt that our marriage was over and that there was no point in me sitting there with a complete stranger discussing the sordid details of my failed marriage. After I took a written test of some forty questions, the counselor informed me that not only was my husband very sick, but that I needed help too! *Of all the nerve!* I thought. I was grossly insulted.

The counselor insisted that I promise to attend some Al-Anon meetings in my community for codependency. He felt sure I had been adversely affected by Bob's drinking behavior. I wasn't ready to take any of the blame, so I finally coerced Bob into paying this counselor a visit. During this particular visit, another counselor was invited to sit in on our session, much to my chagrin because I was getting tired of having our dirty laundry aired before anyone, much less strangers.

Neither one of us went for help to the 12-step groups because we felt that since they weren't even Christian, how could they be good? Thus we allowed the disease of alcoholism to progress for one more excruciating year. By then, my own physical and emotional symptoms were overwhelming. I was truly suffering in every sense of the word due to my despair and lack of control over Bob's behavior. My life as it was became too much for me, and just like a recovering alcoholic eventually must, I hit bottom.

I made a call to contact the counselor at the aerospace firm only to discover that he was no longer there! Instead, the small, quiet stranger who just happened to sit in the corner during our session the year before had taken his place. How could he forget such a crazy couple? He urged me to come in immediately.

OVERCOMERS OUTREACH

This quiet observer was not as shy as I had remembered him. Suddenly he appeared to be a giant, and his voice bellowed loudly across the desk. He pointed out that it was as if I had been hanging by a pole two thousand feet in the air all my life. Then suddenly it was suggested that I let go. No way! From that perspective the thought was terrifying! Yet all of my "hanging on" had been useless. All of my efforts to fix another person had failed. Could I really trust God, let go, allow Him to catch me and take care of my alcoholic? So *this* is what they meant by "Let go and let God!"

I had no way of knowing whether this employee assistance counselor was even a Christian. I had always been convinced that if and when God decided to do anything positive in my life, the source of the help would have a Christian label on it. Yet I sat dumbfounded as I realized as never before that God was talking through this total stranger directly to my heart, and that the Lord's awesome presence filled this office, more so than I had ever experienced in any church sanctuary.

As I sat stunned, my next thought was, *How can I stand by and just let Bob hurt? Doesn't this counselor understand how much of my time and energy have been poured into my cover-up operation?* The counselor began advising me to handle things exactly the opposite of my usual procedures of enabling and covering up. *How could I possibly allow Bob to come crashing to his 'bottom'?* I wondered. In my twisted way of thinking, that would be admitting defeat.

As I continued to listen, though, I learned that in my efforts to control, I had been deciding when and how God could work. I had tried to stuff almighty God into a little box. Amidst all of the confusion, I realized I had lost sight of Jesus Christ in my life, In my anguish, my focus had switched from Him to other people around me. Normally stubborn by nature, I would have never been ready to completely let go until I had tried absolutely everything else I could think of to remedy the situation. Now, my strength was gone.

The tears I had so successfully bottled up all those years began to gush down my face in a torrent. I knew the counselor was right, but how stripped and terribly alone I felt as I stumbled out of his office. "What is my life coming to?" I muttered as I swung my weary body into the car that same evening and headed for my very first 12-step support group meeting of Al-Anon.

What I found at that meeting was not at all what I had expected! We met, of all places, in a Sunday school room at the Methodist church. There

THE FOUNDERS: PAULINE'S STORY

I encountered faces that reflected true joy, and I thought I must be in the wrong place; no one could possibly be this happy if they experienced my lifestyle. And yet I discovered to my amazement that many individuals in that room were coping with even worse situations than mine, but they were finding practical tools that gave them ongoing hope for their own recovery. They were learning to turn their loved ones over to the care of God on a daily basis, and as a result they were finding serenity for themselves. Their emphasis was not on their alcoholic, but upon their own recovery.

I was told that it was possible to experience compassion for my husband even though he was drunk. We learned that alcoholism is a disease, similar to diabetes or cancer. *What would my attitude be if Bob was struggling with cancer instead of drinking?* I wondered. If I could stop judging him and begin to remember that he was a child of God who was hurting and whose brain was fuzzed up with alcohol, I could view him in a new way. During the weeks to come, I found to my surprise that I could actually give him a kiss on the cheek whether he deserved it or not. Within a few weeks of attending Al-Anon regularly, Bob was shocked at the difference in my attitude toward him—and so was I!

Al-Anon was a total surprise for me. Instead of gaining new *fixing* skills (as I had expected), I was supplied with brand-new *coping* skills. My new friends said the support group was for me, not Bob, and that I needed to turn my alcoholic over to the care of God as I understood Him (clearly Jesus Christ in my thinking). At first my mind was so confused that I was able to grasp only the simplest tools offered.

One of the first concepts that saw me through some initial difficult days was the idea of being cheerful but tough. I would smilingly tell Bob to call in sick himself if he wanted to skip work due to a hangover. Also, when I quit pouring Bob's precious booze down the sink, his reaction was a total surprise: he thought perhaps I didn't love him anymore. I must admit some of the shocked looks I noticed on Bob's face were hilarious. I was getting free from the bondage of having my life revolve around another human being. As much as I loved Bob, by that time I had realized how sick we both were, and that somebody had to get well! I had learned that Pauline had to quit being responsible for Bob's actions. These and other new skills helped me find a new way of interacting with my loved one that was infinitely more healthy than my old ways. I was learning that I wasn't trapped in my old ways of approaching life; I could make new choices.

OVERCOMERS OUTREACH

During those first few weeks, I was hurting and trying hard to understand what the 12 Steps were all about. The tears had begun to flow, and I put my new coping tools to work. In returning to my support group meetings each week, I learned that I could find recreation and hobbies for myself and that I could get my focus off of Bob and put it on the Lord again. Before that, my pattern after work had been to say a brief hello to the kids and head for the bedroom, where I would dive headlong under the bedspread, hiding from life and sleeping for hours on end.

My new friends asked me what hobbies I had. I said, "Let's see, I play the piano sometimes."

"What kind of tunes do you play?" they queried.

"The blues, of course!" I answered sheepishly.

"Go home and play happy tunes," was my directive. That would be different all right. I didn't even know any happy tunes.

One night when Bob came home and stumbled down the hallway to crash on our bed, I remembered the suggestions that had been made to me about playing happy tunes on my piano. Since I play mostly by ear, I tried to remember some of those foreign sounds, and the more I played, the more I got into the spirit of it, nearly forgetting that my husband was drunk and being obnoxious. What a strange but wonderful feeling that was! My normal procedure had been to focus upon the despair of my spouse and to get caught up in his misery. As one cheerful song after another pulsated through the house, my foggy husband thought for sure that I had lost my mind! How could I possibly be happy when he was obviously having such a frightful time?

I learned that our whole family had been on a merry-go-round of denial, and that we had mistakenly put our alcoholic on center stage. How were we to know that providing an audience for him just urged him to be more obnoxious? How could we possibly look the other way while he embarrassed us with his behavior? Slowly, I discovered new ways of acting and reacting, or not reacting at all. And my focus began to be upon God instead of on my alcoholic. When I concentrated upon actively routing out my old "stinking thinking" and began to fill my hours with positive replacements, the healing began. I began to take very seriously all of the new principles I was putting to use in my recovery, and my overall mood greatly improved.

It seemed that when I was able to let go of my bitterness and rely upon God to give me the courage to take positive action, fear began to lose its grip on me. By changing my attitudes and learning new ways of

THE FOUNDERS: PAULINE'S STORY

releasing my alcoholic with love to God's care, I went from a reactive, button-pushing mode into concerted healthy action. Instead of concentrating on the manipulation of others, I began to identify ways of making myself happy. I found that I could walk away from an unpleasant scene without feeling that I had to win, blame, or defend myself, or to correct, judge, or fix anyone else. I found that if I lined myself up with God and listened to His will for me, He seemed to take care of others around me, and therefore I didn't have to be responsible for them.

Only a few weeks after I found my Al-Anon group did Bob come crashing to his bottom, but this time I wasn't there to save him. He had to experience all of his own pain, without my interference. He went to his first AA meeting and "put the plug in the jug" (stopped drinking), but that didn't solve our problems because Bob was miserable without booze. A few weeks later I heard that a funny speaker was scheduled to be at the Friday Night Open AA Meeting and I offered to go with him.

Bob's instant reply was, "No way! There's a football game that night at the high school and I'm going to that." Instead of being downcast and disappointed, I realized it might not be God's timing, and besides, it wasn't any of my business. So I backed off.

By the time Friday evening came, it was pouring rain, not very good weather for watching football. "Where did you say this meeting was?" Bob meekly asked me. We attended and that was the beginning of a whole new life for us! We both laughed until we cried as the speaker related his story punctuated with incidents surrounding the insanity of his addicted lifestyle. What was at one time too painful to think about had turned to actual humor in recovery. Just the joy of still being alive felt deliriously good to us. The seed of hope was planted in our hearts that night, thanks to the speaker's transparency and God's goodness.

When we first got into recovery and told our sons about it, they figured we were on some new kick and that it too would pass. After all, they had always been the responsible adults in our household, and Bob and I had been the juvenile delinquent parents. It took a couple of years before they began to get curious about the obvious changes they saw in us.

In addition to helping me with my co-dependency through Al-Anon, the Lord also delivered me from a lengthy addiction to pills. For fourteen years I had been taking just one "harmless" Valium pill each morning. After all, it had been originally prescribed by my Christian doctor, so I wasn't worried about it. My purse or travel bag always contained a well-hidden but adequate supply. I had attempted to quit on my own several times, particularly after Bob stopped drinking, but each time after a few days, my head would fly apart in a million pieces. The anxiety is difficult to describe unless you've lived it; suffice it to say it was a living hell coming off Valium. In order to stop the withdrawal symptoms, I would resume taking them just to function normally. I was resigned to the fact that I would probably be taking them as long as I lived. No one ever realized that I was on anything. Those little yellow pills seemed to be my emotional health insurance and my best friends. They would take the edge off life's daily problems.

While on the drug Valium, I wasn't aware that I had a choice of going through life dancing instead of just surviving. My feelings and emotions were being repressed by my medication. I realized that unless I could truly experience both life's highs and lows, its joys and sorrows, I wasn't really living, but I was merely existing. Yet I didn't have the courage to allow my head to fly apart as it did each time I attempted to skip my daily dosage. And I was too ashamed to ask anyone for help.

Finally, I began to break the tiny pill into smaller and smaller pieces. Every morning I would still take my pill, but over the months it became a tiny morsel in the palm of my hand. After about a year, when I was finally down to one infinitesimal grain, I felt it was time to come clean. I felt safer about it because I was by then working for two psychologists at a local hospital and figured they would be there to help if my head actually flew apart. Yet there was no time in their stressful day to listen to me or tune into my personal agony.

After a few days of going without my little crutch, I began to experience muscle spasms and radical mood swings. I was already getting into trouble at work because my short-term memory was almost gone due to the chemical that had saturated my brain on a daily basis for so many years. I was forced to write absolutely everything down on paper in order to remember it. My office was littered with little notes to myself, and I was trying to keep them all straight. How frightened I was! When I quit the job with the psychologists, I took some time for myself and began to do volunteer work. I felt like Pauline had been totally shattered, and I had to rebuild my life from scratch. God led me to studying at a chemical dependency institute and wouldn't you know, He linked me up with a recovering Valium addict.

My new friend and classmate, Sharon, gave me the courage to press onward in my quaking life without drugs, and after much perseverance

THE FOUNDERS: PAULINE'S STORY

I began to feel reborn. Most of the time I felt better than I had in many years. My worst days without the pills were better than the best days I had while taking them. I embraced the little slogan, "This too shall pass," as I began to experience life on life's terms. I listened intently to stories of others in traditional 12-step groups who described mountains of enormous trauma through which they had emerged victorious due to trusting in God's almighty power! Could I, as a Christian, do any less?

For the next year I began to "come to" and feel more alive. The pains of life were more painful without my drug, but the joys were beginning to emerge and happily catch me off guard. Where had I been living all those years? I had cheated myself not only of experiencing my true feelings, but I was also too numb to sense God's presence in my life. It was both a sad and happy realization for me.

Most of all, I began to experience God's presence just one day at a time, as long as I could continue to focus on the *now*. To think, I had dulled myself to Jesus! As my mind began to clear and I applied the 12 Steps and Scriptures to my life daily, I realized that in order to create even more comfort for myself, I needed to learn to be honest.

One of the first things that happened in my 12-step recovery process was that relationships in my life were healed; that is, with everyone except my mother. Let's face it, this one was impossible! Then one night at an Al-Anon meeting, a woman told about the miraculous healing between her mother and herself. I squirmed uncomfortably in my chair as she talked. Afterward I approached her and said, "That's real nice for you, but it will never happen to me."

Her reply stuck in my mind: "Aren't you selling God awfully short?"

Whew, this was a tall order. And I knew it would begin with me being honest about my feelings about Mom. So one bright morning I stood by our creek and shouted at God, "I hate her, You know! I don't even want a relationship with her. I can't even pray for her. But if it's what You want, You will have to do it because I can't."

Within a few weeks, I noticed that I miraculously began to enjoy phone conversations with my mother. The next time we took her out to lunch, I couldn't believe that I actually enjoyed her company. I didn't suffer my usual migraine on the trip home. Then, the next visit, I found myself putting my arms around her for the first time and giving her a squeeze. I noticed that it made me feel good! The following time when we prepared to leave, I heard strange words pop out of my mouth. "I love you!" I almost had to turn around to see who had said it! The next time we got together, she linked her arm through mine and began to apologize for the very things that had wrapped me so tightly in my resentments all those years. By that time my attitude and response was, "That was yesterday, Mom. Now we've got today!"

And how thankful I am today that I know how it feels to love my mother, especially since she was ninety years old at the time of our reconciliation. We had almost ten good years by the time she passed away at age ninety-nine. With our family joyfully experiencing healed relationships, the miracles went all the way around the table. Our three wonderful sons, Bob, Mike, and Steve, opened their arms to us in our surprise recovery, and new love and respect were born that we never dreamed possible. They welcomed opportunities to share our family miracle with others.

After Bob received his master's degree and became an alcoholism counselor at a local psychiatric hospital, he asked Mike and me to participate in his group for family members. That particular evening in 1979, God really got my undivided attention in an unusual and amazing incident on the highway.

Mike and I headed out on one of Los Angeles' busy freeways at rush hour to meet Bob at the hospital. Just as we were cruising lazily along in the slow lane, an eighteen-wheeler truck came alongside us as we were merging into traffic. I'm still not sure exactly what happened, but suddenly we found ourselves in Mike's little Honda Civic scooting sideways at sixty miles an hour, on brand-new but now mangled tires, practically glued onto the truck's front bumper in a perpendicular position!

"Dear Jesus, help us!" I screamed, as we continued to travel for about eight hundred feet in this precarious manner! I then thought my life was abruptly ending as I watched the guardrail rush by, so I cried, "Mike, I love you!" as my parting words before we were to be ushered to the heavenly gates.

Mike's amazing reply was, "It's gonna be OK, Mom!"

We later learned that the trucker didn't know his vehicle had acquired us as its newest bumper sticker; he merely felt some vibration and figured he had just blown out one of his eighteen tires, so he pulled over and stopped.

"Get out of the car, Mom!" Mike yelled. The driver's side was flattened up against the truck's monstrous shiny grill. A moment later the driver saw us for the first time as he climbed out of the cab. This big truck driver

THE FOUNDERS: PAULINE'S STORY

began to cry like a baby when he saw the two of us emerge without a scratch from the little car plastered on the front of his truck.

As we stood there hugging one another and pinching ourselves, another young man who had witnessed the whole event came running back up the freeway shouting, "It's a miracle, it's a miracle!" He didn't know the half of it. We later learned that the truck's bumper had impacted the very strongest point of Mike's little car.

As we stood before an audience of families later that evening, I remarked, "I feel like I've been hit by a truck!" But looking back, I was hit by much more than that. I was bowled over by the fact that for some uncanny reason, God wanted me to still be alive. For what? What in the world did He have in store for me that would cause Him to send His mighty angels to protect us against all odds so securely on that highway? This event was a turning point in my life, because God displayed how He valued Pauline as a person, no matter how I had screwed up my life.

The evening following this incident, I couldn't wait to share at the Friday Night Family 12-step meeting. My feet were still six feet off the ground and I was somewhere in limbo marveling that I was still alive. That night for the first time I felt total freedom to share at my traditional 12-step group about my Higher Power, Jesus Christ, and how His angels had rescued my son and me from certain death the day before. As long as I live, I will never forget the quizzical expressions on the faces of my new friends surrounding me as they listened intently to my amazing freeway story.

I knew for a fact that some of those wonderful people listening to me were still searching for their "Higher Power." We were aware of the tremendous need to help people like ourselves make the jump from "God as you understand him" to Jesus Christ, God incarnate. Somebody needed to find a way to bridge the gap. But could God use weak vessels like Bob and Pauline for such a task? *No way,* we both thought! And yet God had other ideas.

Now you see why I'm addicted to miracles!

5

BRIDGING THE GAP

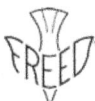

After trying so many other methods through the years to get help, we were stunned at the magnificence of God's power through the simplicity of the 12-step program. To our utter amazement, He spoke the very message we needed to hear through the mouths of some of the most unlikely people. After we hit bottom with alcoholism and codependency in the fall of 1973, we were by then in enough pain to become willing to do whatever was necessary to get well. When God surprised us by using traditional 12-step groups within our community to bring healing and hope, we became anxious to share our miracle with others!

Early in our recovery, we began to attend some traditional 12-step groups that were geared for the whole family. The meetings were a curious combination of people, including both recovering alcoholics and family members. We learned to be vulnerable, looking into one another's faces and sharing true feelings, whether it was intense fear and loneliness or the unexpected joy of being freed from addictions.

Since we sensed no judgment in these meetings, each person could clearly be heard and was accepted exactly the way he or she was; no one seemed to have designs on changing or controlling anyone else. Neither crosstalk (interrupting others to tell one's own story or make a comment during the other's sharing time) nor giving advice was allowed. It was understood that God was free to speak to an individual's heart without human interference. If a person wasn't up to sharing a word, that was totally acceptable too. We began to witness miracles; marriages were restored and communication gaps were successfully bridged. We were overwhelmed with gratitude for experiencing God's total forgiveness and peace of mind. We couldn't wait to share with others these new miracles of healing!

Every Friday night we would drive home from these family meetings asking each other, "This is so great; why isn't the church doing something like this?" As weeks and months went by, our haunting question became, "Why is it we can be so honest at the traditional 12-step support groups and not so revealing at church?" We struggled to answer that one.

Before long, God began to plant a heavy burden within our hearts to share our new-found experience, strength, and hope with individuals in our church. At first, this prospect was terrifying. But it didn't take long before we noticed that the more we had the courage to honestly share, the more it became evident that we were not the only ones struggling with issues of alcoholism and codependency after all! After years of wrapping our pain in a cloak of secrecy, this willingness to be verbally candid was frightening, to say the least. At that time (about 1975), this was a rather radical thing to do in church circles.

The simple tools derived from the family meetings we attended and other traditional 12-step groups really made sense and began to work wonders in our lives. As our foggy brains began to clear and we became more familiar with the Steps, we began to distinctly recognize these principles. We had read each and every one in the Bible! How we hungered to have God's Word clearly applied to each Step!

Though traditional groups were helping millions of people, they were never intended to save souls. Even though the generic "Higher Power" was discussed frequently, the group traditions rightly discouraged any mention of a specific "Higher Power" such as Jesus or other specific religious leader. Therefore, people of all faiths or no faith felt welcome, as they were there for only one purpose—to stop their addictive behavior. But how we longed to share *our* "Higher Power," Jesus Christ, with others who were still seeking Him!

Since we soon discovered other Christians in the program, it didn't take long for us to band together and begin a Bible study in various homes. Some people in the group were still searching for the identity of their "Higher Power." God used this little group and several individuals found Jesus to be the God they were seeking. Yet not all people attending had it so easy. Some became disturbed because in light of the Scriptures, they could no longer create their own concept of God—one that allowed them to live as they pleased. After some heart-wrenching discussion, the group disbanded due to this controversy. Though painful, the dissolution of that group was helpful in the long run in that it forced us to crystallize our thinking: were we going to let the Scriptures be central to our study or not? History—in the formation of OO—shows that we decided to let the Bible lead us in a front-and-center role.

After that first group broke up, we began an earnest search for the missing link between recovery groups and the church. We kept praying that somebody would catch on to the fact that the Steps worked so well because they had their roots in God's Word. We also realized what a vital tool mutual prayer could be for a bunch of fellow strugglers like us who were on a recovery journey. Traditional groups seemed to allow only certain prayers that were repeated or read in a ritualized fashion. There appeared to be a gaping hole between two distinct populations: on one end of the scale, those recovering within traditional 12-step groups who needed a Savior, and on the other end, Christians who clung fiercely to denial, refusing to get any outside help at all. We began to sense a real need.

Recovering, but Still Searching for God

The traditional 12-step groups had literally saved our lives. The atmosphere of total acceptance and love—no matter whether people were rich or poor, married or single, drove up in a Cadillac, came on a bus, on a bicycle, or even walked to a meeting—overwhelmed us and drew us into the circle. Recovering people from all walks of life seemed free and eager to share their sordid secrets as well as pass along their experience, strength, and hope. The "Higher Power's" presence was joyfully celebrated on a daily basis, along with the freedom and forgiveness of self and others. Life became manageable because we believed that absolutely anything can be handled with the help of "God as we understand him." Many of us would be dead if we hadn't found this new way of life.

Even though God (in a generic sense) was talked about a great deal in the meetings, it became clear that traditional 12-step groups were there primarily to offer simple tools for living to produce sobriety or recovery from addictions and compulsions. In a new, more stable state, people are more in a position to make a rational decision concerning their faith.

In a traditional 12-step group, part of the program is to begin to search for who the "Higher Power" might be. This can be quite foreign to people who, for one reason or another, were turned off to religion or faith in God. Just like the original members of AA, we too found that we could no longer place the blame on religious members for our own problems. It became clear that the defiance that such blaming represented was near the core of our problems and posed a huge obstacle to our sanity. The following is what the founders of Alcoholics Anonymous had to say about this person:

> We were plumb disgusted with religion and all its works. ...But it was the morality of the religionists themselves that really got us down. We gloated over the hypocrisy, bigotry, and crushing self–righteousness that clung to so many "believers" even in their Sunday best. How we loved to shout the damaging fact that millions of the "good men of religion" were still killing one another off in the name of God. This all meant, of course, that we had substituted negative for positive thinking. After we came to AA, we had to recognize that this trait had been an ego-feeding proposition. In belaboring the sins of some religious people, we could feel superior to all of them. Moreover, we could avoid looking at some of our own shortcomings. Self-righteousness, the very thing that we had contemptuously condemned in others, was our own besetting evil. This phony form of respectability was our undoing, so far as faith was concerned. But finally, driven to AA, we learned better.
>
> As psychiatrists have often observed, defiance is the outstanding characteristic of many an alcoholic. So it's not strange that lots of us have had our day at defying God Himself. Sometimes it's because God has not delivered us the good things of life which we specified, as a greedy child makes an impossible list for Santa Claus.
>
> ...When we encountered AA, the fallacy of our defiance was revealed. At no time had we asked what God's will was for us; instead we had been telling Him what it ought to be. No man, we saw, could believe in God and defy Him, too. Belief meant reliance, not defiance. In AA we saw the fruits of this belief: men and women spared from alcohol's final catastrophe. We saw them

meet and transcend their other pains and trials. We saw them calmly accept impossible situations, seeking neither to run nor to recriminate. This was not only faith; it was faith that worked under all conditions. We soon concluded that whatever price in humility we must pay, we would pay.[1]

In the traditional 12-step programs, no one forces any preconceived ideas upon anyone else regarding God, so there is a hunger created to find or renew one's faith—at least in the best-case scenario. Some are initially fearful of pursuing "God as we understand Him," but soon learn that in order to fully recover we must "let go and let God." (By "let go" we mean give up the control over our lives and future we so stubbornly retain; by "let God" we mean letting God run our lives and bring about His will for us.) Many people who had previously been alienated from God and/or the church share that as they are able to "let go," God takes them in their weakness and brokenness, accepting them just as they are, when they call out to Him for help. With complete abandon, the simple cry, "God, please help me!" has brought a miracle to multitudes who have tried it. At that dark moment in a person's life when all seems lost, the mind cannot fathom all the blessings our "Higher Power" has in store for those who finally surrender!

CHRISTIANS IN SEARCH OF RECOVERY

Without question, traditional 12-step support groups have proven to be tremendously effective, and thousands of Christians who faithfully attend them have benefited enormously. People who were once stumbling in darkness are being freed. We were grateful for this, but we still felt that there were some important ingredients missing: believers not being able to pray spontaneously, not being able to study God's Word, and—most of all—not having the freedom to call our "Higher Power" by His true name: Jesus Christ! The church tried its best to reach out to folks in the '70s, but fell pitifully short, which was especially disappointing when people coming out of the 12-step groups sought healthy Christian love and acceptance that they unfortunately didn't find in churches.

The AA founders said it has to do with being 100 percent honest in our humility before God and our admission that our addiction has us whipped; otherwise, we're just going through the (religious) motions of recovery and won't experience God's awesome grace in remaking our lives. The AA founders had a lot to say about those who liberally profess their religious faith, and yet just can't seem to get sober:

> Now let's take the guy full of faith, but still reeking of alcohol. He believes he is devout. His religious observance is scrupulous. He's sure he still believes in God, but suspects that God doesn't believe in him. He takes pledges and more pledges. Following each, he not only drinks again, but acts worse than the last time. Valiantly he tried to fight alcohol, imploring God's help, but the help doesn't come. What, then, can be the matter?
>
> To clergymen, doctors, friends, and families, the alcoholic who means well and tries hard is a heartbreaking riddle. To most AA's, he is not. There are too many of us who have been just like him, and have found the riddle's answer. The answer has to do with the quality of faith rather than its quantity. This has been our blind spot. We supposed we had humility when really we hadn't. We supposed we had been serious about religious practices when, upon honest appraisal, we found we had been only superficial. Or, going to the other extreme, we had wallowed in emotionalism and had mistaken it for true religious feeling. In both cases, we had been asking something for nothing. The fact was, we really hadn't cleaned house so that the grace of God could enter us and expel the obsession. In no deep or meaningful sense had we ever taken stock of ourselves, made amends to those we had harmed, or freely given to any other human being without any demand for reward. We had not even prayed rightly. We had always said, "Grant me my wishes" instead of "Thy will be done." The love of God and man we understood not at all. Therefore we remained self-deceived, and so incapable of receiving enough grace to restore us to sanity.[2]

We knew there had to be other people like us sitting in the pew every Sunday who were secretly devastated because of hidden addictions or compulsions, and that they were too ashamed to share them. Sadly, many Christians were reluctant to attend a "secular" 12-step group in order to get well. They sometimes insisted upon finding a quick fix—a book, a tape, or some sort of "Christian" solution. They might have had it all figured out, yet their lives were in shambles! Many churches still choose to ignore such problems and don't seem to provide many practical answers.

Some folks in recovery are working a 12-step program but are not comfortable going to church. In fact, some are content to just let the 12-step group serve as their church, a less-than-ideal situation, to be sure. They figure that Christians are phony and hypocritical, not living in the real world, and certainly are not to be trusted, so they avoid a resource for growth that could help them greatly. As an unfortunate but undeniable result, many people searching for God in their recovery are afraid to go to church.

It became increasingly obvious that a bridge was needed between traditional 12-step groups and the church. Regardless of a person's stance, the bottom line is that we all share common problems and God has provided powerful tools for our recovery. Diverse perspectives can be blended into a freedom we have never known before.

The Bible tells us that seeking God with our whole heart will pay off in a relationship with Him. "You will find me when you seek me, if you look for me in earnest" (Jer. 29:13). We can know Him.

The New Testament book of Acts talks about the people in Athens, Greece, who had built altars, one of which was inscribed "to the Unknown God" (Acts 17:23). About that practice, Saint Paul exclaimed, "You have been worshiping him without knowing who he is—and now I wish to tell you about him: He made the world and everything in it, and since he is Lord of heaven and earth, he doesn't live in man-made temples... He himself gives life and breath to everything, and satisfies every need there is" (Acts 17:23–25).

The vagueness of the Greek altars "to an unknown God" sounds a lot like the generic reference in AA to the "Higher Power," doesn't it? The Athenians were not unlike people in traditional 12-step groups today. Acts 17:27 perfectly describes the open atmosphere of the various traditional 12-step groups: "His purpose in all of this is that they should seek after God and perhaps feel their way toward him and find him—though he is not far from any one of us." Amazing parallels between two cultures more than two thousand years apart!

The parallels continue. In a sincere and earnest search for God, some people may start out by relying upon the group itself as their "Higher Power"; others actually depend upon an inanimate object (e.g., a doorknob) to be the "power" in their lives. What is God's attitude about these practices? Acts 17:30–31 says, "God tolerated man's past ignorance about these things, but now he commands everyone to put away idols and worship only him. For He has set a day for justly judging the world by the man he has appointed (Jesus Christ) and has pointed him out by bringing him back to life again" (parenthetical note added). He wants us to eventually worship Jesus as the Highest Power, not a support group or a doorknob. This is the foundational principle behind Overcomers Outreach.

So an OO group, which combines the best of AA-style groups with clearly Christian principles, is an ideal setting. Traditional 12-step groups are necessary, too, in conjunction with an OO group. There are far too many Christians out there literally dying of alcoholism or other addictions, who wouldn't get caught dead at an AA meeting, 12-step support group, or any outside help that isn't labeled "Christian." When we hear this excuse, we are reminded of the following story. It can enlighten us all in terms of being able to see God's hand in everyday events.

It seems that a certain man lived on a farm. This man was a devoted Christian. On a particular day it began to rain and it rained long and hard. The water level rose until it covered his front yard. A neighbor came by in a four-wheel-drive vehicle and offered to drive the man to safety, but the man refused. He informed his neighbor, "God will take care of me."

The water continued to rise and pretty soon the man was stranded on the second floor of his house. Another neighbor, seeing his plight, came by in a rowboat and offered to take the man to a safer place, but once again the man refused, saying, "God will take care of me."

The water continued to rise until the man had to climb on his roof to escape the rising torrent. Rescuers flew by in a helicopter and lowered a rope to take the man to safety but the man once again refused, giving the same excuse, "God will take care of me."

The man finally drowned.

When he got to heaven, he asked God why He hadn't protected him in his recent encounter with the flood. God responded: "I did send help to you. First, I sent some men in a four-wheel-drive, then I sent some men in a rowboat, and finally I even sent some men in a helicopter!"

The man was crestfallen; he realized he had rejected God's help without even knowing it.

God works in many different ways, and it is our job to trust the Lord and accept that help, no matter in which form it might arrive.

BRIDGING THE GAP

THE BRIDGE OF OVERCOMERS OUTREACH

Today, Overcomers Outreach is helping to provide a bridge to freedom. In response to the needs we see on both sides of the bridge, Overcomers Outreach seeks to point the way to the Highest Power, the creator of the universe, our Lord and Savior, Jesus Christ. "For in him we live and move and are! ... 'We are the sons of God'" (Acts 17:28).

An Overcomers Outreach 12-step support group is a supplementary Christian program designed to help bridge the gap between traditional 12-step recovery programs and Christian churches of all denominations. Continued attendance at traditional 12-step groups in the community is strongly recommended to our members. It has been demonstrated time and time again that those who have the best chance for recovery and get well the quickest are those who are attending these traditional groups in addition to Overcomers Outreach. Life-saving meetings are available almost every day of the week in the traditional 12-step community. For someone coming off an addiction, regular attendance at meetings is essential for his/her very life.

Though the pioneering work was done in 1977, the ministry of Overcomers Outreach was officially founded in May 1985 as a Christ-centered, non-profit corporation dedicated to reaching out to people within the church with problems of addiction, compulsion, or codependency. Its goals are to provide encouragement for those within the Christian community to discover additional help in their recovery through traditional 12-step groups. In addition, it offers people within traditional 12-step programs a fresh look at the "Higher Power" they have been seeking, in the person of Jesus Christ. This spiritual experience can pave the way for their return to the church of their choice.

Overcomers Outreach groups utilize the 12 Steps of Alcoholics Anonymous along with corresponding Scriptures. We believe that the principles found in the 12 Steps of Alcoholics Anonymous were originally derived from The Holy Bible, and we have linked each Step with some of its corresponding Scriptures.

Although a portion of the Christian community considers alcoholism and drug dependency to be a sin or merely a spiritual problem, we believe addiction to be a disease of body, mind, emotion, and soul, and that all aspects of the person need to be addressed in order for quality recovery to occur. Being an Overcomer puts us in a position to be salt and light in the world (Matt. 5:13–16). We can invite our recovering friends who need a Savior to a place where the gospel is presented and our faith in Christ is openly shared. They are free to open God's Word for themselves. Many exclaim, "I didn't know that was in the Bible!" Those of us who already consider Jesus as our "Higher Power" are overjoyed to have a recovery group where we have the freedom to talk about "God as we understand Him" in the person of Jesus Christ.

We have found that there are preferable ways to share our faith with our friends in traditional 12-step groups. It must be done appropriately and with the greatest discretion. Inviting our friends to an Overcomers Outreach group, where the Bible is linked to the 12 Steps, sometimes turns on a spiritual light for those seeking God, and they find Christ as not just a "Higher Power," but a personal Savior as well. They receive not only a better life in recovery here on this earth, but also the promise of eternal life.

The 12 Steps have become precious and priceless in our living from day to day, and therefore the Steps remain intact within the Overcomers Outreach literature (with the approval of AA World Services, of course). Though some Christians avoid traditional 12-step programs because of their referral to a generic "Higher Power," we have no problem whatsoever with that less-than-crystal-clear identifier, as we know our Lord Jesus Christ to be our "Higher Power"!

The OO ministry is a vast support-group network that provides recovery literature and education through regular OO meetings held worldwide dedicated to initiate and maintain Christ-centered 12-step support groups. A national directory of OO meetings is available, as well as many other recovery resources. Information is available on the OO Web site: www.overcomersoutreach.org.

Overcomers Outreach is not a substitute for church, Bible studies, or worship services. It is not a psychotherapy group—we refer individuals to recommended professional counselors when indicated. It is not even a "Christian AA meeting"—but is rather a supplementary program to traditional 12-step support groups, as we advocate continued attendance at these life-saving programs.

We have found that the bridge works both ways—bringing recovery tools to the church as well as pointing people in recovery programs to Jesus Christ as their Highest Power.

6

BIRTH OF A MINISTRY

Overcomers Outreach clearly had its roots in the birth of Alcoholics Anonymous, which was decades previous to the founding of OO. Though today we are not officially linked with AA, certainly we owe a lot to AA's founders in terms of their basic approach and philosophy. We have built on their foundation, adding in the Christian principles to round out the total life-saving approach we believe is most helpful as a supplement to traditional 12-step support groups.

We don't know exactly and fully why the 12 Steps work, we just know that they do. Undoubtedly it is largely because they are derived from the Holy Scriptures. In an era of failed reform programs and half-baked solutions to the crushing problems of our world, they shine like a beacon in the night. Jacqueline Weir, writing in a religious periodical, puts it this way:

> The 12-step programs are God's gift to the modern world. They magnificently demonstrate to a doubting, cynical humanity that God is always present to the humble, sincere seeker. Precisely because addictions are so crippling and so compelling, those who recover through the 12 Steps often must exercise heroic faith. The sufferers, through their helplessness and despair, have to take a chance, to act as if, to make the wager of surrender and trust to a "Higher Power" they do not always believe is there. Often

it requires a leap of faith that has been likened to a shivering man poised on a windy and rain-drenched cliff on a freezing, mid-winter day trusting that when he leaps, unseen hands will save him from an icy death. Perhaps they won't. But he leaps anyway.[1]

This is the faith, spoken about in the Scriptures and lived out by thousands of recovering persons in Alcoholics Anonymous as they come to "let go and let God."

A portion of chapter 5 of the *Big Book* of Alcoholics Anonymous is read at most AA meetings. These words are the very heart and soul of recovery for those getting well in AA fellowships all over the world. They bear brief mention here to understand what the founders had to say about the program's effectiveness. Appropriately enough, this chapter is titled "How It Works":

> Rarely have we seen a person fail who has thoroughly followed our path. Those who do not recover are people who cannot or will not completely give themselves to this simple program, usually men and women who are constitutionally incapable of being honest with themselves. There are such unfortunates. They are not at fault; they seem to have been born that way. They are naturally incapable of grasping and developing a manner of living which demands rigorous honesty. Their chances are less than average. There are those, too, who suffer from grave emotional and mental disorders, but many of them do recover if they have the capacity to be honest.
>
> Our stories disclose in a general way what we used to be like, what happened, and what we are like now. If you have decided you want what we have and are willing to go to any length to get it—then you are ready to take certain steps.
>
> At some of these we balked. We thought we could find an easier, softer way. But we could not. With all the earnestness at our command, we beg of you to be fearless and thorough from the very start. Some of us have tried to hold on to our old ideas and the result was nil until we let go absolutely.

BIRTH OF A MINISTRY

Remember that we deal with alcohol—cunning, baffling, powerful! Without help it is too much for us. But there is One who has all power—that One is God. May you find Him now!

Half measures availed us nothing. We stood at the turning point. We asked His protection and care with complete abandon.[2]

(See the 12 Steps on pp. 304–305.)

For more than half a century, the 12-step program of Alcoholics Anonymous has reached out to addicted persons, offering practical tools of recovery that really work. In 1935 God, in His infinite wisdom, drew a couple of "hopeless alcoholics" together—Bill W. and Dr. Bob. In total desperation, they got on their knees and began to ransack the Bible. In their last-ditch effort to stop drinking, they put James 5:16 to work: "Admit your faults to one another and pray for each other so you may be healed." When the church wasn't listening, two lowly drunks—a stockbroker and a physician—in their powerlessness and hopelessness, were willing to surrender to God and to take the risk of sharing their hearts with rigorous honesty, thus tuning into God's healing power.

To their surprise, they both began to accumulate days of sobriety, then weeks, and before they knew it, months had gone by and they were celebrating a whole year without a drink. To their amazement, one year led to another, and to another. In their excitement, they began to carry the message of hope to others who were still suffering. They soon found that they couldn't hang onto their sobriety unless they were giving it away to others.

Bill W. and Dr. Bob started out "preaching" to other drunks, but soon found that just sharing their own stories, along with how God had intervened in the midst of their difficulty, was much more effective than preaching. Incredible healing began to occur. And soon, by word of mouth, the news of this remarkable movement of Alcoholics Anonymous began to spread to others in need of victory over addiction to alcohol. Since then, millions have been helped because Bill W. and Dr. Bob took the Bible literally and put its principles into practice.

Amazingly, many people in Christian circles question how 12-step programs like Alcoholics Anonymous can possibly be biblical. Without a doubt, the roots of co-founder Bill W.'s basic philosophy were firmly planted in mainstream Christianity. He was greatly influenced by the Rev. Sam Shoemaker, rector of Calvary Episcopal Church in New York

City, and one of the most influential Christians of the twentieth century, besides being author of dozens of books and founder of the "Faith at Work" organization. In addition, the Oxford Group, an informal evangelistic movement dedicated to reclaiming first-century Christianity, was the organization that finally offered Bill W. hope and provided the biblical principles that nurtured his sobriety and profound spiritual awakening.

The basis of the 12-step program is derived directly from the Bible, particularly I Corinthians 13, the Sermon on the Mount (found in Matthew 5–7), and the book of James. Over the years, hundreds of other 12-step programs have formed, using the simple 12-step formula with amazing success. Each week, literally hundreds of thousands of recovering people from all walks of life meet in support group settings to honestly share their experience, strength, and hope.

We are told that the 12-step meetings are a program of "attraction rather than promotion." In other words, we should offer the benefits to others in a no-pressure manner and not force their participation, but rather let them naturally choose to include themselves based on their attraction to the movement. All we know is that thousands of people are being delivered from their addictions due to this gentle approach. We have discovered that we're not bad people who need to be good, but sick people who need to get well.

How did the 12 Steps actually come to be? Of course we believe that God inspired their formulation in a general sense, but in a more specific sense, Bill W. wrote about the actual origins of the 12 Steps:

> At length I began to write on a cheap yellow tablet. I split the word-of-mouth program up into smaller pieces, meanwhile enlarging its scope considerably. Uninspired as I felt, I was surprised that in a short time, perhaps half an hour, I had set down certain principles which, on being counted, turned out to be 12 in number. And for some unaccountable reason, I had moved the idea of God into the Second Step, right up front. Besides, I had named God very liberally throughout the other Steps. In one of the Steps I had even suggested that the newcomer get down on his knees. When this document was shown to our New York meeting, the protests were many and loud. Our agnostic friends didn't go at all for the idea of kneeling. Others said we were

BIRTH OF A MINISTRY

talking altogether too much about God. And anyhow, why should there be 12 Steps when we had done five or six? Let's keep it simple, they said. This sort of heated discussion went on for days and nights. ...Our agnostic contingent finally convinced us that we must make it easier for people like themselves by using such terms as "Higher Power" or "God as we understand him." These expressions, as we so well know today, have proved lifesavers for many an alcoholic. They have enabled thousands of us to make a beginning where none could have been made had we left the Steps just as I originally wrote them. Happily for us there were no other changes in the original draft and the number of Steps still stood at 12. Little did we guess that our 12 Steps would soon be widely approved by clergy of all denominations, and even by our latter-day friends, the psychiatrists. This little fragment ought to convince the most skeptical that nobody invented Alcoholics Anonymous. It just grew—by the grace of God![3]

The co-founder of Alcoholics Anonymous, Dr. Bob Smith, a medical doctor, was also emphatic about the true Christian thrust of 12-step recovery. Everyone he worked with in Alcoholics Anonymous was given a required reading list, to include the King James Bible, particularly the Sermon on the Mount, the Lord's Prayer, the book of James, and 1 Corinthians 13. In addition, Dr. Bob strongly recommended daily reading of the well-known devotional *The Upper Room*.

According to Bill Pittman, author of an intensive study of Alcoholics Anonymous entitled *AA: The Way It Began*, "...Bill W. did not wish to be known as a saint, a prophet, an author, or the inventor of a new religion, but just as another alcoholic trying to stay sober one day at a time."[4]

God was able to use AA's founders so greatly just because they knew they must remain humble in order to maintain their sobriety. Experience had told them that they were "just one drink away from a drunk." While working their program of recovery, they couldn't afford to be searching for power or notoriety, because they knew they would die or go insane in the process. Instead they became God's instruments to introduce recovery to people of all faiths—or no faith at all.

OVERCOMERS OUTREACH

Decades after AA's founding, author Catherine Marshall had some interesting comments about the relationship between Christianity and the 12-step movement:

> Sometimes laymen who approach Christianity with few preconceived ideas can be surprisingly specific and helpful. A case in point are the twelve steps toward God outlined by Alcoholics Anonymous. Out of great need and hard experience, the men who were the founders of this movement hammered out the steps. When I first read them years after my own entering-in experience, I was astonished to find that this path to sobriety was precisely the road I had traveled on my way to a personal commitment to Christ.[5]

Noted author J. Keith Miller hypothesizes about how God raised up the traditional 12-step movement in lieu of the church's initiative: "The 12 Steps have been too tough for the church to handle, so God took 'the stone the builder rejected' and started traditional 12-step programs."[6]

MEETING THE NEED

In 1975, it was with fear and trembling that we approached our church's pastoral staff with the proposal that we start a Christian support group for alcoholics, addicts, and affected family members. We shared our testimonies and showed an educational film on alcoholism.

Two long years went by. Soon, God gave us a Scripture passage that literally changed our perspective:

> I will climb my watchtower now, and wait to see what answer God will give to my complaint. And the Lord said to me, "Write my answer on a billboard, large and clear, so that anyone can read it at a glance and rush to tell the others. But these things I plan won't happen right away. Slowly, steadily, surely, the time approaches when the vision will be fulfilled. If it seems slow, do not despair, for these things will surely come to pass. Just be patient! They will not be overdue a single day."
>
> —Hab. 2:1–3

BIRTH OF A MINISTRY

It seemed the Lord's unmistakable message to us was to wait for His perfect timing.

By then, the need for a support group had become abundantly apparent in our church. Our pastor of Care and Circles of Concern suggested that we think about starting a special Sunday night circle for recovering people. And so the first Overcomers group began in 1977 as a Circle of Concern at Whittier Area Baptist Fellowship in Southern California. Our senior pastor, Dr. Dan Baumann, admitted honestly that he didn't feel equipped to handle these types of problems and began to welcome the idea of such a support group in his church.

The first Overcomers meeting was held in the home of Dick and Jeannette U., in La Mirada, California. About seven or eight curious people showed up. We continued to meet one Sunday night per month in various homes. In preparation for the first meeting, we used Bible concordances and Thompson Chain Reference Bibles, discovering many Scriptures both in the Old and New Testaments that corresponded with AA's 12 Steps. We could hardly contain our enthusiasm! We would start out with some hymns and praise songs to warm up; then for our study time, it seemed logical to begin with Step One of AA, linking it to the corresponding Scriptures we had found. The Bible verses were passed around, and as individuals read them and compared them with the first Step, everything came into focus. All the participants were asked to do was comment on what that particular Scripture meant to them in light of the Step. No one felt pressured to perform, but just to speak what the Holy Spirit revealed to them through God's Word.

The heart of the meeting was the personal sharing. To our delight, rigorous honesty came to life there, just as occurred in our traditional 12-step groups. We closed the meeting with sentence prayers concerning one another's needs and then finished in the traditional manner of all 12-step groups, with The Lord's Prayer and a triumphant chorus of the slogan "Keep Coming Back—It Works!"

Our little band of searching people had a whole month to decide what to do at the second meeting. It made sense to take a look at Step Two, so back to the Scriptures we went, to glean applicable verses. As the next meeting approached, people could hardly wait to return to their safe place of refuge in Overcomers where they had permission to be real. As the months went by and we continued to follow the same simple format of Bible study, sharing, and prayer, the growth in individual lives was astonishing. People from other churches and from varying denominations began to attend. Many people found Jesus as their "Higher Power" for the first time. Families were reunited. The 12 Steps proved invaluable in individuals' efforts to overcome addictions and/or compulsions, and caused many to find sobriety for the first time. The power of the Holy Spirit was evident at each meeting.

During the first year, about fifty different people became involved. Some would drop out along the way, but others became regulars. Before long, our highly enthusiastic members insisted that a meeting once a month wasn't enough. So we began to meet twice a month for a brief period, but that only made us hungry to meet every week. Soon the first weekly gathering of Overcomers was held, and the meeting room at the church began to fill to capacity every Tuesday night.

The freedom to talk about Christ as our "Higher Power" and worship Him, to link God's Word with the Scriptures, and to pray together was exhilarating. Due to the honest sharing, much healing was taking place. And we noticed that our prayers were not about some issue or distant person, but concerned the people within our group, along with our own needs. We learned quickly not to share our prayer requests with people outside the group, so everyone soon felt secure in their anonymity.

As people became well and began to put the 12 Steps and Scriptures to work in their lives on a daily basis, their enthusiasm knew no bounds. Because rotation of leadership was stressed, different people led the meetings each week, and these lay leaders began to blossom and grow at an astonishing rate. We were eventually forced to develop a simple, written meeting format that was similar to that used in traditional 12-step groups. As people became more firmly grounded in recovery, they had a desire to start additional Overcomers meetings in their own churches. Taking the Overcomers concept with them, several other Overcomers groups and related 12-step spin-off recovery groups were formed by the emerging group leaders whom God had put in place.

About that time, our new pastor would occasionally drop by a meeting because he recognized the group as a safe place to just be himself. He would say, "Hi, I'm Lee and I'm a sinner." He was amazed that the leaders had no formal training. All he knew was that there were miracles happening and that God's Spirit was evident because He was allowed to work.

GOD AT WORK

As the original group and several spin-offs flourished, coincidences began occurring in our lives, laying the groundwork for the eventual

BIRTH OF A MINISTRY

formation of a comprehensive recovery ministry. Despite our limited vision at the time, God had a plan. Little did we realize its scope!

During this time Bob was introduced to a man who encouraged him to go back to school and work toward a graduate degree in counseling alcoholics. The Bartosch family will never forget the day when 47-year-old Bob, complete with cap and gown, received his master of science degree at LaVerne University. What a far cry he was from the husband and father we'd known just a few short years before!

We continued to hold down regular jobs (Bob as an insurance agent, and I [Pauline] as an administrative assistant). The 12-step meetings were our lifeline to sanity. We gobbled up all the literature and educational information we could lay our hands on, learning about what had been happening to us all those traumatic years. As time went by, our consuming interest in the field of alcoholism and addictions got the best of us. We attended four different week-long summer schools on alcoholism and drug abuse at the University of Utah in Salt Lake City. What a breakthrough it was when we learned that alcoholism was a disease of body, mind, emotion, and soul. We gained new hope because we knew that God is able to forgive sins and also heal diseases (Ps. 103:3).

At that stage we were about five years in recovery, and our lives had improved about 1,000 percent as healthy relationships were developing. Surrounded by new friends from every walk of life who loved and accepted us exactly the way we were, we reveled in the unparalleled support from these wonderful people. And no one seemed to have more fun than people in recovery!

One Sunday evening the Overcomers meeting was being held in our home. We closed the meeting with a circle of prayer, with Bob asking God to open more doors of opportunity to reach people. Just then, the phone rang. It was an associate of Dr. James Dobson from "Focus on the Family." Somehow they had obtained an article that I (Pauline) had written describing our family's recovery from alcoholism. They asked us to appear on the "Focus on the Family" radio program the following week and share what God had done in our lives through the traditional 12-step groups. We were dumbfounded at this awesome opportunity. The show aired on almost 2,800 radio stations in all fifty states and overseas. As a result, responses began to pour in.

After that, a producer of a Christian TV program called "JOY" heard about us. Soon an invitation was issued from Trinity Broadcasting Network for us to appear on the show with host Jim McClellan. Having never authored a book, the only document we had was a study entitled

OVERCOMERS OUTREACH

12 Steps and Scriptures that Bob had developed and simply photocopied on Long Beach Alcoholism Council stationery. During the show, Jim held up the rumpled copy for the cameras to focus on with his usual gusto. We sheepishly offered to make additional copies and send them to any viewers who might be interested. Since we naively figured at the time that this particular religious audience might not have need for our type of material, we had no way of knowing what would happen next. More than three hundred requests from fifteen states came in to the TV station requesting our photocopied study. Since we both had steady jobs at the time, our biggest task waited for us in the evenings when we began to send out the simple material and answer the letters that came pouring in.

The most prevalent question the respondents asked was, "Where can we find such a group as yours in our area?" We knew that there were one or two other Christian organizations out there that were dealing with alcoholism at the time, and we tried to find out as much as we could. We promptly discovered two distinct schools of thought: 1) those who recognized the 12 Steps as one of God's tools to help people, and 2) those who rejected the 12 Steps because they had their origin outside the church.

The other question we got was, "How can we start an Overcomers group in our church?" We kept thinking that someday we probably should write down all the concepts God had given us, so the next time we were invited to appear on the "JOY" show, we stopped by a local print shop and made a simple cover with an acronym that had been developed in 1979 by Jess Maples (Overcomers group leader at Eastside Christian Church in Fullerton, California). It read: "FREED"—Fellowship in Recovery, Reconciliation to God and His Family, Education about Chemicals and Addiction, Edification through Faith in Christ, and Dedicated Service to Others. The first page had a table of contents and the rest of the pages were blank. We had a pretty good idea what would be included on those pages, but it was yet to be developed. And so when Jim offered the book, we had cautioned him not to open it on camera because there was nothing in it!

As we responded to the numerous letters pouring in from all over the country from people who wanted to start Overcomers groups, we realized that this wild phenomenon certainly hadn't been in our plans. We hadn't dreamed of it, even in our wildest imaginations. Our vision had been limited to one group in our local church. You would think that with such blatant signs we would have been able to hear God's voice beginning to

BIRTH OF A MINISTRY

call us to start a ministry. Yet we needed more signs to finally be able to read the handwriting on the wall.

Beginning to Sense God's Call

In 1984, Bob began to suffer burnout on his job as executive director at the Alcoholism Council in Long Beach. During his five years heading up the Council, he had been naively attempting to sober up every drunk in Long Beach all by himself. In return, he painfully watched as more and more people succumbed to the deadly disease of alcoholism.

Finally, in June of that year, the stress caused Bob to visit our doctor, who informed him he had three options: 1) suffer a heart attack, 2) succumb to a stroke, or 3) quit his job. None of those appealed to him, but after hanging on as long as possible, he finally let go and gave notice of his resignation. Soon Bob was spending more time in God's Word and his 12-step meetings, wondering what God had in mind for him next. Neither of us was ready, however, for the brokenness that was to follow.

Just as Bob was beginning to feel better in August of 1984, we decided to head for a relaxing fishing trip in the mountains near Lake Tahoe, California. That first morning, Bob cast his line from the muddy shoreline, and just as I (Pauline) was preparing to toss mine out, my feet suddenly slipped out from under me. With a thud and a sickening snap, I realized that my ankle had just broken. On hands and knees, I ascended the adjacent hillside toward our car and Bob raced me to the nearest hospital, which was twenty miles away.

I was treated and released with a bandage and temporary splint, but no crutches (which would have come in handy). Awkwardly hopping along with Bob as my stabilizer (as usual), we entered a sandwich shop to have lunch, where we were seated next to a nice-looking young couple, Ken and Gail Harris. Seeing my hop-a-long plight, they offered to loan me their son's crutches, which were in their garage at home.

Later that day, Ken and Gail appeared at our campsite with crutches that, miraculously, would accommodate only someone 5' 5" or less. I was precisely that height, and so I couldn't help but exclaim, "God sure does work in my life, even down to the details!"

When Ken and Gail responded with "Amen!" we realized we had found new Christian friends. In fact, we discovered that Ken was the pastor of a local church. Ken and Gail insisted that we come to their house and share leftovers for dinner. But as we approached their beautiful log home in the woods, my eyes traveled toward the steep stairway to the

67

entrance, which would be a problem on crutches. I counted them, and there were exactly twelve steps!

Ken unknowingly played further into the heavenly message when he assured me, "Pauline, just take one step at a time on those crutches and you'll be OK." I realized God was walking me through another one of His miracles.

God's guidance didn't dry up after that trip. After arriving home, my patience wore thin as I hobbled around on my broken ankle. But as I searched the Bible for reassurance, God kept pointing out Mark 1:17 where a verse popped off the page: "...I will make you...fishers of men" (KJV). By then I wasn't too interested in any kind of fishing trip.

The next incidence of brokenness was excruciating and affected our entire family. Our eldest son, Bob, was rushed to the hospital after being hit by a three-hundred-pound satellite dish. While he was helping to install the equipment, the huge dish had slipped and fallen on Bob's hip and upper leg, shattering the bones. After the surgery, the doctors were amazed at how all the bone fragments fit back together like a jigsaw puzzle, but the following weeks were sheer agony. We wondered why these events of brokenness were happening all at once: Bob resigned his job for health reasons, I broke my ankle, and Bob Jr. suffered compound fractures. Yet as it turned out, it was through Bob Jr.'s brokenness that we came to a point of being much more open to God's call toward ministry. And another bonus popped up; our son Bob's wife, Debbie, trusted Jesus as her personal Savior just weeks after the accident.

Another event that pointed the way toward God's special ministry was an Al-Anon retreat that I attended right about then. On Saturday afternoon of the conference we were all asked to have a quiet time, talking only to God. I wrote the Lord a long letter in the hushed sanctuary of the church. "Lord," I wrote, "what's next? Even though I'm quite comfortable in my job right now, if You want me to do something different, help me to be willing!"

After being back at my job just three days, to my utter surprise I somehow sensed that it was time to move on. So in February of 1985, I gave my two-week notice. *What now?* I wondered.

We shared the events of recent days with our pastor and his response was, "Well, now you're both out of work. What are you going to do?"

Our reply was, "We don't have the slightest idea!"

We were uncertain as to our next step, but at least in the meantime we had more time to send out *The 12 Steps and Scriptures*, answer the

BIRTH OF A MINISTRY

letters that continued to pour into our mailbox, and to take never-ending phone calls from all over the country.

God Sends His Message

One evening we were out with some dear friends, Dave and Mary Jean Becker, on our way to a speaking engagement to give our testimonies. The Beckers remarked, "Wouldn't it be great if you could devote your time to get Overcomers groups started all over the country?" These dear Christian people offered to give money every month toward such an endeavor. We pictured ourselves trying to survive on donations from our friends. It was a sweet gesture, but we just couldn't picture living on donations.

Just two days later, we happened to run into another couple at a restaurant who had been extremely instrumental in our lives. Sig and Evelyn Esselstrom shared that God had given them a message that we should consider starting a ministry for alcoholics and their families. We balked. Where would the resources come from? They insisted, "If God is in it, He will provide everything you need."

Within the remarkable month of February 1985, we had multiple offers of both prayer and financial support to get a ministry started. Some folks offered sizable monthly pledges; other Christian friends simply gave us encouragement and suggestions. But the most valuable ingredient during that time was earnest prayer being offered by scores of interested believers. Every day produced more risks, decisions, and challenges. We began to receive phone calls day and night from people needing help. Although we felt scared at the prospect of stepping out into uncharted territory, we sensed the intense guidance of the Holy Spirit of God.

At that point, the new pastor of Care and Concern at our church, Dr. Dale Ryan, became intrigued with the miracles he saw coming from the OO group. He noticed that not only were people being helped with addictions, but also many of these people were reaching out for help with additional problems that were often uncovered in the group sharing process. Soon an A.C.A. (Adult Children of Alcoholics) group spun off, made up of individuals who had been raised in an alcoholic home and had been deeply affected.

The church's Circle Ministry offered to assist us with printing and postage. We spent hours and days in two connecting bedrooms in our home collating, stapling, and addressing a huge mailing of *The 12 Steps and Scriptures*. It wasn't long before the responses flooded back. The most frequent response was, "This booklet is an answer to prayer!" We couldn't help but wonder how such a simple little unsophisticated piece could be so instrumental in helping so many hurting people. All we knew was it was working!

Finally, on February 22, 1985, we met again with our church leaders to discuss the feasibility of formally developing a ministry. That same evening, we also met with a Christian physician, Dr. Willard Hawkins, and with a Christian psychologist, Dr. Earl Henslin, who had approached us with a sense of urgency regarding the need within the Christian community to start a recovery ministry.

Then, on February 25, 1985, we went to Bob's weekly breakfast with good friend and mentor Henry Warren. All during this time of job transition, Henry and Bob had been meeting for breakfast once a week to help Bob develop a new resume and to set career goals. Week after week went by with no replies to his job search. That morning, Bob finally began to share with Henry the idea of starting a Christian recovery ministry. At that moment, Henry pulled a long list out of his pocket of the strategic steps that God had given him to share with Bob when he seemed ready. Henry exclaimed, "I was waiting for you to come to this conclusion, Bob!" After witnessing the phenomenal success of the several Overcomers groups in existence at the time, Henry convinced us that it could work in any church, large or small. This list turned out to be the basic framework of the ministry.

The month of March 1985 provided even more confirmation of God's call. Surrounding us at our first steering committee meeting were twelve dedicated individuals, humbly seeking God's specific direction. It became so obvious that God was in it that the committee voted unanimously to meet three more times that month to discuss the ministry's approach and destination, identifying needs, setting goals, developing a rational statement of purpose, deciding preliminary budget, and planning our kick-off dinner. Whittier Area Baptist Fellowship offered to be a temporary conduit for donations until the ministry could be incorporated, and a Father Martin film and projector were purchased for our numerous speaking engagements.

One of the more fascinating discussions during the early meetings was regarding the name to be chosen for the ministry. Considered were Overcomers Christian Fellowship, Overcomers Ministries, and Overcomers, Inc. But when Jess Maples and I (Pauline) simultaneously came up with Overcomers Outreach, the name seemed exactly right!

BIRTH OF A MINISTRY

MINISTRY IS LAUNCHED

In May 1985, with the assistance of its founding board, the ministry of Overcomers Outreach was officially launched in Whittier, California, The kick-off dinner drew 120 curious guests. By then, sixteen Overcomers groups were going strong. Our church decided that Bob should be licensed as a minister. OO board officers were selected and by-laws were developed. Some of the goals we set included education regarding chemical dependency; establishing a network of Christian support groups; developing a newsletter and referral directory; and having a speakers' bureau and a youth program. All of these goals were eventually realized.

On August 19, 1985, God gave me the design of the FREED "Dove," and it was soon registered as Overcomers Outreach's official logo.

We began to expand our outreach in earnest. The first youth team was sent out in October 1988 to share their testimonies at a church youth group in Bellflower, California. Soon thereafter, Curt Grayson put into place the T.N.T. (Tried 'N True) teen program for young people between the ages of twelve and twenty who were either living in an alcoholic home or were struggling with their own addictions. Three hundred youth gathered for the first T.N.T. Youth Conference held on November 10, 1990, at Eastside Christian Church in Fullerton, California. Many teens approached the workshop presenters during the weekend with such comments as, "I've never been able to talk about this before, but..." and "Thanks for letting me know I'm not the only one going through this. Now I know there's hope for me."

In 1991, Alice Clements, several other consultants and I (Pauline) completed the O.K. Kids Workbook for children between the ages of five and twelve. Alice and her helpers tested an O.K. Kids pilot group for three years in Whittier, California, finding that the group drastically changed the lives of children forced to live in an alcoholic or dysfunctional home, paving the way toward harmonious relationships. Mike D., a young recovering alcoholic/addict father, testified that it was through the help of the O.K. Kids support group that his little daughters learned about the disease of addiction and new ways of relating to one another in the home with a recovering parent. Additional O.K. Kids groups started, focusing on teaching children *The 12 Steps and Scriptures* along with basic principles of relating to a loving heavenly Father.

The H.I.M. Ministry (Hospitals, Institutions, and Missions) was initiated in 1990, with Bill Ritchey coordinating teams of recovering people to share their testimonies at various treatment centers, prisons, and

OVERCOMERS OUTREACH

missions. As a result, dozens of Overcomers groups have started in those facilities. God miraculously used the brokenness in the lives of some of His wayward children in order to create His ministry, filling a vacuum in churches both large and small. No longer must hurting Christians suffer in silence attempting to maintain a cheery facade that all is well while they are dying inside.

The truth really does set us free!

The office situation was getting cramped. By the fall of 1985, there were twenty-two Overcomers groups in existence and we were still working out of our Jack-and-Jill (adjoining bedrooms) "office," sharing one typewriter in shifts. By January 1986, our home office was usually humming with faithful volunteers and we used the church's folding machine and paste-up equipment for OO's quarterly newsletter. But after a year and a half of working out of the bedrooms, it became apparent that we needed to seek outside office space because our phone was ringing twenty-four hours per day!

With renewed encouragement supplied by Christian friends, in October of 1986 we rented a small upstairs office three blocks from our home, despite concerns from the frugal Overcomers Outreach board. For the first year, it was just the two of us and a volunteer crew. A grand Open House was celebrated on December 28, 1987, as we dedicated the office space to the Lord. With eighty-six groups in nineteen states, we also began to realize how much we needed additional staff members.

Then we were invited to be interviewed on "The Biola Hour" radio program, among our other radio and TV appearances. Quite unexpectedly, the Biola switchboard lit up like a Christmas tree afterward, and we were suddenly deluged with mail and forced to add another phone line at the office.

It was great to be out of our house and in real office space, but after only one year, we were stepping on each other in our cozy new upstairs office. Dear friends Dave and Mary Jean Becker helped us "lay hands" on the adjacent office's connecting door (which had been hidden behind a bookcase) and pray for more space by God's help. We then took a deep breath and called the landlord. It was available so we got the adjoining office.

It wasn't long before the ministry began to snowball. By June 1987 there were 125 groups in 24 states. In July 1987, Mary Jean Becker announced that God had led her to quit an eight-year position, humbly offering herself as office assistant. This gesture was too amazing for words.

BIRTH OF A MINISTRY

Later on, the office across the hall was vacated by an insurance company and temporarily replaced with some rather shady characters. Dave and Mary Jean helped us "lay hands" on that office also, and God allowed them to remain just long enough until they got into trouble and Overcomers Outreach had saved enough funds to branch out once again. After that, it didn't take too long before the last remaining upstairs office in our building was claimed for the Lord. A door was cut through to make the mailing department.

CONTINUED EXPANSION

While we once chuckled at the prospect of Overcomers Outreach becoming an international ministry, with God's guidance and timing it indeed began to branch out into all directions of the globe. This was not the result of a public relations campaigns, advertising, or grants, but was the result of Overcomers Outreach remaining a faith ministry, where there was much prayer and focus on taking one step at a time under the guidance of our Lord. Many times the Overcomers Outreach board has found themselves having to say no to lucrative offers in order to maintain the ministry's integrity, focus, and vision.

During its first ten years, Overcomers Outreach celebrated each year of ministry with an annual banquet. At each event, we heard tremendous testimonies from recovering people, raised funds to keep the doors open, and usually reported an increase in the number of Overcomers Outreach Groups worldwide.

OO TODAY—A BRIGHT LIGHT IN A DARK WORLD!

Overcomers Outreach's central office has returned to its initial birthing place in Whittier, California. It is now housed in the former home of two of OO's early founding board members, Sigurd and Evelyn Esselstrom, who are both now with the Lord. Without Sig and Evelyn's early encouragement, spiritual influence, endless hours of volunteering their expertise, energies, and faithful financial assistance, OO might well not have been launched in 1985. They were two of God's special angels who just quietly encouraged us with constant prayer and their words, "If God wants Overcomers to happen, He will provide for every need." They were right! Little did we know, when we just happened to run into Sig and Evelyn's daughter, Lenore Remland, in the fall of 2008 that she would invite us to bring the OO ministry from its tiny office in the San

OVERCOMERS OUTREACH

Fernando Valley to her parents' precious but empty house in Whittier, just a few miles away from its original home at the Bartosches'. Today, the OO Office is located on this sacred hilltop, overlooking a panoramic view to the Pacific Ocean. God's plans can be amazing—beyond anything we could ever imagine. And God's work is up and running. We're currently taking phone calls, e-mails, and Web site communications from all over the world. Hits on the OO Web site (overcomersoutreach.org) indicate that many people from around the globe are tuning in and reaching out for the specialized help offered at Overcomers Outreach. OO is currently operating under the capable direction of CEO Jeff MacLeod and the board of directors. New technology has made possible an exciting, comprehensive Web site (developed by our creative director), which includes an online national OO Group Directory, online OO meetings, and even a chat room. Since Jeff has many years of extensive experience serving as a ship captain in the Merchant Marine, he is right at home steering the OO ship. Hundreds of people are referred to OO groups by such Christian organizations as Focus on the Family, The Billy Graham Evangelistic Association, Trinity Broadcasting Network, American Family Living, and many others. The OO office personnel suggest referrals to appropriate support groups, treatment centers, and Christian therapists who are knowledgeable about the disease of addiction. Communications of every variety arrive at the office from people seeking help, and each one receives a prompt personal reply.

We continue to develop and upgrade educational OO pamphlets that deal with every addiction and suggest appropriate sources of help. Simple literature is offered so that people will become more aware of the facts concerning addictions and compulsions. Many treatment centers, as well as private therapists, send their recovering patients to OO for aftercare, actually making their job easier in the process and helping to prevent relapse in their patients. A vast network of OO support groups now encircles the globe. Most groups employ a rotation of leadership and utilize OO's simple FREED guideline booklet as their meeting structure. Both the addicted person and family members are welcome to attend. Anonymity is strictly adhered to, making the meeting a safe place to share our hearts. God's presence is most apparent of all as He speaks a message of hope through the mouths of His children.

The mission of Overcomers Outreach is to serve as an important bridge between 12-step programs and churches of every denomination. OO proclaims our "Higher Power" as Jesus Christ, our Savior and Lord.

BIRTH OF A MINISTRY

People in churches have a safe place to share their hearts and seek help for their particular addiction, and to be directed to an appropriate traditional 12-step group for needed additional help. And many in traditional 12-step programs are quite surprised to discover their "Higher Power" by name—perhaps for the first time in an OO group—and make their way to a church of their choosing where their Lord Jesus Christ welcomes them with open arms! The future of OO holds bright promise of sending a resounding message of hope to people all over the world, for the Christian and non-Christian alike. Only God could have designed this Christ-centered, meaningful, effective recovery program, drawing His somewhat resistant children together in His name. Through OO, He is healing the wounded, giving sight to the blind, and opening our eyes to the exceedingly abundant life He has planned for every one of us, no matter what our circumstances may seem to be. We can be free indeed, one day at a time, through the power of Christ!

PART II

FROM THE PROFESSIONALS

7

FROM THE PASTOR: HEART-MENDING AS THE CHURCH'S TASK

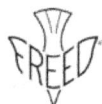

BY ANTHONY L. JORDAN, D. MIN.
SUPERINTENDENT, SOUTHERN BAPTIST CONVENTION
Oklahoma City, Oklahoma

I am neither a psychologist nor a psychiatrist. I am not a professional in the field of chemical dependency. As a matter of fact, I am a lifetime tee-totaller. The truth is, I was pastor of a large Southern Baptist church in the heart of the Bible Belt for many years. These are not very impressive credentials from which to write in the area of dependency and recovery.

But before you stop reading, realize these are exactly the credentials necessary in order for me to address the subject at hand. My purpose is twofold: first, I must challenge the "old wineskins" of the church (outdated assumptions) in regard to ministry to the chemically dependent and their families. I hope this article will reveal the need for the evangelical church to use "new wineskins" (new approaches and mindsets) in ministry. Second, I desire to open the eyes of the hurting to the love that is now available in the church.

Turn in the Bible to Luke 4:18–22, and listen to the words of Jesus as He describes His ministry assignment. I believe He was describing the ministry of the church as well. Jesus spoke these words at the inauguration of His public ministry in the synagogue in His hometown of Nazareth. We are to be the incarnational living-out of the ministry of Jesus. The local family of faith—your church and mine—is to bear the marks of His life and ministry.

Jesus' opening words are very comforting to me. "The Spirit of the Lord is upon Me, because he hath anointed me to preach the gospel to the poor; he hath sent me to heal the brokenhearted, to preach deliverance to the captives, and recovering of sight to the blind, to set at liberty them that are bruised, to preach the acceptable year of the Lord" (Luke 4:18–19 KJV). Notice that He didn't put a period after the word "preach." The words that follow reveal a broad responsibility. His assignment, and thus ours in the church, is to become instruments of healing for the brokenhearted. In essence, He has called the New Testament Church to be heart-menders. The church is to be the place where the brokenhearted can find a healing balm for their fragmented lives.

It was in the reading of this passage that the Lord began to speak to my heart. I heard His still, small voice asking me, "Will you be one of those who will mend broken hearts? Will your church become a place where the brokenhearted can go to get their hearts mended?" Every pastor and Christian layperson knows the correct answer to these questions. The challenge is, are we following His calling in our lives and church ministries?

Under closer scrutiny, I had to admit that far too often people with heartaches shun the church. Even those within the church who are enmeshed in pain and shame often leave without revealing their hurts. This is never more true than in the case of those suffering from addiction. The same is true of their families. But why?

I do not purport to have all the answers to such a significant question. However, I do believe God has shown us some of the answers to that question. I am convinced that the church can become a heart-mender. We can become a safe haven for the chemically dependent and their families to come out of hiding and find healing. Even in a church traditionally not noted for social ministry, the brokenhearted can find love, acceptance, and help—if we will change.

If we are going to mend broken hearts, we must first see people as Jesus saw them. This is not as easy as one might think. For many of us, there are some real barriers to seeing people as they really are.

The first barrier for many church people is a stained-glass-window view of life. I fit that description perfectly. I was raised in a godly Christian home. Mom and Dad were Sunday school teachers. Mom played the piano and organ for our church. One grandfather was a pastor and the

FROM THE PASTOR: HEART-MENDING AS THE CHURCH'S TASK

other a deacon. I was surrounded with biblical teaching and Christian living. I never once in my entire life questioned whether I was loved and accepted. You can imagine my astonishment to discover that everybody did not grow up in a family like mine. Frankly, increasing numbers of the families in our society can be described as dysfunctional. Addictions have taken their toll on families and individuals. Yet many of us in the church have not seen the magnitude of the problem because we view life through stained-glass windows.

Let me explain what I mean by sharing a bit of my own journey. I can vividly remember my first encounters with alcohol because there were so few. My first taste of alcohol came as a small boy. No doubt, my dad had enlisted the help of a Methodist friend to go to the liquor store in town to buy a bottle of whiskey. (After all, everybody in town knew Baptists don't drink.) I had a bad cold and dad had the remedy: he mixed a drop or two of honey and fresh lemon juice with a tablespoon of whiskey. The moment it crossed my lips, I determined I never wanted to taste that stuff again! It made a lasting impression because since that day I have not drunk alcohol.

Strangely enough, the first time I ever saw anyone somewhat inebriated was at a Sunday school party. A young wife in Dad's class called to request help with her husband who had been drinking on his way home from work. Her spouse insisted on coming to the class party. Dad assured her that they could ride with us to the party and that he was welcome. My eyes must have been the size of saucers when the husband stumbled out the door on his way to our car. Dad lovingly guided him along. Later on, Dad led him to the Lord and today he is a leader in that same church.

Perhaps my greatest eye-opener came in seminary. As a student, I was required to have a practical ministry project. My assignment was to spend two hours, one night per week, at the Baptist Rescue Mission in New Orleans' French Quarter. Quite an experience for a stained-glass-window Christian! I was stunned at what I discovered there. The men were not ignorant, uneducated bums, as I had assumed they would be. Many of them became alcoholics while serving in some of life's most respected occupations: medicine, ministry, architecture, and engineering. Many had fallen through the cracks of our churches without our even knowing it. They found themselves on the bottom, living lives of drunkenness and emptiness. Where was the safety net inside our stained-glass-window churches? I asked myself.

OVERCOMERS OUTREACH

I, like so many, was blinded to the brokenness around me because I viewed people through my stained-glass-window perspective. By God's grace I had been spared the tragedy of a dysfunctional family lifestyle, but that did not exonerate me from the responsibility to minister to the brokenhearted. Many of us in the church today view people as I did. We don't see people in their hurts; maybe that's why we aren't mending broken hearts like we should.

We have also built stained-glass walls in our churches. Because of this, there is tremendous secrecy in the church. We drive to church in our fine cars, dress in our finest suits and jewelry, sing the hymns, and listen to the sermon, while hiding incredible pain and shame in our lives. We are afraid to let anyone in the church know our hurts.

Do people hide their pain and shame because of calloused attitudes in church? Do we give off vibes that say it isn't OK to have hurts and failure? I'm afraid so. I've concluded that in most of our churches it is OK to admit we are sinners as long as we don't get too specific about our sin. We are comfortable when a person confesses a generic sinful condition of life, but our comfort zone is violated when a person begins to confess addiction to alcohol, drugs, sex, etc. When we hear who a person really is, we don't know what to do with that person!

People fighting the pain and shame of addiction need to perceive an attitude of safety and acceptance, not one of condemnation and shame, from people in the church; otherwise, the stained-glass wall is too high for them to crawl over. They will stay hidden and often fall away, drowning in their hurt. It is not inconsequential that the words of Jesus recorded in Luke 4 were described as "gracious" (v. 22, KJV). I am convinced that, although our preaching must be without compromise, the truth of the gospel must be proclaimed graciously, not judgmentally.

A last hindrance to our seeing people as Jesus saw them is our stained-glass doors. We look through these doors to the outside world and think it is their fault for not entering our houses of worship. Tragically, the truth is that they don't come into our churches because we have locked the doors! We inside the church have the healing balm of the gospel of Jesus Christ. We can offer the brokenhearted hope in the midst of their problems; we are to be dispensers of grace, yet we don't open the doors and go out to those in need. People in the world on the outside are fearful to walk through our stained-glass doors. The treatment they receive when they do try to enter is so cold and distant that those stained-glass doors may as well have been locked from the outside.

FROM THE PASTOR: HEART-MENDING AS THE CHURCH'S TASK

I discovered this truth when I began to see the world through the eyes of Jesus and sought to meet people's needs. The more encounters I had with the chemically dependent, the more I discovered an open hostility towards the church among them. It got me to thinking. Even those in AA found it difficult to walk through the doors of the church. Why?

For many, their rejection comes from an all-too-real experience base. They have tried the church and received rejection and misunderstanding. (There are other reasons; I also believe that many of the positive images in the church remind them all too clearly of what might have been if they had not taken the course of chemical dependency or other addictions.)

It is time for the church to stop looking through our stained-glass windows, walls, and doors. If we are to become the healing community of Christ, our vision must be corrected. When we see people through the eyes of Jesus we will have made the first step toward becoming heart-menders. That is a key first step.

The second step of becoming a heart-mender requires us to touch people like Jesus touched them. Gary Smalley and John Trent tell a wonderful story in their book entitled *The Blessing*, which incarnates this idea for me.

> A little four-year-old girl became frightened late one night during a thunderstorm. After one particularly loud clap of thunder, she jumped up from her bed, ran down the hall, and burst into her parents' room. Jumping right in the middle of the bed, she sought out her parents' arms for comfort and assurance. "Don't worry, Honey," her father said, trying to calm her fears. "The Lord will protect you." The little girl snuggled closer to her father and said, "I know that, Daddy, but right now I need someone with skin on!"[1]

This is the cry of individuals and families devastated by addiction. They cry, "Friend, what I need from the church is somebody with skin on."

What keeps the church from touching these hurting people caught in the web of addiction? My next statement may shock you. The greatest hindrance to fleshing out the ministry of Jesus to those in bondage to addictions is the pastor. Let me tell you why. He is the shepherd; he is the leader of the flock. Therefore, if he does not see people through the eyes of Jesus and willingly open the doors of the church to them, they will not find help.

Please do not misunderstand me. I have been a pastor for many years. I love pastors. I understand them and know the tremendous pressures they live under every day. Yet the church will not advance any further than the pastor who leads it.

Frankly, most pastors are overworked and underpaid. They are not looking for another ministry to add to their workload. They have enough people draining their energies and complicating their lives. Moreover, most pastors do not have the knowledge to deal with the chemically dependent. Words very familiar to those in the world of addiction are totally foreign to most pastors. They have little training and few resources on which to draw in ministering to those in addiction or recovery.

I have been where most pastors are. Back before my eyes were opened in this way, I knew people were in desperate need of help. I also knew it was my responsibility to lead my church to minister in Jesus' name to them. But what could I do with the limited time, knowledge, and resources available?

The answer came to me when reading Ephesians 4:11-12: "And he gave some, apostles; and some, prophets; and some, evangelists; and some, pastors and teachers; For the perfecting of the saints, for the work of the ministry, for the edifying of the body of Christ..." (KJV). It was like a light turning on inside me. The answer had been there all along. I don't have to minister to the addicted and their families all alone. I simply need to become the facilitator for ministry by creating a climate of acceptance and provide training opportunities to those called to this ministry. So I began to pray for God to send someone to me with a heart for ministry to those with addictions, and I asked Him to provide the resources for such a ministry. God did an incredible thing when He answered my prayer!

My answer came at our weekly pastor's conference. On this particular Monday, a woman was given five minutes to tell about her desire to minister to people in alcohol and drug addiction. She was a church counselor; I'll call her Josie. Could she be the answer to my prayer? I made an appointment to meet her. It was a divine appointment. I shared with her my desire to discover a way to build a bridge between the church and AA. I told her of my prayer for the Lord to open the door of ministry to the chemically dependent through our church. Josie listened intently and then pulled from her purse a booklet with the word "FREED" on the front. She turned to the back of the book and laid it before me. Eureka! There

FROM THE PASTOR: HEART-MENDING AS THE CHURCH'S TASK

it was—a bridge with the church on one side and Alcoholics Anonymous on the other. It is the booklet produced by Overcomers Outreach, which builds Scripture into the 12 Steps of AA.

This encounter with Josie began a journey that is still going on in our church. Through Overcomers Outreach and the ministry of just one woman who really cared about the brokenhearted, our church was able to begin not only our ministry to the chemically dependent, but we started more than twenty other ministries in sister churches.

The church can incarnate the ministry of Jesus. We can touch the brokenhearted the way Jesus touched them. He has given us a very simple plan to get the job done. His plan will not add stress to the pastor, but it will expand his ministry. It requires neither enormous financial resources nor expensive professionals. It does, however, demand people with a desire to be heart-menders. These people are often those who have experienced brokenness and found the healing power of Jesus in their lives. Those in the church who are in recovery are the best heart-menders.

I conclude with a word to my fellow pastors. Your church can be the heart-mending center of your community. It will require, however, seeing the broken people around you through the eyes of Jesus. You will be called upon to lead your church to touch people with the same compassion and love Jesus had. But the rewards are immeasurable on this side of heaven.

The chemically dependent and their families are all around you. Some are hiding in the pews of the church you serve. Many are outside your walls, afraid to come inside. You cannot personally minister to all of them. I hope you will discover, as I did, that my responsibility is to create a climate for ministry. God will create the person to lead in ministry.

Where do you go to mend a heart, one breaking from addiction? May the answer always be, "The church!"

8

FROM THE PHYSICIAN: HEALING BODY, MIND, AND SPIRIT

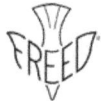

BY WILLARD E. HAWKINS, M.D., F.A.A.F.P.
Family Practice Physician (Retired)
Nixa, Missouri

As a practicing family physician for many years, I have been very concerned with finding a way to effectively deal with specific underlying causes of disease, rather than merely treating the symptoms.

It is increasingly obvious that many diseases of unknown origin are directly related to excessive anxiety and stress. Lowering stress levels for people suffering from these psychosomatic conditions invariably relieves their physical symptoms. The challenge is to find a way to equip these individuals to live a less stressful lifestyle.

Anti-anxiety and anti-depressive medication, along with empathetic, cathartic counseling, may be useful for short-term relief, but these methods are impractical for long-term management. Far too often, a physician's attempt to solve the problem may instead precipitate a long-term addiction to the very medication that was originally intended for short-term use. Many victims of psychosomatic disease are prone to abuse chemicals, including prescription mood-altering drugs, which complicate their problems, and eventually direct intervention and treatment are required. In such cases, chemical abuse is the primary portion of the illness, and has become the first priority for treatment. Medical problems such as hypertension, liver disease, diabetes, and peptic ulcer, along with emotional problems such as depression, anxiety, insomnia, obesity, and compulsive behavior cannot be successfully managed until sobriety has been established and treatment has begun.

Of all the chemicals that are abused, alcohol is by far the most popular. Alcoholism was defined by the American Medical Association in 1956 as a disease. It affects body, mind, emotion, and soul. The disease is progressive in nature, always getting worse, never better, unless arrested. It is prudent to realize that many alcoholics die prematurely or go insane. Research and treatment center experience with alcoholism shows that it is clearly caused by a combination of factors that are all physiologic in nature and occur in the body, not the mind.[1] Alcohol depresses the central nervous system, interfering with the normal control functions of the brain.

No longer is alcoholism considered entirely a moral failing. It is diagnosed and treated as an addiction, a disease with physical symptoms, and more often than not, physical roots. The good news is that it is treatable!

An alcoholic is a person whose drinking causes a continuing problem in any area of his or her life, and yet he or she continues to drink. These problems could be in relation to the person's marriage, family relationships, or job performance. More often than not, the person's state of health is adversely affected.

We have known for years that alcoholic men who do not give up the bottle have a death rate five times higher than the average. The rates are even more dramatic among men under the age of forty-five, who have mortality rates ten times as high as their sober counterparts.[2]

However, a medical study, authored by Dr. Igor Grant in the *Journal of the American Medical Association*, conclusively claims that alcoholics who stay off the bottle—even after more than ten years of hard drinking—can live as long as their nonalcoholic counterparts. He maintains that "giving up drinking will literally save their lives."[3] It allows them to physically recover and lead full lives. But the importance of recognizing the early warning signs of addiction cannot be over-emphasized. Unfortunately, the best-known symptoms only occur in the latter stages of the disease.

A practicing alcoholic unknowingly crosses an invisible line into addiction. No longer is he or she drinking to get high or experience euphoria, but only to take the edge off of life, to feel normal. Drinking is no longer a social pastime, but an allergy of the body coupled with an obsession of the mind. It becomes larger than life, tormenting and

FROM THE PHYSICIAN: HEALING
BODY, MIND, AND SPIRIT

destroying its victims. The alcoholic has lost his or her choice about drinking. One drink is always too many—and a thousand are never enough—for an alcoholic.

Anderson Spickard, M.D., noted Christian physician and co-author of *Dying for a Drink*, stresses that "because addiction follows a predictable pattern and has a pronounced inheritance factor, it is not inappropriate to call alcoholism a disease. However, it is never simply a physical disease; rather, alcoholism is a paradigm disease of the whole person."[4] Hard information is now available to show that alcoholics are genetically predisposed to this disease and that their blood chemistry and brain electricity demonstrate a pathological response to the ingestion of alcohol that is different from a normal person.

The use of alcohol by a person genetically predisposed to this disease precipitates a physiological process in the body, typified by progressive mental mismanagement and an increasing emotional distress that can reach suicidal proportions. The drug lowers inhibitions and allows the person to indulge in ever-increasing destructive and antisocial behavior. Dr. Spickard emphasizes that "long before a heavy drinker becomes an alcoholic, his relationship with God is badly damaged. Heavy drinking quenches spiritual understanding and often leads the drinker to violate his own moral principles."[5] As the pre-disposed drinker continues his or her lifestyle, he or she develops more and more shame, guilt, self-pity, and self-hatred, which is largely repressed and unconscious and is often projected onto others, especially their immediate family.

Actually, alcoholics know very little of themselves and their own behavior because they are not confronted by their own actions as others are. This is due to a combination of factors characteristic of this disease, including denial (inability to recognize the problem), blackouts (when the brain ceases to function properly and all memory is erased), repression (keeping reality at bay), and euphoric recall (remembering only the good times of drinking). As this process continues, the drinker becomes more deluded, with increasing impairment of judgment and memory. He develops conscious and unconscious ways of forgetting painful experiences as a matter of survival. Eventually, he loses touch with his emotions and reality altogether. A spiritual impoverishment develops that makes the alcoholic's destruction complete.

Alcoholics will deny any efforts to confront them with their bizarre behavior and will view any attempt to interrupt their drinking habits as meddling. Once alcoholics are in the throes of addiction, they are unable to recognize the fact that they are ill. Since they have no spontaneous insight into their own needs, and since the disease makes it so difficult to approach them, it is crucial that people close to them understand the nature of the problem. If the illness is to be arrested, it is imperative that the significant others in the alcoholic's life learn to resist the natural impulse to help him by fixing the messes that his behavior produces. For it is only by a buildup of crises that the protective wall of denial can be penetrated, allowing the alcoholic to recognize his or her need for help. It is strongly suggested that family members make a commitment to attend regular meetings of Al-Anon, in order to accumulate the tools necessary in dealing with the alcoholic.

Many years of suffering and self-destructive behavior may ensue before this person hits bottom and surrenders to treatment. If he does not surrender, he will almost certainly die of the disease, as many do. This is when the family members can take the initiative and consider a professional intervention. A loving, planned, formal confrontation of the alcoholic with specific facts of his destructive behavior is a method of raising the alcoholic's "bottom" to manageable levels rather than allowing further self-destruction and deterioration in the normal course of the disease, when he will eventually hit bottom on his own. The intervention may well save a life, although there are no guarantees whatsoever. It has been proven to be an effective approach for one to take who loves the alcoholic and wishes to see him or her recover. It is crucial to remember that an intervention must be done by a professional interventionist, or the results could be damaging instead of helpful.

Above all else, there is hope for any chemically-dependent person. Experience has shown that sobriety can be best maintained by working the 12 Steps of Alcoholics Anonymous, regularly attending 12-step support group meetings, and using a sponsor for advice and direction in the recovery process.

FAMILY DISEASE

John Friel, Ph.D., director of "Lifeworks," an intensive family therapy clinic in St. Paul, Minnesota, maintains that "alcoholism is a family disease. It is passed from one generation to another via the genes and the dynamics that exist within families. Alcoholism can kill the alcoholic. But it's the behavior that does all the other damage."[6]

Donald Goodwin, M.D., former chairman of the Department of Psychiatry at the University of Kansas Medical School, also claims that

FROM THE PHYSICIAN: HEALING
BODY, MIND, AND SPIRIT

"alcoholism runs in families. That's probably the oldest observation ever made about alcoholics. Children of alcoholics are three to five times more prone to alcoholism than the rest of the population. There is an apparent biological link to alcoholism. If there's alcoholism in a blood relative, you're at high risk. So any drinking you do should be watched. It should be as well known to you as if you have a parent with adult diabetes and you have to watch what you eat."[7]

Families that are marked by high-stress, obsessive-compulsive behavior (e.g., overeating, workaholism, perfectionism, excessive religiosity, etc.), along with chemical abuse are known today as "dysfunctional." The homes they form fail to function as safe places for their children to grow up in because the parents are impaired and thus unable to be there emotionally for the kids. Emotional, physical, sexual, and religious abuse are common forms of negative fallout from the more severely impaired parents. Early on, family members usually attempt to rationalize the behavior by inventing excuses. Later, the behavior and the irrational rationalizations become a "normal" way of life. No one dares to talk about the real issues. Children raised in these families learn to never trust others. Trusting others would mean investing confidence, reliance, and faith in another person, virtues that are in short supply in dysfunctional homes.

Children raised in severely dysfunctional homes develop a firm denial system about both their feelings and their perceptions of what is happening in their lives because there is no validation from parents or relatives. They try to bring stability into their lives, cope with the crazy-making behavior, and survive the abuse by detaching from their own feelings and perceptions and by focusing on other people and situations outside themselves. Failing to develop an internal self-esteem, they look to environmental cues for their validation as persons of worth. They have learned to fix uncomfortable situations and to please people at all costs in futile attempts to avoid the painful chaos of their lives. This mindset produces a lifestyle of such stress, anxiety, and fear that psychosomatic illness is virtually assured. These are the patients who fill our medical offices and hospitals today. As this family dysfunction proceeds from one generation to the next, a highly dysfunctional society eventually evolves. It is my belief that this perfectly describes our society today.

As I became acquainted with the dynamics of the dysfunctional family and the role it plays in laying a foundation for disease, my interest in learning to intervene in this process became intensified. I began to inquire about each patient's family of origin in order to identify specific needs that could be addressed to start the process of recovery for them. As a result, I became aware of my own history of dysfunction as an adult grandchild of an alcoholic and as a codependent enabler of an alcoholic in my immediate family. I was introduced to the 12-step recovery process of Alcoholics Anonymous, Adult Children of Alcoholics, and Al-Anon. I have studied and worked the 12 Steps, read intensively on the subject, attended seminars, and, ultimately, did an intervention on the alcoholic loved one in my own life, which led to sobriety and treatment.

Along the way, God brought a specially-gifted psychotherapist into my life. Dr. Earl Henslin (who writes the next chapter in this book) and I were to become the closest of friends and colleagues as we collaborated in developing a method of diagnosing, intervening, and treating our patients who were suffering from psychosomatic, compulsive, and addictive disease. We identified their family of origin issues and networked with others in the healing professions to develop a recovery process tailored to their unique individual needs and circumstances. Convinced of the holistic nature of both the patient and the illness, we attempted to deal simultaneously with their physical, emotional, and spiritual needs.

As Christian therapists attempting to network within the church to develop the spiritual aspect of our recovery process, we were disappointed to find that many churches and their leadership were woefully ignorant of recovery issues as we had come to know them. There was a distinct tendency to over-spiritualize the issues. A denial of the physical and emotional needs existed, as well as a distrust of our therapeutic approach. This was especially true in regard to the use of psychotherapy and the 12-step recovery concepts we were advocating. Instead of being a healing haven for these crippled Christians, the church seemed to be shooting their wounded by shaming them into denial of their pain, and by avoiding legitimate recovery programs for them. We believe that ignorance and denial of family dysfunction, compulsive behavior disorder, and substance abuse on the part of the church was the core of the problem that was keeping the Bride of Christ from playing her vital role in the recovery of her Saints.

While pondering and praying over these matters, God brought Bob and Pauline Bartosch into my office as new patients. In taking Bob's history, I learned that he was a trained pastor and was also a recovering alcoholic with a real heart for helping Christian families to recover from chemical dependency and other family dysfunctions. At the time, he and

FROM THE PHYSICIAN: HEALING BODY, MIND, AND SPIRIT

Pauline shared our frustration in trying to network with the church in a legitimate recovery process. In fact, they had already begun a 12-step "Overcomers" group in their church, using biblical back–up for each step, and naming their "Higher Power" as Jesus Christ.

In 1985, when Bob and Pauline officially started the fledgling organization of Overcomers Outreach, it was with excitement and a grateful appreciation to God for His provision that I became active on the board of directors. Today I regularly refer patients to OO groups, as well as to the traditional 12-step meetings, as necessary components of the recovery program.

At long last, we have a model for dealing effectively with the underlying causes of many diseases, rather than just treating their symptoms. We are grateful to God for these insights and concepts and especially for the vehicle of Overcomers Outreach to bring the good news of recovery of body, mind, emotion, and soul to those who are still suffering.

9

FROM THE PSYCHOLOGIST: 12-STEP PROGRAMS MAKE MY JOB EASIER

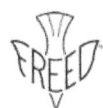

BY EARL R. HENSLIN, PSY.D.
Christian Therapist and Author
Brea, California.

For the past twenty years, I have been involved in the helping profession. I became aware of the fellowship of Alcoholics Anonymous while on my very first job working at a detox center (inpatient treatment facility for alcohol and other substance abusers). Part of my responsibility was to take patients to AA meetings, but I soon realized I was benefiting greatly from the meetings myself. Even though I had been a Christian since I was twelve years old, I had never experienced such honest sharing and acceptance like I witnessed in those meetings.

One night while I was working the eleven P.M.–seven A.M. shift, a man came in who, according to his wife, had been on a binge for the last thirty days. He looked like he had fallen or been kicked down a flight of stairs because he had a strip of black and blue marks about two inches wide across his lower back. His tongue was swollen, seemingly either from him having bitten it or from having a seizure. His breathing was labored and raspy from his nicotine addiction and from the sedation of the alcohol. After the nurse and I had admitted and medicated him so he could go through the detox process, I began to thumb through his chart. This must have been his seventh or eighth admission to such a facility. Then I saw that he identified his religion as "Christian."

OVERCOMERS OUTREACH

At that point in time (1972), a Christian did not dare turn to the church for help with alcoholism; one especially did not mention involvement in a 12-step program. To do so was to invite shame and criticism. There were no Overcomers Outreach meetings where it was okay to name Jesus Christ as one's "Higher Power." The 12 Steps of AA were not seen as a resource for the recovering Christian alcoholic, drug addict, sex addict, eating-disordered person, etc. The primary intervention offered by the church was prayer and Bible study, with no acknowledgment of the horrible struggles of the compulsive and addictive disease present in nearly every congregation.

It was my job as a detox technician to check the vital signs of each patient throughout the night. This man's condition was so precarious that I looked in on him frequently. This was during a time before inpatient and outpatient treatment of alcoholism became commonplace. Hospitals did not really want alcoholics. Back then, detox was primarily conducted by other AA members who would keep a fifth of booze under the seat of their car and give the alcoholic a little to drink, as they gradually weaned him or her off the alcohol. Suddenly, at 3:06 A.M., I could no longer hear the labored breathing of this new patient who was in a bed behind the wall of my desk. I ran into his room and discovered he had stopped breathing. I called the nurse and an ambulance to take him to the emergency room of the hospital. The police and ambulance came within minutes, but it was too late; he was dead. An autopsy later revealed that he had suffered a cerebral hemorrhage. A blood vessel to his brain, most likely stressed and weakened by so many withdrawals from alcohol, had finally burst. My job, at 4:30 A.M., was to inform his wife and two teenaged sons that their husband and father was dead.

What I learned in those few hours has stayed with me for the rest of my life. Alcoholism is a serious disease that can lead to premature death if it is not aggressively and seriously treated. It is an illness that impacts every member of the family. I began to wish that there was some way to make it safe for people within the church to find the kind of support and help that is found on a daily basis in more than 113,000 12-step groups all over the world. I wondered if the key to this man's sobriety could have been finding a group of other Christians in recovery who were able to openly identify Jesus Christ as their "Higher Power." Rather than feeling great shame and believing that he was a bad Christian for having an addictive illness, he could have found other Christians with an addictive disease who could identify with his illness and struggles.

FROM THE PSYCHOLOGIST: 12-STEP PROGRAMS MAKE MY JOB EASIER

Shame is one of the biggest issues that begins to change for Christians in recovery. The moment they enter the door of an OO meeting and hear others tell their stories, they begin to understand that even a born-again believer can have an addictive illness. They realize that it is acceptable to bring their stories out in the open and share their struggles with other Christians. For many, it is the first time they experience acceptance and a refreshing lack of judgment.

After working at the detox center, I was offered a job to help open and develop a half-way house for recovering alcoholics and addicts. Eve D., the founder of the half-way house, had twenty-three years of sobriety from alcoholism at the time we began working together. Her story was similar to so many Christians who struggle with addictive disease. She had been in a continuous shame spiral, continually walking down the church aisle and giving her addiction over to the Lord, only to return to her drinking when withdrawal began.

A friend introduced Eve D. to the fellowship of AA, where she found the tools that she needed to turn her disease over to God, and learned how to rely on Him one day at a time for sobriety. In her excitement of finding a release from her obsession with alcohol, she went to tell her pastor. Her pastor told her, "You need to leave AA immediately; it is an occult organization." Fortunately, Eve decided to continue in AA and chose not to share her recovery with her pastor again.

Thankfully today, there are more pastors, physicians, and therapists who are educated and informed about recovery issues, and possibly in recovery themselves. Yet thirty years ago that was not the case. From working with Eve D. for the next two-and-a-half years, I essentially received a graduate education in the disease of alcoholism and the importance of working a solid recovery program. Later, when I entered the psychotherapy field, it became critical to the therapy process that clients become grounded in a 12-step program in addition to attending individual counseling. The change that occurred in the people who were working a 12-step program was drastically different from those who were not. Many times I felt sorry for those clients who came in for psychotherapy and did not fit into AA or Al-Anon! Changes that took months and years for those not working a program happened in days and weeks when my clients began to experience God's love and acceptance through the strength, hope, and encouragement offered in AA and Al-Anon.

It has been more than twenty years since I was first introduced to Bob and Pauline. They excitedly shared about their Overcomers Outreach group at their church. I was excited to hear that they viewed Overcomers Outreach as a bridge between the 12-step community and the church. I was impressed that Bob and Pauline both continued in their own 12-step groups, in addition to their OO group. Both of them were clear about the role that AA and Al-Anon were playing in their ongoing recovery.

It seemed like a missing piece of the puzzle had at last been found. I immediately began to refer all my Christian clients to OO meetings. I found as they worked both their regular AA, Al Anon, O.A. (Overeaters Anonymous), S.A. (Sexaholics Anonymous), etc. groups and attended OO, where they could freely acknowledge Jesus Christ as their "Higher Power," that their recovery program deepened and relapse rates appeared to decrease. Shame issues that had been so strong and powerful in their disease began to change just by being in a recovery group with other Christians.

Unfortunately, what also became apparent was that some Christians attempted to use OO as their only support group. The same excuses and rationalizations came into play that I would ordinarily face:

- "They use bad language in those traditional 12-step meetings."
- "They don't talk about Jesus in those meetings."
- "Someone in my AA meeting uses the group itself as their 'Higher Power.'"

These excuses generally resulted in their justifying that they did not need an AA, Al-Anon, Codependents Anonymous, etc., meeting in their overall program. Usually, within a short while, relapse would occur and they would be back into their disease. It became abundantly clear that both groups are needed for the recovering Christian. To stay sober through OO alone was usually not sufficient; likewise, AA was a key element because of almost seventy years of experience, wisdom, traditions, and tools that have been refined and passed on from one recovering person to another.

As a psychotherapist who has been involved in individual, marital, and family counseling for many years, I see numerous reasons for my clients to be involved in traditional 12-step groups and OO. They include:

1. The unconditional love and acceptance inherent in traditional 12-step groups and OO are foundational to recovery. When I walked into my

FROM THE PSYCHOLOGIST: 12-STEP PROGRAMS MAKE MY JOB EASIER

first 12-step meeting, I found a love and acceptance that I had never experienced before. Shame, judgment, and criticism were strong parts of the dysfunction I had experienced in churches and within my dysfunctional family. Here, I could share my story and heart and not be interrupted; plus, after a meeting people would come up and give me a hug. Talk about heaven! People in the program did not care what I had done, what I had accomplished or achieved. They were only concerned for Earl. I was still accepted, even though I was struggling with my eating disorder. No need to perform here, just learn to accept God's love and grace as evidenced through the fellowship of other recovering people. It felt strange and wonderful all at the same time.

2. In traditional 12-step groups and OO, feelings and issues are heard without criticism, judgment, or shame. In a meeting, it is OK to share whatever feelings or issues that I might have. It does not matter if I feel angry, sad, or fearful; I have the freedom to express whatever I need or feel.

3. The 12-steps of AA are at the core of traditional meetings and OO; actually working those 12 Steps is the key to recovery. The rubber meets the road, so to speak, in 12-step meetings and in OO. By working the program, I began to learn the crazy paradox of how unmanageable my life was, and how I needed to turn it over to God each day, each hour, each minute, etc. I am helpless and powerless over my life on my own, yet now I have the responsibility to take action by using the tools of recovery. There is a sense of responsibility that keeps growing the longer a person is in the program. The ability to accept that responsibility, and let go of changing, blaming, and controlling others is a key to spiritual and emotional maturity. As a psychotherapist, this is one of the keys to any type of growth. To move from blame and control to only changing what I am able to change, and accepting what I am not able to change, is a key step.

Another significant part of the 12 Steps of AA is that they encourage self-reflection and introspection, but not to the point of self-centeredness or self-preoccupation. Doing an inventory and then identifying those people whom I have wronged and being willing to make amends is a powerful part of the 12 Steps. Every individual, marriage, or family can benefit by working the Steps. I believe that we have all grown up in families that have some type of dysfunction. As a result, there is a lot to learn about being responsible for myself and taking responsibility for when I have sinned in my relationship to God, myself, and others. The Steps hold the key to learning how to ask for forgiveness, give forgiveness, make amends to the people we have wronged, and also that our own recovery does not depend on someone granting us forgiveness. The 12 Steps help give us practical tools, based on guidelines from God's Word, about how we are to relate with each other—and with Him—while we are on this earth.

I find that the people I see in counseling who work the steps in a recovery group are taught practical tools that are not always learned in psychotherapy. The two processes—psychotherapy and 12-step work—are mutually compatible. As an example, when a couple comes in for counseling for their marriage, and they begin to face the anger and resentment that has built up between them, without a recovery program, the counseling process is much longer and more difficult. Participants in 12-step programs learn to take responsibility for themselves and not blame others for their problems. They also learn that they cannot change another person and can only change themselves. As they wade through the old anger and resentment, they begin to face the underlying issues and their own dysfunctional family past, rather than staying at a level of defensive anger with each other. When the couple does not work a 12-step recovery program, it takes longer to get to the core of their problems.

4. In 12-step groups and OO there is no shame in having an addictive disease. One of the most difficult steps for many Christians is to accept that their addictive illness is real. In the Christian culture there has been the belief that if you pray hard enough, you will be delivered from alcoholism, sexual addiction, eating disorders, work addiction, etc. God does provide deliverance, and is still in the business of miracles; however, research shows that of those individuals who have had a dramatic spiritual experience, only 5 percent have been delivered from their addictive disease. Unfortunately, we in the Christian community have considered that to be the norm, when the reality is that 95 percent of us will need to learn to stay sober one day at a time, with the Lord's help—which, quite frankly, is still a miracle

FROM THE PSYCHOLOGIST: 12-STEP PROGRAMS MAKE MY JOB EASIER

to me. More than sixty years ago, AA recognized that alcoholism was a complex disease process that was spiritual, emotional, mental, and physical. Recovery means having to pay respect to all dimensions of the illness.

Until recent years, the number of physicians, counselors, and pastors with training in addictive disease has been woefully inadequate. Physicians treat the medical symptoms. Counselors treat the family of origin in hopes that if a person deals with the core issues enough, he will not need to drink, eat, work, or use sex in an addictive manner. Pastors treat the spiritual aspect, believing fully that if people become committed-enough Christians, they will no longer feel the desire to practice their addictive illness. Each one is trying to help but is only dealing with one facet of the disease rather than treating the whole problem. In 12-step groups and in OO, the struggle with addictive disease is recognized as a one-day-at-a-time struggle. Help is only a phone call, meeting, or prayer away. In these groups, the addict finds help, meets people with similar struggles, and recognizes that he or she is not alone. For me to be able to walk into a group and say, "Hi, my name is Earl, and I am a compulsive overeater," begins to break the shame connected with having a compulsive disease that is beyond my ability to control.

5. Sobriety is the first step in recovery from an addictive disease. Plainly and simply, psychotherapy will not be effective unless sobriety is found. When an individual with an addictive illness is in counseling, the first goal for the therapist is to get the client into a 12-step program that will help him find sobriety. Ironically, the process of individual counseling, working on deeper issues, will often trigger the client to use more of whatever substance he or she uses to numb the pain. Whatever new insights were gained in therapy will be lost once the individual is back into his/her addictive illness. The issues we face, which impact our daily lives, are not solved by counseling alone, but through the powerful combination of counseling and step work.

6. In 12-step groups and OO there is an acceptance that recovery is a life-long process. We are never healed of the human condition. When I first started in counseling, I remember talking to a psychiatrist who diagnosed everyone with the following diagnosis: chronic human

imperfection. That pull inside of us toward evil says that we are still no different from Adam and Eve. By embracing Jesus Christ's penalty-payment on the cross, we are saved from eternal separation from God, and do not have to face the consequences of our sinful nature. With the Holy Spirit within our hearts, we have access to one of the greatest change agents in the universe. Yet with all of that, I may still have the pull within me toward addictive living and/or a codependent over-concern for others. What I need is the continuous help of God and others to find the way to stay grounded spiritually and emotionally so that I do not self-destruct. Within OO and 12-step groups, spiritual and emotional growth is accepted as a life-long process. I do not ever reach a point of being 100 percent fixed or cured. I am accepted no matter how scared, lonely, or anxious I might be. This sounds frightfully similar to how God views us in Christ, doesn't it? Left to my own devices, I am dangerous to myself and others. Yet with a vulnerable and open relationship with God, there is hope for all of us. I need a meeting where I have a safe place to share, and yet I still remember that I won't be cured of my chronic human imperfection until I leave this earth and am joined with Jesus.

As you can see, I am convinced that a tremendous amount of healing and recovery occurs through the dynamics of 12-step groups, yet many people—many Christians—are reluctant to participate. I recently saw a T-shirt at a Christians in Recovery conference that read, "Denial is not a river in Egypt!" Denial is what keeps people stuck in their addictive disease.

Is denial sinful? Yes!

Is denial an outgrowth of the progression of the disease of addiction in the family, both for the addicted individual and the codependents that surround them? Yes!

Many years ago, when I met Bob and Pauline, I realized that OO could be the tool for breaking denial in the Christian community. The group became a safe place for me, and my denial began to change into a deeper awareness of my helplessness and powerlessness over myself, people, places, and things. As J. Keith Miller put it at an OO conference, "Denial is part of the 'sin disease' that we are all born with—the sin of self-centeredness where I believe that I can run my life better than God can."

FROM THE PSYCHOLOGIST: 12-STEP PROGRAMS MAKE MY JOB EASIER

As we work the Steps, denial begins to slip away; helplessness and powerlessness become real feelings, and not just something that is in our heads. As denial begins to melt away, the secrets hidden within ourselves, within the family, and even within our churches (as more Christians begin to work their own programs) will be uncovered. I no longer need to avoid saying, "I'm sorry" or "I am responsible." A real spirituality begins to flow where I become more transparent and real before God and others. It is no longer comfortable to just play church. The Scriptures come alive and convicting of steps that I need to take toward God, myself, and others.

Denial maintains the status quo, the disease in all of us. A church body finds it easier to overlook signs all around them and to not see the signs of addiction, codependency, family dysfunction, abuse, etc. When recovery issues begin to be faced within a church, the secrets begin to come out. Just by people facing their own issues and working their own program, a healing process begins within a body of believers. Needless to say, this is not a comfortable feeling for many people within a church, but it is crucial for its health.

With the fall from grace of so many Christian leaders in the past few years, it would appear that we have limited our gospel. Yet when we take a step out of denial we are also taking a step deeper into the gospel of Jesus Christ. Is our gospel strong enough to be at the deepest and darkest levels of our lives? Yes! The erosion of denial within a Christian community is a dangerous threat to everyone within that church. No longer is it so easy to "look good" in church. Tears come a little more readily, and there is a sense of urgency to share openly in Bible studies and adult fellowship classes in the same way we share at a 12-step meeting.

I believe it is definitely of God that the recovery movement has been growing within the Christian community. Jesus wants the message of His love and grace felt at the deepest and darkest levels of our lives. He knows that hidden under the addictions, under the co-dependencies, and under whatever other dysfunctional behavior is a wounded little boy or girl who is scared and lonely. An inner child, who desperately wants connection with others and a safe place to share, lives inside each of us. The decrease of denial in a body of believers brings an entirely new movement of the Holy Spirit. That church in which such openness occurs will never be the same! It will either grow or slowly shame its members into a passive spirituality, an image-conscious way of life. Denial can be

OVERCOMERS OUTREACH

Satan's most powerful tool to limiting the full expression of the gospel of Jesus Christ.

Welcome to Overcomers Outreach, a group of fellow strugglers on this journey of life. You are welcome here. All you need is the desire for sobriety, especially from the intoxication of people, places, and things that may interfere with your relationship with Jesus Christ, yourself, and others. You are in the right place!

PART III

CHANGED LIVES:
Overcomers Share Their Experience, Strength, and Hope

10

FATAL ATTRACTION: MY LOVE AFFAIR WITH ETHYL

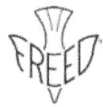

BY JACK J.

I was sitting at the end of a long table awaiting the beginning of the court-ordered D.U.I. (Driving Under the Influence) class. It was nearly eight A.M. on this Saturday, June 9, 1984, and I was still basically intoxicated from a long night of drinking. My hands shook, I was unshaven, and my clothes were disheveled.

At home that morning, I had used ample amounts of mouthwash as I prepared to leave for the class, but I was running late and couldn't take the time to clean myself up. Now as the class was about to being, about twenty men and women were sitting all around the table, awaiting a long day of penance for getting arrested for driving while intoxicated. What bad luck!

One man to my left said, "I hope this class isn't boring, because this is the last place I want to be on a Saturday."

I muttered, "Me, too." The clock read 8:05 A.M.

When the class started, I stood up, walked to the chalkboard, and introduced myself as the instructor for the D.U.I. class.

There was a long silence as unbelieving eyes gazed upon me, startled and bewildered by the appearance of their instructor.

The man to my left where I had been sitting stated, "My word—I can't believe it. I thought you were one of us!"

OVERCOMERS OUTREACH

Can you imagine? Someone thought that I was a participant in this D.U.I. class; that I was one of them. Me, a certified drug and alcoholism counselor, with a Ph.D. in counseling, a field instructor for graduate students at the state university, the clinical director of a mental health agency, a successful professional, and most of all, a professing Christian who proclaimed Jesus as Lord! I was a bit shocked myself.

Where did it all begin? How did this journey evolve, one that would find me more identified as an alcohol abuser or addict than a doctor who was to teach a class on the dangers of ethyl alcohol and the evils of drunk driving? Why couldn't I see in myself what was observable and diagnosable in others? Delusion, denial, and years of perfecting intellectual defenses blinded me not just to my alcoholism or drug abuse, but to the deeply-rooted character defects that grew into my being during my forty years of life.

Thankfully, something would happen to me that June day in 1984 that would break down the thick walls of denial. The Scripture reflects this: "...God is Light; in him there is no darkness at all. So if we say that we are his friends, but go on living in spiritual darkness, we are lying. But if we are living in the light of God's presence, just as Christ does, then we have wonderful fellowship and joy with each other, and the blood of Jesus His Son cleanses us from every sin" (1 John 1:5–7). Yes, I was in darkness and not only out of fellowship with God, but with others as well. I needed to see the light, but how would this happen?

The only friend and lover I had who stuck by me through the years was Ethyl—ethyl alcohol. Of course, it was like the enemy that comes to steal, kill, and destroy—initially bringing pleasure for a season, then wrecking her havoc on my life. My first drinking as a teenager began a life-long pathological relationship that kept me addicted and afflicted.

Over the years this relationship would keep me in darkness. I was living a lie, blinded (literally at times) in chemically-induced amnesia incidents called blackouts. At other times, I would act out my inner pain and rage in reckless abandon leading to physical harm. I was injured in accidents and on one occasion my insanity led me to take on a gang of youths at a seaside resort that would lead to my hospitalization with my face destroyed beyond recognition. Sexual sin, licentious living, and self-centered narcissism were all fed by this disease that was destroying my body, soul, and spirit.

Oh, what a cost this friend and lover would require of me! Through it all, my heart's desire was to serve the Lord in ministry but this addiction

FATAL ATTRACTION: MY LOVE AFFAIR WITH ETHYL

and my ongoing character defects robbed me of God's vision and His purpose for my life. Enter a wife and son, but the drinking soon stripped me of them too. I was left confused and sick. I was in darkness; blinded from the truth.

A second marriage lasted only two years. I sabotaged all my hopes, desires, love, and dreams by this thief that continued to rob and blind me. I considered my drinking to be a way to medicate my pain, to feel, to celebrate, to be alive, and yet I still walked in darkness.

Now, a third marriage and a baby daughter, a career enhanced by graduate degrees, success, new dreams, but my deepest and most enduring relationship was still with a chemical, not with God or people. "Better living through chemistry" was the motto I adopted. Sure, in the beginning that's exactly what it offered. I was a shy and melancholy youth who always felt defective, alienated from others, unloved, lonely, and afraid. But my first experiences with drinking changed all that...for a season. I bonded to this friend and lover, alcohol, but never did I think I would have to add the "-ism" to that word someday. Alcohol was the magic elixir I used to medicate life or celebrate life, for good times or bad. It became my lifestyle, and in a deeper spiritual way, it became my "Higher Power," my idol, my god.

As I continued to walk in darkness, I was about to lose my third wife and my precious little daughter. My soul—mind, will, feelings, emotions, personality—was sick, and had been for years. I tried marriage counseling, pastoral counseling, psychiatry, psychotherapy, and everything the mental health professionals recommended, including various anti-depressant medications. I enjoyed the pills and the booze; they had a nice synergistic effect. My body was now pathologically under the curse of this disease: bleeding ulcers, migraine headaches, high blood pressure, hiatal hernia, skin disease, impotency, and, of course, the loss of irreplaceable brain cells, executed by the excessive ingestion of alcohol. I was on medication for all of these illnesses along with medication to counteract the negative consequences of those medications. Where would it end—the grave?

Only a week prior to my final debauchery (my eye-opening D.U.I. class experience), my wife had rushed me to the emergency room of our local hospital with intense pain and pressure radiating from my chest. My esophagus had gone into spasms from the alcohol, and I had difficulty breathing. My therapists, doctors, ministers, colleagues, friends, and family and, most importantly, myself, still had not identified this disease of alcoholism! All of them could identify the pain: physical, emotional, mental, and spiritual, but the cause, rooted in addiction, was still eluding them. No wonder no one could see the truth. Here I was, a Ph.D. in counseling, certified in addictions, a specialist in chemical dependency, running alcohol and drug programs. Here was a professional, with all the knowledge about the disease, yet I was dying from it, unbeknownst to others or to myself. A wall of denial encompasses the alcoholic as well as everyone around him.

Many times when I was watching Christian television I had prayed that God would stop my drinking. I prayed and fasted, went on retreats, and attended church prayer services for healing. I rededicated my life to Christ and went to church several times a week. I read the Bible. Why was I still afflicted? I tried to control my drinking; once I even stopped drinking for three months! (Of course, I called it a "Lenten fast" and I promptly ended that on Easter Sunday.)

Never once did I call my problem by its true name: alcoholism. At times I began to question myself, *Could I possibly be an alcoholic?* but I ruled that out, since I was functioning so well in my job and all. (Or at least I thought I was!) Back then I didn't see the powerlessness over alcohol and the unmanageability of my life.

By this time my wife said she was hurting and in pain because of me, and that she couldn't take it anymore, but even she never guessed that I suffered from alcoholism. I had deluded others and myself into believing that my problems were due to other people, places, and circumstances. Drinking seemed to be a helpful way to deal with these life difficulties. How could alcohol be the enemy?

I ended the D.U.I. class early on that Saturday. I felt physically sick, seriously depressed, confused, and confounded. *What is wrong with me?* I cried out in my soul. *Oh, God, help me, please. I can't go on like this anymore!* I agonized.

Just then God had a serendipity for me—one of those unexpected miracles served up by the Lord out of the kindness of His heart. I saw a book sitting on the desktop of one of the graduate students I supervised. I was drawn by its title: *It Will Never Happen to Me*, by Claudia Black. Without thinking, I opened it up at random and there, staring at me, was a poem entitled "My Daddy."

This poem changed my life. It was about a man's daughter who was crying out to her father because he was no longer in her life due to alcoholism and the resultant divorce. This man's "little princess" pleads

FATAL ATTRACTION: MY LOVE AFFAIR WITH ETHYL

to the Lord from the bottom of her heart about the pain of losing her daddy to this disease.

When I saw the name of the girl who wrote the poem—Renee—the light went on. I emerged from the darkness and was confronted by the truth staring me right in the face. My own daughter's name is Renee. I realized gravely that this poem would become a prophecy of what would happen to her if I didn't face my addiction.

Tears began to fall and I cried for an hour as I read and re-read this poem. All my education and knowledge couldn't do for me what this poem had done. I prayed and asked the Lord to help me know what to do next. Suddenly I walked over to the phone book, looked up Alcoholics Anonymous, and called. The next day, June 10, 1984, I attended my first AA meeting. Attending AA was like coming home. I was now beginning to walk in the light and to understand the truth, to put feet to my prayers to get to the place of my healing.

The early days of my recovery were extremely difficult, filled with feelings of loss, grief, and anger due to the dying process of my addiction and the letting go of my old friend, Ethyl. I knew the relationship with alcohol was based upon a fatal attraction as my old friend and lover turned against me in the disease of alcoholism. This pathological relationship robbed me of a call to ministry, two wives (and nearly a third spouse), several good jobs, homes, and many friends. Because of my need to seek geographical escapes to fix my life problems by looking for greener grass in another city or state or another employer, I nearly lost everything. I was robbed of my self-respect, my relationship with God, peace of mind, finances, my health, and almost my life. The insanity was that I still was grieving that I had to put the cork in the jug and say goodbye to my drinks, my social lubricant, my medicine, my cup of celebration.

I went to 12-step meetings and the Lord began to speak to me through the people and the program. The process of healing and recovery had begun, and thank God, there was no going back. When tempted to give in to the euphoric recall of the fun and pleasure associated with past occasions of drinking, or the opportunity to escape the mundane or painful existence that at times comes to us all in the human condition known as life, I stopped, put my "stinking thinking" on hold, and reached for my wallet. I took out my first twenty-four-hour chip (an award for twenty-four hours of sobriety) I had received the night of my first AA meeting, and then I took out the photos of my wife and daughter. I held them, treasuring the gifts they were to me from God. I knew that little blue plastic chip represented my sobriety and the gift of recovery and life. I knew that one drink would rob me, possibly forever, of what that chip and those photos represented to me. For my sake, the sake of my loved ones, and for my Lord, I knew I couldn't turn back.

I had a small pocket-sized leather-bound New International Version Bible that I took with me whenever I was driving in my car. When the mental obsession and physical compulsions to drink manifested within me, I would squeeze that Bible in my right hand and cry out, "Jesus, I'm holding on to Your Word and its promises for me—I'm holding on to You. Rescue me; save me. Oh, my God, help me."

My going to meetings and crying out to my Lord and Savior brought me through those early difficult days of recovery. I was healing, but I knew something was missing in my program. It was in 1985 during my first year of recovery that I was watching a program on Christian television called "JOY." Two guests were being interviewed about their ministry to alcoholics, and they shared their testimonies of personal recovery. I couldn't believe what I was hearing. I identified with this man who talked so freely of his own battle, as a believer, with alcoholism, and his wife's corresponding pain and confusion because of his drinking. I got out of my chair and went to the TV and turned up the sound. I sat glued to the program as they mentioned a booklet called *FREED*. Bob and Pauline Bartosch had just given birth to the ministry of Overcomers Outreach. I picked up the telephone and called for more information and a copy of the booklet.

With that information and their help, I started Overcomers meetings for the addicted and the afflicted in two churches, and in treatment centers of hospitals that offer inpatient care with a Christ-centered focus. OO has enabled my wife and me to gather with fellow Christians who have been wounded through addiction. We address our 12-step recovery and life problems from a common belief and faith in our "Higher Power," Jesus Christ. What a complement OO is to traditional 12-step programs! It is truly a rich blessing to pray and share without shame and condemnation with people who honestly struggle and look to the Scriptures and the biblical principles of the 12 Steps. This time together enables me to be empowered by my Christian faith, to continue the spiritual, mental, and emotional transformation of "taking off the old man and putting on the new," of "renewing the mind" that Christ calls us to. This is a process I must do daily. Even though I'm a Christian in recovery, I'm not bullet-proof to a future relapse.

FATAL ATTRACTION: MY LOVE AFFAIR WITH ETHYL

I no longer have a drinking problem, but I do have living problems. The alcohol is gone, but I still have the "-ism" related to the "I-self-me" problem that is rooted in my character defects, in my sin. Thus, through the brokenness of addiction, I learned I couldn't be my own savior, let alone my own "Higher Power." I learned that education and knowledge don't impress this insidious disease. It doesn't hesitate to kill the unlearned or the Ph.D., the Christian or non-Christian, the rich or the poor.

Today I can walk in the light and in the truth because God has provided a way through these recovery programs. I have even found that with Christ "all things work together for good to them that love God, to them who are called according to his purpose" (Rom. 8:28 KJV). As I am grateful to the Lord for my spiritual transformation and ongoing journey of recovery, I can now apply what I have learned to my work and ministry.

Life is now manageable, as long as I allow God to manage it on a daily basis. The intense pain within my soul, the dreadful depression, the shame, the rage, the unquenchable "I want" that drove me, is gone. My impulsiveness, impatience, and lack of self-respect are gone. Oh sure, I have more character defects to work on since God isn't finished with me yet, but that's why I have a program of recovery. I can live with myself now, rather than thinking about ending it all. And my loved ones tell me that they, too, can live with me, even though perfection is far from my grasp.

Yes, in Christ all things are possible—even for an alcoholic Ph.D. running programs in chemical dependency and blinded to his own disease. God's wake-up call for me was a poem called "My Daddy," and because of it, today I have this new life.

I pray that all of us hear our own unique wake-up call from God before it's too late.

11

DON'T QUIT BEFORE THE MIRACLE HAPPENS!

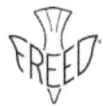

BY DEBBIE K.

Before I even had my first drink, I was attracted to alcohol. My first clue came when I was a child. When everyone else asked for a puppy for Christmas, I wanted one of those Clydesdale horses on the beer commercials. After my first drink I knew I was hooked, and those childhood feelings of being different from others only became worse.

I grew up in a Christian home and both my parents were in leadership at church. They were model Christians at church, but at home it was a whole different story. After church, before we even had our matching Sunday dresses changed, my dad would start yelling. He seemed to be angry about something all the time. My sisters and I took quite a few beatings from him. As he took off his belt to spank us he'd say, "This is going to hurt me more than you," but I knew it wasn't true. Instead of taking a drink to deal with life, my dad would hit us kids. I could feel his rage with every swat of the belt. This was the beginning of my learning not to feel—to shut out all emotions.

To deal with my loneliness, I became the class clown and the center of attention. But humor can only go so far, and it wasn't laughs I was looking for. Love is what everyone needs.

When I was ten, my family moved from Chicago to Michigan to start a new life. Suddenly, what few loving relationships I had with Sunday school teachers were ripped away. Moving from the city to the country was quite devastating, but Mom had said to people, "Debbie will love the country; she's our little country girl." So instead of showing my sadness, I tried to live up to her expectations. Even if I had shown my sadness, there would have been no one there to comfort me.

By the age of twelve I had discovered alcohol. I don't remember my first drink, but I do remember the change that seemed to happen overnight. Suddenly I could forget that Dad hit me, that Mom was in another world, and those terrible feelings of depression were eased. My grandparents lived next door so I started visiting frequently, and carefully ravaged their liquor cabinet. (Of course there was no alcohol in my house, because my parents were strict Christians!)

For the first time in my life I could survive family dinners without the horrible fear of getting backhanded by Dad because I said something wrong. Of course, I still might be hit, but I didn't dread it with the booze in my system. It didn't take long for a few sips of alcohol to run into a daily need for many gulps! I learned to steal from my mom's purse and had the older kids buy my alcohol. My lunch money turned into a liquid snack for after school. Being a good athlete and above-average student, I was able to maintain a facade that no one could see through.

The other side of this was my love for God. Growing up as the scapegoat in an abusive home led me to a strong desire for God, for someone to help me. It seemed like I loved God before I ever loved anyone or anything else. Yet as my addiction to alcohol grew, so did my guilt. This began the cycle of either being "Debbie the party animal" or "Debbie the super Christian." I either won awards for bringing the most kids to Bible School or for chugging the most beer.

When I was thirteen or fourteen, I read *The Cross and the Switchblade*. This book had the biggest impact on my life, more than any other factor. I longed for the love and attention those teens received while sobering up at Teen Challenge. I decided someday I would become a drug addict, get cleaned up, and then have a ministry for teenage drug addicts. I believed this with all my heart and it became a self-fulfilling prophecy. This vision for ministry often kept me alive in the years to come.

Finally the day came when I moved out of my house and went to college. I became very involved in Fellowship of Christian Athletes (FCalifornia) and played drums in several Christian music groups. One band traveled all over the Midwest doing concerts. Since I was designated as the person with the worst childhood, I became the main speaker for the group. I thought I was unique because I could relate to

DON'T QUIT BEFORE THE MIRACLE HAPPENS!

any audience, no matter where we played. Orphanages, churches, youth centers, or the city park: I had something in my story for everyone. The problem was I still had no solution for my own issue. My relationship with Jesus was as sincere as it could be, but my addictions had me in a firm stranglehold.

During this time, my relationships were either shallow or hostage-type (where one partner is dominating and controlling, and the other is overly submissive). I always had one best friend whom I held onto for all my love, attention, and intimacy. After a few years of staying sober for religious reasons, I took that first drink. Once again, I felt the relief I so badly needed. Alcohol numbed out the fact that I was about to graduate from college with no clue about what I wanted to do with my life. I also wanted to block out the fear I felt because my hostage friend and I were about to part ways. It didn't matter that my parents had just gotten a divorce and I didn't know where either one lived. It also didn't matter that a guy I had dated for three years was caught sleeping with a fourteen-year-old girl. All that mattered was that I could forget all my pain and be the center of attention for awhile.

Eventually the guilt overcame me and I felt like a dying person. How could I play in these Christian bands, but be drunk before the bus was packed up? I became severely depressed and stopped eating for about two months at a time. Thus started another addiction. By obsessing on food and my weight, I could forget the other realities of life. For many years I became trapped in the hell of anorexia, with my weight going up and down, my health on the edge, and a deep, deep hatred for what food did to my body. Whenever anyone tried to make me eat, or held me back from throwing up the piece of lettuce I may have eaten, they ended up with a black eye! I would go to any lengths not to eat.

By the time I graduated from college I was an emotional mess. I decided to move to California to get my life together. What a joke! Within three months, I discovered the world of cocaine. For the next three years, I was an all-out drunk and drug addict. Although I don't remember my first drink at the age of twelve, I do remember the day, twelve years later, when I told God to leave me alone, that I was no longer His. Then I threw myself into the unbelieving world.

From this point my story is the typical one of pitiful, incomprehensible demoralization. For two years straight I partied from ten P.M. until four A.M. Then it was off to a drug-induced sleep for a few hours before having to show up at work by eight A.M. I was one of those drunks who could say, "I am never late for work, therefore I am not as sick as everyone thinks."

During this time, I started going to therapy for my eating disorder (as if I didn't have any other problems). My counselor, whom I credit for saving my life many times over, told me about a group called Overcomers Outreach and gave me a phone number to call for help. I laughed at her at the time, but for some reason I carried that number with me everywhere I went.

One night, in desperation at a bar, I called Pauline Bartosch, waking her out of bed since I had called so late. Given my lifestyle, I didn't know that most people were in bed by midnight, but she talked to me through her grogginess anyway. She encouraged me to meet her at an Overcomers meeting.

With a friend in tow, I showed up at my first Overcomers meeting—high. I couldn't go through the door without a few lines of coke (cocaine) up my nose. I thought I pulled it off quite well, since by then I knew how to be a Christian and to be high at the same time. Later I found out the size of my pupils had totally given me away!

At the meeting, I was amazed to hear other Christians talk openly about their addictions. Of course, I believed they had just cut down the amount they were using and were all lying about it to look good. And this one-day-at-a-time thing really bothered me. One day at a time, right! For the rest of my life? Nevertheless, I could see they had something I didn't have. I kept attending the meetings because I had no one else to talk to and because they seemed to accept me. I also attended a few AA meetings, but I wasn't ready to get sober yet.

For about the next two years, I attended Overcomers meetings while continuing to use drugs and alcohol. I did everything in my power to make those people kick me out so I could get on with my demoralization, guilt-free. But they kept saying, "Keep coming back!" And the most important thing I heard was "Don't quit before the miracle happens!" Every week those people would applaud me for my two or three days of sobriety and listen to my war stories. I couldn't decide who was crazier, me or them!

During this time, my life didn't mean much to me. I lived on the edge and enjoyed shocking everybody with my wacky exploits. It was the only way I knew of getting attention. Eventually the roof caved in. Within a two-week period, I had a series of numbing events. My mother showed

DON'T QUIT BEFORE THE MIRACLE HAPPENS!

up uninvited from Michigan to find out what was wrong with me because her sweet Christian girl had called her drunk one night. Ugh!

In my insanity, I decided this was a perfect time to commit suicide, but instead, I ended up in the hospital the next morning. (Talk about trying to convince Mom everything was OK!) Then one week later I had to move out of my apartment since all my roommates ran for the hills to get away from me. That night, with nowhere to stay and what little I owned packed in my car, I headed to my Overcomers meeting. After the meeting, I was involved in a terrible car accident in which two people were killed. As I looked at them lying on the street covered by bright orange blankets, I knew this was death—and it wasn't what I wanted. I was seriously scared.

I also knew that some miracle had saved my life in that accident. Again I remembered the OO saying: "Don't quit before the miracle happens!" Was this my miracle?

One week later I was fired from my job. I couldn't believe my boss fired me. I was the top salesperson—irreplaceable in my mind's eye! But he said he couldn't watch what I was doing to myself anymore and was trying to get me to wake up and face reality. I left devastated and broke.

But like all good alcoholics, I landed on my feet, wobbly though they were. For the next few months I slept in hotel rooms, on park benches, or on people's couches. My fair-weather friends and I continued to party. After awhile, I got a job and rented a room with a fellow cocaine addict.

For another whole year I drank and went to Overcomers. My favorite hangout was Venice Beach with the homeless bums; we understood each other. By this time I really wanted to get sober, so I went to spend the night at Venice Beach to scare myself into sobriety. It was different, all right! I learned to be street savvy and scrounged pizza out of a Dumpster. *Maybe this isn't such a bad life!* I thought. The next morning I proudly arrived at the Overcomers office to give details about my latest exploit. They gave me a few polite smiles, but deep down I knew it wasn't funny anymore.

At my next Overcomers meeting, I heard a guy who had three months of sobriety talk in a way he never had before. My heart leapt because I knew he "got it." The miracle happened for him. I could see it, and I had seen where this guy had come from. For the first time, I had hope that it could happen for me.

OVERCOMERS OUTREACH

On August 1, 1987, I made a clean sweep of my life. I moved into a new home, started a new job, and drank my last beer. I've been sober ever since. With time, I saw the miracle happen. I believe God saved my life through Overcomers Outreach. My defense for not going to AA was that it was a cult, but I would go to Overcomers—thank God! Eventually I attended AA, and still do to this day.

Isaiah 51:3 says, "And the Lord will bless Israel again and will make her deserts blossom; her barren wilderness will become as beautiful as the Garden of Eden." God has comforted me, just like this verse says He would do for Israel. God is in the process of restoring all that was lost. Overcomers was my one connection to God through all this insanity and I am eternally grateful to the Christian therapist who sent me there.

Over the years, I have learned to trust God to walk me through the things I could never face before, sober. With time, I have been able to use the gifts God has given me to help others. I no longer feel so different from everybody, even though I would still like to have a Clydesdale horse!

Today, I am happily married with two beautiful children. I continue to share my experience, strength, and hope daily. Thank God I didn't quit before my miracle happened!

12

FOOD WAS MY LIFE

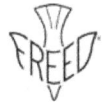

BY DORIS R.

I grew up in a Christian home in a small town in Southern California. I was taken to church and Sunday school by my parents, and as a very young child I believed and received Jesus as my Savior. I always knew that He loved me unconditionally. My parents loved me too.

But tragedy struck when I was ten years old when my father died of cancer. I didn't know it was appropriate for me to grieve; I thought that word applied only to adults. So as a young child I began to stuff all my feelings of fear, anger, loneliness, sadness, shame, etc., and continued to do so as I grew up.

My best friend was God, and we had a very close personal relationship.

My second best friend was food, and this relationship was unknowingly encouraged by my family. My mother would say, "Doris, I just baked some chocolate chip cookies. Have some; it will make you feel better." We lived with my grandparents following my dad's death and Grandma would say, "Doris, I just took a coffee cake out of the oven, have some." Grandpa would say in the evening, "Doris, wouldn't you like some ice cream? I'll get some from the freezer for you."

My family believed that fat children were healthy children. As a result, no one was alarmed when I began to gain weight. I knew that whenever I started to feel feelings, they seemed to go away if I ate. This became my pattern and by the time I was sixteen, I had dresses in sizes seven, nine, eleven, thirteen and fifteen and I wore whatever I could fit into that week. I was always on a diet, up thirty pounds, down ten, up fifteen, down five, up five, down fifteen—thus went the constant yo-yo of my weight. I knew I ate differently from my friends, because if I took one bite of something sweet, I couldn't stop eating it until it was gone. Once I started, I ate the whole thing.

In college, while living in the sorority house, I was presented with a beautiful chocolate cake for my birthday. I can remember carrying it to my room thinking, *Wow, what a gift. I've never had my very own birthday cake before!* I put it down on my bedside table. Later that evening, when my roommates and I came in from our dates and they went to sleep, all I could think about (and smell) was that chocolate cake in the room.

Before long a wonderful idea popped into my head. *Doris, it's your birthday, why don't you have some?* So I got up in the middle of the night, snuck downstairs to the kitchen with my cake, found a plate, knife, and fork, and went into the bathroom where I cut a piece and ate it. Then I thought, *Wow was that good! It's your birthday, Doris, you deserve another piece.* So I ate a second piece, then a third, fourth, fifth, and sixth. I stopped and took a close look at the cake. I remember seeing only about one quarter left, so I decided at that point to eat the whole thing. It was best not to waste any.

I went to bed feeling full, fat, and sick to my stomach. When I awoke in the morning, my roommates' first question was "Doris, what happened to your birthday cake?"

I explained.

It seemed only minutes until my entire sorority knew that I had eaten my whole birthday cake, all alone, in the middle of the night, in the bathroom. I had not shared the cake with my friends on the third floor. Then the whole school seemed to hear the bizarre story. I was incredibly angry at myself. I felt guilty, ashamed, embarrassed, and fat, and I just wanted to scream, *But you don't understand—I intended to have only one piece, but I wound up eating the whole thing.*

Compulsive eating was the story of my life. During my twenties and thirties, I went into full-blown addiction, but did not know what it was. Sometimes I could control what I ate, but most of the time food controlled me. I was obsessed with food. I would go to the refrigerator at least a hundred times a day to see if anything had changed, or to my favorite bread-box, just to look inside. But it was always the same thing: once I started eating something, I couldn't stop.

I began eating in secret—eating very little in front of my family and friends, but privately I would binge. Then I began switching foods. I switched from chocolate candy to hard candy and licorice because it took longer to eat, from ice cream to sherbet, because I really didn't like sherbet quite as well. I also had another way of eating: taking bites of other people's food. For example, I would never order a piece of pie in a restaurant, but would say, "Oh, I really don't care for any, but I'll have a bite of yours." My husband and children got pretty tired of this, but that was the way it was.

As my addiction escalated, I hid food everywhere. I hid it in closet drawers, in purses, in the china cabinet. The trunk of my car looked like a candy store—I had sacks of every kind of candy imaginable. Somehow I didn't see this as being abnormal. This was simply what I needed to do to survive on a daily basis.

In 1982, my husband chose to get help for his disease of alcoholism. I was introduced to Overcomers Outreach and a traditional 12-step group (Al-Anon) and realized my codependence. I had a lot of guilt and shame, anger and sadness, loneliness and hurt, and yet it was a relief to know that not only did I not cause him to drink, but I couldn't control his drinking, nor could I cure it. I had to let go and let God work. I began to realize that his recovery would be his responsibility, with God's help.

As I began to take the focus off my husband, my disease of compulsive overeating strangely began to escalate. I remember in August of 1985, sitting in an Overcomers Outreach meeting as a darling girl shared about her recovery from food addiction. I realized that she was talking about me, and for the first time a ray of hope appeared. On the way out to my car, a thought came to my mind, *If you admit you are a compulsive overeater, Doris, you will have to stop eating compulsively.* The light was beginning to dawn.

Yet somehow I wasn't ready and I stayed in my disease for another whole year. By then I knew I needed help because now my disease was so serious I was eliminating all food and eating only sugar. I couldn't go five minutes without a piece of hard candy in my mouth and I knew I was dying.

One evening in January 1986, my husband and I were going out for dinner. I thought he was taking a shower, so I decided I would have some ice cream. I'll never forget my husband's face when he opened the door and saw me with my tablespoon scooping ice cream into my mouth from a gallon container from the freezer in our garage. He stared at me and said, "Doris, you are sick. You need help. You have the same disease as I do. You use food; I use alcohol, and you will die if you don't get help."

It was my moment of clarity. God spoke to my heart. The next day, January 20, 1986, I went to my first OA (Overeaters Anonymous) meeting and began my recovery.

Today, I know that Overcomers Outreach, OA, and Al-Anon have helped me change my life. In these support groups I am no longer alone, but I am responsible for my own recovery with God's help, which I do one day at a time. I use the 12 Steps of AA, substituting "food, people, places, and things" for "alcohol." I have the tools of the program such as making phone calls, writing, reading, and giving service, which aid me. I have a sponsor who has guided me through the last six years of my recovery and I have had the privilege of sponsoring a number of women in the program.

Most days I'm grateful, because I know that God has allowed the circumstances of my life to draw me closer to Him and that He gives me strength to stay abstinent, one day at a time. I have lost weight, though my focus is not on the bathroom scale; it's on balanced living. I have learned to accept and trust that in God's perfect plan, He is in charge, not me. I now say, "I can't, God can, and I think I'll let Him."

Gratitude is the hinge on which the recovery door swings and I praise God that He led me to Overcomers Outreach as well as other 12-Step groups where I received the help I needed.

It's been my privilege to help begin an Overcomers Outreach group in our church. Not only that, my husband and I served on the OO office staff for three years. Today my life is full, and I no longer have abnormal cravings for food. In fact, my cup is full and running over!

13

SKEPTICAL ATTORNEY FINDS HIS "HIGHER POWER"

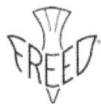

BY MIKE H.

It all started innocently enough, with a call from another lawyer whose clients needed help. Could I steer them through the legal maze created by their son's death in an industrial accident? With typical humility (something we lawyers are not long on), I assured him I could, and soon met with them at his office.

Clients who have recently lost a loved one are always a challenge, but these folks were different somehow. They seemed to be at peace in the middle of the usual maelstrom created by financial hardships, difficult decisions, and grief all brought on by the unexpected death of a loved one. They told me that Jesus Christ was their lawyer, but they knew He worked through lawyers like me also. Stifling a weak joke about Jesus' legal qualifications in that state, I told them I appreciated their faith and would try to help them. I was not a Christian at the time, though I was married to one.

The matter proved routine because of my experience and connections and we soon met at a settlement hearing. It was there that Betty and Larry (those aren't their real names) handed me an open letter they had written that described their son's accident, his death, and their beautifully answered prayers. Asking God for a sign that His hand was in these circumstances, they had looked out the windows of the hospital where their son lay dying and saw a beautiful double rainbow displayed in the Denver skies.

When I got home that night after a typical Thursday whirlwind of appointments and court matters, capped by an evening AA meeting, I was describing this rather unique couple to my wife as I undressed. In the inside pocket of my sport coat, I found their open letter. Without a single thought about it being a confidential client document, I handed it to my wife and said something like, "Here, you're a Christian. Maybe this will make more sense to you than to me!"

I watched her tears flow as she read it, but we didn't talk much about it. At this point, I was about two years sober and our new marriage in sobriety was still mending. (I was much more into action than feelings, and spirituality came hard for me.) My wife, Ruth, knew this, and respected my awkwardness by avoiding discussions about spiritual issues and religion. Oh, sure, I believed in God, but "God as I understood Him" at that time was somewhere between a golfing buddy and a celestial Santa Claus. I was proud of my progress, though, having entered treatment two years before, although as an atheist (a thoroughly beaten and confused atheist, I might add).

Ruth broke her silence about this matter a few days later, when she told me that the letter had deeply affected her. It had awakened a need to get back to church and to enroll our five-year-old in Sunday school. I agreed to go with them, but only once! My "church" was a Sunday morning AA meeting and I planned on keeping it that way.

We picked one of the three hundred Wichita churches near our new home, a large church where we wouldn't be noticed, and off we went. We arrived late and, to my chagrin, were seated in the second pew from the front. Almost immediately the choir marched down the aisle in front of us. I glanced up from my song sheet and looked directly at the unmistakable face of the man who had authored the open letter as he strode by with the choir.

To say I was stunned is an understatement! First, the letter had mentioned their church by name, and this wasn't it! Second, the odds of our chance meeting like this were astronomical. Beads of cold sweat trickled down my armpits and forehead as I came to the fearful conclusion that I had been set up by a Power greater than myself. *It's too late to become a Christian at forty*, I thought. That day, I hurriedly made my exit, resisting the pastor's altar call, even when he said, "Let's sing the last verse again." (It was some hymn where the refrain said "Come!")

SKEPTICAL ATTORNEY FINDS HIS "HIGHER POWER"

He sensed that there was someone there who was resisting the call of the Holy Spirit, and that someone was me.

I learned in the next several days why some call Christ "the hound of heaven." Everywhere I went, I felt the fearful presence of God all around me and within me I kept hearing the word "come." Finally, my resistance spent, I knelt down in my study and asked Christ to come into my heart. To my amazement, we met at the cross. I sensed simultaneously His agony, His love, and the incredible cleansing power of His blood. I learned later, when meeting with Betty and Larry, that they had been praying for my salvation since our first meeting, and had only begun to attend that church a couple of weeks before our chance meeting there the Sunday morning I showed up.

The same pastor who bade me "come" a couple of years previously was the one who handed me the Overcomers Outreach literature in early 1988. In a churchy sort of way, he told me to get busy, that our church needed a Christian 12-step group like this. He had met Bob and Pauline at a California seminary conference and was impressed with their organization and their vision.

At the pastor's insistence, Ruth and I attended a Christians in Recovery conference in Oklahoma City that fall and we were hooked. The sense of the reality of Christ and His loving commitment to all of us was awesome and inspiring. Our group in Wichita started in late 1988, and out of it have spawned several other groups in Wichita and around the state of Kansas.

Early on, I viewed Overcomers Outreach as just a Christian AA and Al-Anon. Experience has proven me wrong. It is much more. Since starting an Overcomers group only a couple of years ago, we have been privileged to see God bring people to Christ, and restore a broken relationship between a father and son. We have seen Overcomers as a refuge of hope for those suffering from depression and divorce. We have seen adult children from dysfunctional families begin to feel, to grow, and to love. We have seen well-meaning Christian parents learn to release their addicted children and trust them to Christ's boundless love. As Pauline often says, we too are addicted to miracles.

Jesus comes to every meeting, just as He promised (Matt. 18:20). And in the experience, strength and hope shared at every meeting, we experience the reality of our Lord's words in John 16:33, "I have told you all this so that you will have peace of heart and mind. Here on earth you will have many trials and sorrows; but cheer up, for I have overcome the world."

Today, as a recovering alcoholic who discovered my "Higher Power" in the person of Jesus Christ, I am overcoming as Jesus said we would, one day at a time.

14

ADDICTED TO LUST, ALCOHOL, AND DRUGS

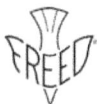

BY BILL R.

I'm Bill—an alcoholic, sexaholic, and adult child of two alcoholics. When I hit bottom in September 1983, I was curled up in the corner of a garage in a back alley in a little northern California coastal town. I was in full-blown delirium tremens, having opted to try sobriety instead of suicide.

My mother's religious background was Mormon; my father's was Catholic; they represented fully opposite poles of the religious scale, the conflict of which added to the isolation of our alcoholic family. We children were left to make up our own minds about religion, and what moral training we received was confusing and often contradictory. What experience I had with religion tended to be negative, and trying religion without a relationship with the Lord didn't help. By the time I entered recovery from my alcoholism, I was very anti-religious. It was not uncommon to hear me curse the church openly. Many of my understandings about God were misdirected at best. In trying to fill that spiritual void in my life, I had used a number of "Higher Powers," including pornography, alcoholism, and addiction to other drugs, as well as occult beliefs from reading New Age literature.

Virtual insanity dominated my life by the time I hit bottom and finally surrendered. Alcoholism can be traced back three generations on both sides of my family tree; it should not be a surprise that I drank in an abusive, out-of-control manner from the beginning. My first real binge occurred when I was sixteen. A buddy of mine and I stole a fifth of vodka from his parents. I learned the next day that I had been a real pig, having had much more than my share by drinking most of the bottle myself. Once I started drinking, I was unable to stop if there was any alcohol left, unless I passed out. I felt so good, so free of burdens when I drank, that I didn't want that feel-good feeling to ever end. This was to be the pattern of my drinking for the next sixteen to seventeen years.

I was a blackout drinker from the time I was nineteen, and I have total gaps in memory for periods up to forty-eight hours. I have experienced other forms of psychotic breaks on at least three occasions due to mixing alcohol and drugs, which produced irrational fears and hallucinations.

A variety of other drugs came into my pattern of use and abuse as I was introduced to them, the most significant of which were marijuana and amphetamines. I enjoyed the mind trips that marijuana induced, and the amphetamines helped me stay awake longer so I could drink more. I used many other drugs during my drinking/drugging career. If there was a pill or a powder offered me, I would often take it without questioning what it was. In the end, I did not draw a sober breath for almost six years. Surprisingly, I never had a drunk-driving charge, and was never locked up in a mental ward, though I should have been a number of times.

It was like there were two people living inside me, the alternate personality coming out when under the influence. But I take full responsibility for my actions, because no one forced me to put a bottle to my mouth or to put the other drugs into my system. The insanity comes in because every time I became inebriated, I thought I would be able to control myself. Such is the denial about personal powerlessness.

At the end of my drinking and drugging career I was becoming suicidal. I was actually on the way to get a rope to hang myself in the garage when I called out to God in an act of desperation. I had heard about Alcoholics Anonymous but had always thought it was for people other than me. Like many others, my definition of an alcoholic or addict never included behavior like mine. That short, desperate prayer was answered immediately, and I knew that I would find help at AA. Four or five days passed before I attended my first meeting, however, because I was still going through the severe detoxification period and all I could do was remain curled up in a fetal position in a corner of that garage.

I felt very welcome at my first AA meeting, and I was encouraged to keep coming back. The stories I heard there convinced me I was in the right place, that these people understood what I was going through. They also told me I couldn't get drunk or loaded if I didn't take the first drink or the first drug. This gave me a new level of understanding in simple terms I could comprehend. People I met at AA also helped me get into a 12-step house where the spiritual aspects of recovery were emphasized in general ways. I was encouraged to seek after an understanding of God through prayer and meditation. Rather than being told what to believe, I was urged to look to the "ultimate creator of the universe" for my knowledge of God. It was six months before I would begin to get a clear understanding of that.

Along the way, I was tempted by a variety of philosophies and theologies, but none of them seemed right. I understand now that the Holy Spirit was leading me to the truth even then. When I did hear the gospel, it was outside of church proper, but I knew it was the truth. My seeking had not been in vain; knowing God is possible through Jesus Christ. That truth struck to the very depth of my soul, and I asked the Lord to come into my life and was born-again on the spot. I also experienced a marvelous deliverance at the time but did not realize it until after my public baptism at a local church two weeks later.

I had been experiencing "cellular cravings" (a friend of mine thought I was talking about cell phones but, no, I mean desperate, biologically-based cravings) from time to time since I came into recovery. This type of craving would come over me if I smelled the faintest hint of alcohol in the air. Starting about three inches behind my navel, tremors would radiate out like an earthquake until I was shaking all over, often drooling on myself. It seemed like every cell in my body was craving alcohol. This type of craving is common among late-stage alcoholics, so I am not surprised that the longer a person drinks, the more difficult it becomes to get sober. When I accepted the Lordship of Jesus Christ, I believe I was changed instantly on a cellular level. The night after my baptism, I went out for pizza with the singles group from the church. One of the guys in the group ordered a wine cooler, which was passed to him right under my nose. Two weeks earlier, that would have sent me into a frenzy. I would have been trying to get away from the alcohol, such was my desire to not drink again. There were no cravings this time. All I experienced was a foul odor. I had been delivered!

I would like to tell you that I never think about drinking anymore, but that just isn't true. At times when I am under stress the thought of a drink still comes to mind. I have found that I am not immune from ecstatic recall—those times when all I can remember is the feel-good feeling that used to come with drinking. That is what hooked me in the beginning and that is why Alcoholics Anonymous still plays a part in my life today. It is there I find true understanding when I share these feelings, and share them I must, or they seem to have power over me.

I would like to tell you that my church was fully supportive of my recovery program, but that wouldn't be true either. However, my pastor and the deacon who was involved in discipling me never discouraged me from attending AA. There were people in both the church and AA groups who told me that all I needed was their organization (and not the other) and everything would be OK. (I need to stress that these were individuals, not AA as an organization.) I believed both had something useful to offer me. Unfortunately, I felt like the two groups were in a tug-of-war and I was the rope. The rope seemed to be in danger of breaking at times.

Pornography had become an addiction for me as much as any chemical I had taken in the past. In the same way that alcohol led me into the use of other drugs, pornography led me into other unhealthy sexual activity. Among those activities was compulsive masturbation, use of prostitutes, and a tendency to compulsively molest the women I dated. Needless to say, I didn't have many repeat dates. I just couldn't keep my hands to myself. Those relationships that did develop past the first date tended to be very unhealthy because the women were probably victims of past sexual abuse, and I was just another victimizer in their lives.

When I came into recovery for alcoholism, I was encouraged to give up the other chemicals as well, but I never mentioned pornography to my counselors because I didn't think of it consciously as an addiction that needed attention, at least not at that time in my life. Pornographic magazines and videos drifted through the recovery home I was in, and I recognized at some level that I needed to be abstinent in that area of my life if I wanted to be truly sober of mind and body. When I became a Christian, sexual purity was firmly encouraged. I found it fairly easy to be sexually abstinent apart from pornography.

I returned to college, understanding this to be the Lord's will in my life. Although I attended a Christian college, there were numerous opportunities to slip sexually as well as with alcohol and other drugs. Working on campus security gave me plenty of opportunities to see how our Christian youth can easily go astray when on their own, often for the first time in their lives. In the course of the several years I was on campus, I had to bust more than a few students for smuggling infractions. I caught

ADDICTED TO LUST, ALCOHOL, AND DRUGS

Playboy magazines and serious hard-core porn, as well as alcohol and other drugs, including "crack" cocaine. All too often the administration of the school and the churches turned a deaf ear when I tried to raise warnings. Such is the denial system of the church.

I very much wanted to begin a support group for Christians in recovery at the campus, but was thwarted at every turn. I finally met a pastor who was supportive of my efforts, even though he was sure there was not a problem at his church. I was sitting with him in his office sharing my belief that the 12 Steps were scripturally-based and that I planned to personally begin research in that area during the following summer vacation. Pastor pulled an envelope from his desk that contained a yellow booklet called *FREED* and several other pamphlets pertaining to Christians in recovery from addiction and codependency. When he asked if I had heard of the Bartosches and Overcomers Outreach, I had to admit my ignorance. I knew from a quick glance at the literature in my hands that further prayers were being answered and that guidance was being given to me. The pastor arranged a meeting with Bob and Pauline for the following week, and I went home to review their material.

Next to my salvation experience, my first Overcomers meeting was among the most wonderful events in my life. I came away knowing I had found people who understood my struggles about being a Christian in recovery because they were going through the same thing. After reporting back to my pastor about the meeting, I was assured I would have the support of his staff and the church if I would start an Overcomers group there. A month later, group number 12 had its first meeting.

The personal benefits for me were staggering. I had felt torn between the church and 12-step groups for so long, but now I felt as if a bridge had formed under me to support me in the ministry to which the Lord had called me. I finally sensed some balance was beginning to occur in my life, at least more so than before. I knew the Lord still wanted me to use Alcoholics Anonymous in my program because I was being ministered to there by the Holy Spirit in ways I didn't get elsewhere. The church assisted me in knowing God better through study of His Word and through corporate worship, and Overcomers seemed to fill the gap between the two. The Holy Spirit witnessed to me that all three aspects were, and still are, important to my Christian walk.

Among the things lost to my addictions was a wife and a daughter through divorce, which occurred seven years before I hit bottom. I began to accept the idea of remaining single my entire life if that was the Lord's will, although I did struggle with the sexual area of my life. A year and a half before graduating from college, a series of events occurred that led me to understand that I would eventually marry again, but that I had not yet met the woman who was to be my wife. It was necessary that I begin praying for her, because she was in danger at the time, I sensed. I had no doubt about the power of prayer to bring about deliverance, and I prayed earnestly for my wife-to-be.

At the same time, I prayed the Lord would prepare me to be the man she needed me to be when we finally came together. When we met a year later, I found out that during the time I prayed for her she had been escaping from her ex-husband to avoid physical harm. Friends had helped her hide until he left the state.

I would like to tell you that our life together was perfect from the start, but that would be far from the truth. Although attraction developed between us quickly, I was the hesitant one. I wanted to make sure I wasn't running ahead of the Lord's will for me. When we did marry, a few problems arose almost immediately. From the beginning, I had been honest and open with my wife about my past—all of it, including the pornography addiction. In trying to have a normal sexual relationship with my wife, all sorts of old lusts came back to life. I thought I had been delivered of these sexual lusts along with alcoholic lust, but it didn't work that way because so much of our sexuality is both mental and emotional. The first two years of our marriage were very difficult. I experienced a lot of shame about my feelings, which I had a very difficult time sharing with anyone, let alone my new wife.

But God is good and when I was ready He brought the right people into my life at the right time to teach me new tools of recovery through God's Word and the fellowship of Sexaholics Anonymous. I was also introduced to literature that not only reinforced my understanding of sexual addiction, but helped me to recognize many of my family's dynamics at work. I saw my wife display classical symptoms of being codependent to a sexual addict, even though she didn't know me during my acting-out years and I wasn't using pornography again.

I had to hit a new type of bottom and accept my personal powerlessness and unmanageability at deeper levels than ever before. The blessings I discovered were truly profound, as I realized new depths of the Lord's love for me. Preparing to have these defects of character removed from my sexual self is proving to be much more difficult than dealing with my alcoholism ever was. These issues strike at the very core of my personal sense of identity, so long has sexual lust been a part of my life.

The battle is not over yet! Some days are better than others, but I thank God each day for the program of recovery He has given me through the 12 Steps and His Word. Each day has its own struggles as well as blessings and victories. I am not perfect by a long shot, but through a balance of traditional church, Alcoholics Anonymous, Sexaholics Anonymous, and Overcomers Outreach meetings, I find most days to be challenging and fulfilling.

The Lord has given me a second opportunity in more ways than I ever dreamed possible. Having been told some years earlier that I was sterile due to an industrial accident, we rejoiced when our son was born in 1992. Trust is growing and my relationship is improving with my daughter from my first marriage. One of my two step-sons made us grandparents three times, and I love being Daddy and Grandpa. God is truly good!

I have a message of hope to carry to those who still suffer, and I carry that message in and out of 12-step meetings and the church. I also have time-proven principles to practice in all my affairs.

15

DEALING WITH MY HUSBAND'S SEXUAL ADDICTION

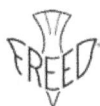

BY LINDSEY E.

A blazing August heat wave overloaded the transformer that supplied the air conditioning to the hermetically-sealed 27-story skyscraper in which I worked. Within minutes our office felt like a scorched desert and I found myself fighting my way through a throng of people rushing towards the elevator and parking garage under the building to go home.

Not until I was on the freeway did I realize I was headed home in the middle of the afternoon, and what this might mean upon my arrival. As I came closer to my destination, I noticed a cold freeze beginning in my toes and spreading upward through my body. I pulled into the carport underneath our apartment and parked next to my husband's truck. For my own sake, I revved the car a few times, like a lighthouse blasting a fog horn, warning a ship of imminent danger. Hoping it was heeded, I gingerly walked up the stairs to our door.

How I hated standing before that door and facing the unknown behind it. I hated the man who slept next to me each night and made me suspicious every time I entered my own house. I hated the secrets and lies, but I hated the things that broke our safe routine even more. I hated change, although I knew that without change our marriage would die—and with it, I felt I would die too.

OVERCOMERS OUTREACH

I turned the key with both hope and reluctance, and as I entered my eyes scanned the room. As the door swung away from me, the momentum sucked out my breath and I thought I would suffocate. To anyone else it looked like a cozy, lived-in living room. But to the wife of a sex addict, the clues were filled in like a completed crossword puzzle. The newspaper was folded on the floor, the personal ads tucked inside, boasting tall blondes and busty redheads able to measure up in ways that I evidently could not. I set my purse on top of the TV and felt the heat radiating from it, betraying the blank screen now on its face. I put my palm on top of the hot VCR (with the X-rated video still inside) and prayed it would thaw the numbness now swallowing my being.

I only noticed that the shower had been on upstairs when the familiar hum of the water running stopped. I wanted to make a quick getaway and pretend I had not walked in, but fear paralyzed me. Like a rabbit caught in the blur of a car's headlights, I froze, as shame oozed over me like glue. I waited, praying for a quick death, but it did not come. I had lived through this scene too many times before; I knew it would be a slow, agonizing process.

My husband, whom I'll call David, told me of his foot fetish on our first date. Together we laughed at this unusual preoccupation. At the time, we both thought using ordinary magazines to masturbate was a harmless, if somewhat dark, pastime. It was not until after we were married that we both realized the power and compulsivity of David's behavior was not normal. We rarely had sex then, and since have gone as long as three years without it because of David's inability and lack of desire to have an intimate and committed relationship with me.

After three years of marriage, David's addiction was having a major impact on our relationship. The addiction was escalating. The magazines had become pornographic and he was using X-rated videos, calling phone sex numbers, and had moved on to cruising through parks to watch women while masturbating in his car. My greatest fear was that a policeman at our door would inform me that my husband had been picked up for lewd conduct.

One day his inability to stop, and my awareness of the mounting lies, brought everything to a grinding halt. I asked him to move out, but instead he checked himself into a hospital in Minnesota specializing in sexual addiction—the only one in the country that we knew about at the time. Our therapist had trained there and felt that David needed this drastic measure to bring a sobering end to the downward cycle.

DEALING WITH MY HUSBAND'S SEXUAL ADDICTION

David's hospitalization lasted five weeks, and halfway through I attended the family week to learn about my part in the vicious cycle of addiction. The program helped me see that his addiction was not my problem, but obsessing about it was. I had felt like I was wading through a foul and murky duck pond, and that the hospital offered fresh spring water. We were told the first two years would be hell, and if our marriage survived, it would take another two to work through the intimacy issues. The thought of going four more years felt overwhelming—little did I know that the long desperate road to emotional health would lead me to the brink of suicide.

My own inner battle was one of self esteem. I kept thinking that if I was thinner, prettier, or more athletic, David would not do this. If I was more of a woman, he wouldn't need to resort to his deviant ways of relating to women. I battled anorexia for a year and starved to be his only desire, but I was met only with anger at my frailty. From there I tried to fill the love-starved void with food and began a long battle with bulimia.

David had so much repair work to do with his own life that those first two years led us on separate journeys. I felt like an airplane, circling around my own issues, trying to work through the codependence that kept me trapped and to stabilize my emotions that were now diving straight down. David, on the other hand, was out on the runway trying to repair the cracks in it. At every turn something else was broken—the runway lights were out as he staggered in the dark trying to find out where he had been and where he was going. He worked on repairing the windsock of his life, which hung in shreds, lifeless with no direction.

The desire to begin recovery, or to stay in the mire of his addiction, was my husband's choice. But I would also come to realize that I had the choice to stay with him and journey this path together or to abort the landing and move on. I do not believe recovery is a straight road and that once you're on it there will be no slips. We have had plenty of curves and switch-backs.

I found that after David came home from the hospital, I started having sleepless nights and began to battle my own ghosts. In therapy, I started learning how my mother's controlling, manipulative ways never allowed me to break free of her. Every attempt at separateness was met with withdrawal of love and support and, fearing her lack of approval, I would give her first place over my husband. I learned how my angry, rage-filled father controlled me with fear and how my perfectionism was bred by a desire to gain his love and approval.

OVERCOMERS OUTREACH

I felt like a tissue-paper collage in the rain as the days all blurred and the colors ran together. My memory has lost a year; it seems I was never thirty-five. The events of that year all spiraled down into a mass grave.

I remember my first panic attack as I shopped in a grocery store. The sudden need to leave overwhelmed me as I threw things into the cart and veered down the aisles. I felt like I was suffocating, and my eyes were locked on the door as I checked out. Once inside my car the tears started flowing as I hypnotically drove home. The pressure bearing down on me pushed the breath and life out of me. Calming down after a call to my therapist, I started putting away the groceries and found I had fifteen rolls of paper towels, thirty cans of cat food, six bottles of wine, and a few items I actually intended to purchase. I lived in fear the next few days, aware that it could happen again. I've had many different types of panic attacks since then, some paralyzing me for as long as eighteen hours with a nauseating, swirling feeling.

As the intervals between attacks grew shorter, I felt myself slipping further down the dark hole that was trying to suck me in. Even though I was a Christian, fear and shame kept me from sharing what was happening at home. None of my family, friends, or co-workers knew why David entered the hospital and they were shocked that everything wasn't as perfect as we made it seem. I felt sentenced to solitary confinement by a jury of my own fears and doubts.

Two years down the road, at the deepest part of my depression, I was on my fourth anti-depressant drug. I felt mortally wounded and trapped. I did not feel God or the church would sanction a divorce. Besides, I was too ashamed to pursue that option. My perfectionistic and self-righteous attitudes did not leave a way of escape. I would not admit that I couldn't handle life with a man like this, that I had made a mistake in thinking that I could change him. Yet I knew that I no longer wanted to be the martyr; I was discovering that I had needs too. I did not want to live the rest of my life in a celibate marriage.

Thoughts of suicide were what I embraced each morning and played out in my mind each night. The nights were the hardest, as I typically slept only one or two hours. All of the drugs I had been given over the months accumulated in the kitchen cabinet and had a drawing power like a swimming pool to a small child. During this time my therapist was like a lifeline around my waist, holding me above the water.

The new beginning came for me when both my therapist and employer encouraged me to take a vacation alone. I rented a condominium

DEALING WITH MY HUSBAND'S SEXUAL ADDICTION

in Hawaii, and even though the initial step was hard to take, once I was there, life bloomed again for me as fragrantly as the ginger flowers did below my balcony. I slept for almost two days and started eating again. I even gathered the courage to go scuba diving.

I was entranced by the silent atmosphere under the water as I watched the sea turtles dance along the reef. I felt transformed. Diving transported me from a dark gray world of pain to a world of silent beauty. The deafening quiet forced me to use my eyes, which had been glazed over for a long time. The more trapped I had felt, the tighter I had closed my eyes. Now I swam effortlessly with a calmness I had not known in years. A confidence unfolded within me that remained in place even after I shed my wet suit.

For me, my trip to Hawaii was an awakening to the fact that I was a survivor. I would not let the church or David's addiction ever push me into such a state of helpless agony again.

I set a time limit on how much longer I was willing to invest in my marriage. I felt that if David failed to gain control of his addiction within the year, and if the sexual dysfunction in our marriage had not been resolved, I would leave. That left a few short months to pull out all the stops and see if we could find healing.

I still struggled with depression, though. Before my trip to Hawaii, I had sent a letter to my parents and brothers telling them I needed some time and space away from them and to please not call me. The only way I knew to break free of Mom's control was to pull out of that relationship totally. It was horrible, yet at the same time very freeing. I did not have a sense of impending doom every time the phone rang. I did not have to fear the phony Sunday afternoon barbecues, and I didn't have to worry about David's withdrawn behavior while we were at my parents' home. I felt a tremendous sense of relief. David and I were now in this alone and I could deal with our issues without interference from my family of origin.

Yet as the months progressed, very little headway was made between us. Our therapist started us doing sexual exercises that brought familiarity, yet a sense of safety. We could only do so much touching and holding each time, so David never felt any pressure to perform. But the process grew tedious for me when I didn't see David initiate the exercises. I felt like a beggar. David's comments, such as, "Your body is disgusting" continued to destroy my self-esteem and I felt embarrassed and ashamed to be with him.

OVERCOMERS OUTREACH

One night after doing the exercises, I got up because I couldn't sleep. The next day, David told me he had masturbated after I left the room. He did not want to do the exercises, which at this point were barely more than a back rub, and he did not want to have sex with me, yet he had no problem with acting out in his addiction. The frustration and constant roller coaster brought me to the point of wanting to separate again. My August deadline was approaching and nothing had really changed.

I worked for a Christian ministry at the time, and my boss was not willing to watch a divorce occur without trying to help. He wanted to meet with David and me one night for dinner. He asked David if he would be open to deliverance-style prayer with a pastor he knew. David agreed that he would. The pastor agreed to work with us only if I was present in the sessions too. David was reluctant, and I felt likewise, but the pastor said that if I didn't see and hear it for myself, I would be skeptical of what had gone on and would tend to dismiss anything David would tell me.

We had two sessions with the pastor, and in my deadline month we had our third and final deliverance prayer session. Those sessions were an eye-opening experience, to say the least. Many of the demonic spirits that had been afflicting David for years were addressed, and they spoke to the pastor and us. We spoke to them in Jesus' name, and although David did some back-sliding with regard to the demons' influence, I regarded those sessions to be powerful and helpful overall. I still cannot fully comprehend the spiritual realm we encountered, but I do know that the "shared spirits" that David and I had—suicide and depression—were dealt with then for me. Since then, I have never had another day of depression or struggled with suicidal thoughts, and I was able to go off the anti-depressants within weeks!

David and I had never addressed his addiction spiritually. He had gone through therapy, the hospitalization, seminars and workshops, and read books and attended 12-step support groups and group therapy, but we had never pursued deliverance-style prayer. We had had prayer back in 1988 before we even started therapy, but the couple meeting with us did not discern any demonic influence and felt David just had a poor self image. With that settled in my mind, I had not thought of seeking prayer again as a way to heal our marriage or stop his addiction.

I know that what I heard and saw during those deliverance sessions was real, and that the demonic world had had a tremendous influence in David's addiction. I also knew that according to the Bible, the enemy would try to take back the ground gained, and that David would need to

DEALING WITH MY HUSBAND'S SEXUAL ADDICTION

stand firm against the onslaught that would come against him. I knew he would have to turn his will over to God and choose whom he was going to serve.

Following the sessions, I had a change of heart about our marriage, and really believed this would be a new beginning for us. I decided that I wanted to give our marriage another try, and see if David was now able to turn away from his addiction.

Sad to say, David opened the door to the enemy only a short month later. I was at a missions conference in Australia, and when I called, David said he had had an overpowering desire to go to a prostitute. While I was gone, he began calling the phone sex numbers. Over the next seven months we had ups and downs, but things seemed to be getting better and he told me he had not made any more phone calls.

Later, during a joint therapy session, I told David that I felt we should be making more gains in our sexual exercises. Within days we made love for the first time in three years. Over the next two months every area of our lives seemed to be better. I was thrilled to think that we had restored intimacy into our marriage and that this therapy had been the missing link all these years. I felt much closer to him; I felt like a wife instead of an acquaintance or roommate. We were enjoying our time together and looked forward to our times of intimacy. I was sharing feelings and fears and joys openly and honestly. It felt great after five years of therapy to finally be heading down a healthy path with my husband. David suggested we look at condominiums and make our future a little more secure, and I was thrilled!

Then one day David opened the phone bill and it seemed quite high. As we looked over the charges, there were many calls to numbers in Hollywood, Beverly Hills, and the San Fernando Valley. We didn't know anyone in these areas, and after a gut-wrenching two hours, David finally admitted that he had been calling escort services and answering personal ads looking for his ideal fantasy woman. He said he had never met any of these women because they wanted two hundred to three hundred dollars, but the way he said it made me question if it wouldn't be a possibility in the future. There were seventy-two phone calls to fifty-seven different women. He admitted that the girls had our number and he had instructed them that if I answered the phone to hang up. While we were talking, the phone rang and it turned out to be an escort service he had called that morning.

OVERCOMERS OUTREACH

I left the house and called our therapist. He asked me what I wanted to do and I said I must leave; I had to get out. He told me to hang up and call my dad. Dad was at my door the next morning at eight A.M. and never let me stop until I had moved and was on my way to starting over.

I was devastated that David continued to lie and deceive me after what I really believe was his deliverance. He had not changed; he had only become better at deceiving me. His lies killed any hope of reconciliation in my heart. I wished him well regarding his recovery and long-term deliverance from sexual addiction, but I no longer wished to be married to him. Our chance to have a close-to-normal marriage was gone forever. I had to face that fact.

During a meeting with our pastor just before our divorce, the pastor said words to my husband that sum it up for me: "David, in the beginning of your marriage, Lindsey was very codependent and co-addictive. She had no regard for her own heart and allowed the sin of your addiction to wound her, over and over again. As she has progressed in recovery, she has come to regard herself in a healthy way. David, her saying, 'I'm going to divorce you' is actually saying, 'No more wounding!' I am in full support of her and her action. Your sin has caused her to lose hope and trust in you, and no marriage can survive the continuous breaking of trust."

I finally signed our divorce papers, and felt a sense of both great sadness and relief. In my journal I wrote: "Divorcing you is not the death of a dream, it is the lifting of a life sentence."

While David was in the hospital in 1989, I heard a radio show on a local Christian station where Bob and Pauline Bartosch were sharing their stories and talking about Overcomers Outreach. I called the number they gave out and was shocked when Bob answered the phone himself. He was so friendly and encouraged me to come to the local Overcomers group he and Pauline attended. I felt so welcomed and immediately felt it was a safe place to share and cry and grow. The conferences they sponsor have been a tremendous blessing in my life.

Especially as a Christian, Overcomers helped me to see that I could be a Christian, have problems, and be able to share about them. I did not need to be ashamed and hide like I had the first three years of my marriage. God wants us all to have healthy emotional lives. I have found that in Overcomers I have had the opportunity to hear many peoples' stories, and though they may be different from mine, the tears and pain are just as real. I have found brothers and sisters in the Lord who can hold me up in difficult times and I can do the same for them.

As one missionary in Australia wrote me, "(Lindsey), at this time I pray you can lean on God's sovereignty (and know that) no one (not even a rebellious husband) can frustrate God's ultimate plan for (your) life." Those were the most comforting words I ever received.

God has not abandoned me on the garbage heap because my marriage has failed. I need to trust that He knew, even on my wedding day, that this would happen, that the changes in my character, the compassion I now have for other hurting people, and the brokenness I am experiencing are all part of His plan—a plan that includes a future and a hope!

16

A PREACHER'S KID OVERCOMES DRUG ADDICTION

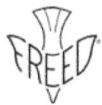

BY LARRY W.

I was born into the home of a Protestant minister and raised to believe that Jesus Christ was my personal Savior. Somehow I was confused about what He was saving me from. Instead of needing to be saved from sin, I felt I needed to be saved from the discipline of a cruel and punishing God, as I then understood Him to be.

As I was growing up, I learned that food was a good way to "stuff" my feelings. I spent my mid to late teenage years weighing in at over three hundred pounds. I ate to stuff all the hurts caused by growing up in a dysfunctional family.

I also ate to stuff the feeling of being "less than." I had no friends at school because I was not socially acceptable at my heavy weight. I had no friends at church because I had no desire to associate with church people.

I finally met someone I liked at church. He seemed to accept me for who I was. He didn't have any preconceived ideas of my being a preacher's kid. I was just a person to be friends with. This "friend" introduced me to drugs and I started using when I was seventeen years old. I was just a casual user at first, getting high about once a month.

This pattern lasted for three years until I joined the Marine Corps. It was there that I learned how to "drink like a man." I also learned how to combine alcohol and drugs so as not to impede my performance. It took me four months to master this art and shortly thereafter I went into the Marine reserves. After I completed active duty, drinking was no longer glamorous to me. I guess I continued to drink to avoid the painful feelings of being in solitude once again.

I went back to college, attending a fine upstanding Christian university. While in school, I majored in video games with a minor in table games.

I met my future wife in college. We would "use" and drink together. We got married when I was twenty-three years old. During the previous two years, I had increased my using, just so I could be comfortable in my own skin. I thought that getting married would be good motivation for me to stop using. I found out it wasn't. In fact, it was the opposite: my using would escalate five-fold over the next two years.

Cocaine and speed were directly responsible for my first job loss. I was fired for stealing to support my habit. My drug habit was also responsible for the bill collectors bothering us and the repossession of my truck. I was able to lie (to myself and my wife) to explain away all the money missing from our bank accounts. Along with doing drugs, great amounts of time and energy were spent keeping my lies straight.

When I lost my job, I accepted a sales position that required that I work up to fourteen hours a day, seven days a week. It was a perfect excuse to increase my drug use, and it didn't help that my boss was a cocaine dealer. It wasn't long before I felt that I had no choice but to start dealing. I took out several loans from Christian credit unions (they don't ask questions of preachers' kids) and invested the money into a massive amount of cocaine and drug-related paraphernalia. I did all of the footwork to make sales, but ended up using the drugs all by myself.

All of my connections had disappeared because I was behind in payments. The money I had borrowed was gone. My boss called me into his office to tell me that I had been using too much. He told me that I had to go home and tell my wife that I was an addict. I informed him that he was obviously mistaken and hell would freeze over before I would tell my wife any such thing. He said that if I didn't tell her, he would!

Telling my wife that I was an addict and that we were tens of thousands of dollars in debt was the most painful thing I've ever had to do. Needless to say, she didn't take the news with great enthusiasm, but she did surprise me by not walking out the door right away. She waited a few months.

A PREACHER'S KID OVERCOMES DRUG ADDICTION

I was lost; I didn't know where to turn. My wife and I tried to work things out over and over again but she finally left me. I even went to a Billy Graham crusade and rededicated my life to Christ. I thought that would take care of everything, but it didn't.

My mother had heard from a co-worker about a group called Overcomers Outreach. She passed this information along to me. Since I had attempted every other Christian solution, I decided to give this a try. My wife came back in order to go with me to the Overcomers' meetings.

I had serious apprehensions walking into that first meeting. I thought that I wouldn't like anyone there because I didn't associate with church people. To my surprise, they listened to my story, smiled, hugged me, loved me, and told me to keep coming back. I did keep coming back, and I quit using—for about three months. Even after I started using again, I continued to go to meetings and just lied to the group about being clean. I carried on this way for almost three months until my wife found out.

The second hardest thing I have ever had to do was sit in front of the Overcomers group and tell them that I had been lying to them. They struck me as fools because they smiled, hugged me, and told me to keep coming back. I later understood that they were not fools, but people who knew where I was and understood me. They had unconditional love for me, but I was too messed up to recognize it.

A few months later they surprised me again by asking me to be a part of the rotating leadership in the group. I was both flattered and petrified, but I accepted. After four years, I finally took a hint from the OO Preamble and started attending AA and NA (Narcotics Anonymous) meetings. The wisdom and experience given by these programs, coupled with the spiritual aspect given to me by Overcomers, proved to be a healthy combination for living everyday life with serenity and a true "Higher Power" to look to.

My program is by no stretch of the imagination perfect, but one day at a time, I have managed to put together more than eight consecutive years of clean time. Overcomers gives me a little self-respect, a lot of hope, and a world of love and acceptance. Because of this modeling of what God's love must be like, I have relearned the concept of salvation.

The cruel and punishing God of my youth is gone and has been replaced by a loving God with whom I have a close personal relationship.

17

HER MASTER PLAN

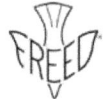

BY RUTH W.

I grew up focused on the future, on that golden someday when life would be better for me. Raised in a highly abusive family, I created a coping mechanism for myself, a master plan called What-my-life-will-be-when-I-leave-home.

At the age of eighteen, I did leave home to attend a well-known Christian university. I was exhilarated, for I was finally free! I was ready to start living out my life according to the master plan I had so carefully built in my mind. The main components of this picture were: being thin, finding the "ultimate love of my life" (of course he would be a Christian), and then settling down with a psychology degree to help fix all the hurting children of the world. Also included were many happy parties where everybody could drink as much as they wanted to, since all would be Christians and thus nobody would have a drinking problem—or so I thought.

The first crack in my perfect picture came when I gained almost twenty pounds during my first semester. Furthermore, there had been no applicants for the ultimate-love-of-my-life position. By Christmas, I was in such a deep depression that, in a fit of hopelessness, I tried to end my life. As a result, I attended counseling, which was mandated for me. During this time, I learned some basic survival tools, and at the end of the following semester was pronounced "functional."

OVERCOMERS OUTREACH

I truly felt like I was doing well because I was back on track with completing my picture. I had found amphetamines (speed) as a weight control device and thus was quite thin. Also, I now had access to alcohol, since I had finally gotten in with the "right crowd" at the Christian school. The best part, though, was that there were plenty of possible candidates for the ultimate-love-of-my-life job.

In my junior year of college, I finally met the perfect candidate. I instantly knew he was the perfect man for me, as he was just the correct balance of Christian and party animal. However, in order to help him moderate his drinking, I decided to give up my use of speed. This was no great sacrifice, since by then I found myself experiencing amphetamine psychosis. My efforts were rewarded! He quit drinking and introduced me to marijuana. What I didn't know was that he had also started using amphetamines.

I graduated with a double degree in psychology and married my husband. I felt so accomplished standing at the altar, my hand securely resting in the hand of my chosen one. I remember snickering inwardly at the pastor's admonishment to keep Christ at the center of our marriage. *I don't need God*, I thought. *I have my husband.*

After the wedding, I settled down to complete the rest of my master plan. However, I kept having this nagging feeling that something just wasn't right, so I kept really busy during the day and got stoned or tipsy at night. Suddenly, it seemed life just turned on us. Bank after bank kept misplacing our money and messing up our accounts. My husband ran into a lot of bad luck in losing money. Once our truck got "accidentally" repossessed. Furthermore, somebody got hold of our bank card and was withdrawing money from our account.

Needless to say, I was in serious denial about some rather obvious issues. Then my husband came home one evening and admitted he was the cause of our financial difficulties, and that we were in terrible financial trouble because of his cocaine addiction. I was utterly shocked!

This new development in my life was absolutely unacceptable to me. Since this was nowhere in my master plan, correction had to be made immediately. I proceeded with vigor to try every possible method to make my husband stop using. Time and time again each one of them failed. Finally, defeated, I decided to return to live with my family of origin. What hurt the most was that I still loved my husband; however, I just couldn't live with a ripped picture.

For the first time in my life, I felt completely hopeless. I contemplated suicide again, but was too emotionally exhausted to even bother. I had hit bottom.

HER MASTER PLAN

God's timing, though, as always, was perfect. The very next day my husband told me about a group called Overcomers where Christians with our problem could go to get help. I don't know why I went; it must have been God's grace that made me go. On the way to the meeting, I kept thinking that I had truly sunk as low as I possibly could; surely I couldn't be going to one of those kinds of groups. It helped that it was a Christian group. My greatest comfort came from the knowledge that—thank God—I didn't belong there. I was just going for my husband.

What an unforgettable moment to walk into my first OO group! I was overwhelmed by the peace and happiness I saw. My husband and I were welcomed without judgment or pity. I let down my defenses and sobbed with relief. For the first time in my life I felt hope. Even though the entire experience left me completely baffled, I was hungry for more.

For the first year in Overcomers Outreach, I attended the meetings just to help my addict husband get clean. I was convinced that without my constant prodding and motivational speeches, he would never make it. I would listen carefully at the meetings for him, and remind him throughout the week of the important things I had heard there. (In retrospect, it truly was a miracle that my husband got clean at all, considering all my interference.)

Since in my mind I wasn't the addict, during this time, I still continued to drink and smoke pot on an almost nightly basis. However, all that good listening at the meetings did not go to waste. Little by little I started to grasp some of the program. Gradually, I started seeing some of my own issues. Before long, I got involved in an incest support group and reentered therapy for myself.

The day before I confronted my father about the incest, I successfully learned to purge (force myself to vomit). I was elated, for I had been unsuccessfully trying to purge most of my life. For the first time in a long time, I saw hope for accomplishing, at last, part of my master plan. I thought I had found a no-lose way to be thin. I quickly lost the weight on which I had blamed so many of my problems, but because of what I had learned in Overcomers, I knew I was sinking into another addiction. For almost two years I sat in the group, admitting I was a bulimic, yet unwilling to take the first step.

I believed that someday I would quit, especially if I ever got pregnant. Inwardly I knew I had little to worry about in that area, since my eating disorder had hopelessly messed up my reproductive cycle. Imagine my surprise when, one morning, a home pregnancy test turned out to be positive!

OVERCOMERS OUTREACH

I was petrified when, a few months into my pregnancy, I discovered I was completely unable to stop purging. It had been OK for me to damage my own body, but I couldn't destroy the little life growing within me. I was so frightened that I went to Overeaters Anonymous (recommended by a fellow Overcomer). In that group I found the tools and the grace to stop purging. Today, in light of that craziness, I consider my son an absolute gift from God.

It was through this experience that I came to terms with my other addictions, including my codependence. At this point I also joined Al-Anon. It was difficult, but rewarding, to begin working the 12 Steps for myself. It was through working the steps and learning about alcoholism in Al-Anon that I finally had to face the terrifying truth that I was an alcoholic. I could see the clear signs of the disease; however, this time I didn't speak about it to anyone, not even my husband. I was too afraid, for I knew that I would never be able to live without alcohol. So I kept denying the facts. I convinced myself that I only sounded and thought like an alcoholic; I wasn't actually one of them.

When I started sneaking extra wine at night, and kept changing my glasses into ever bigger goblets, I knew—thanks to the OO program—that things were just going to get worse if something didn't change. This time, because of five years in Overcomers Outreach, I didn't have to hit a low bottom. Rather, knowing where I belonged, I began attending Alcoholics Anonymous.

Giving up alcohol has been the most difficult thing I have ever done. It was just as hard as I had envisioned it would be. But the surprise has been the newness of life and the freedom I have received in sobriety. My new way of living is bringing forth a wonderful change in my life. I am amazed on a daily basis at the person God is changing me into. He has removed from me the obsession to drink and has given me the willingness to grow and change.

When I received my one-year AA chip, all I could do was sit and stare at it. Finally, I looked up and chuckled, "Something is wrong with this picture!" Then it hit me: for the first time, something was right with it. Praise God!

I continue to change my picture one day at a time. Actually, I am allowing God to create His picture within me. I am now willing to follow His master plan for my life. I am deeply grateful to Overcomers Outreach for introducing me to a new way of life.

18

DRUG ADDICT SET FREE TO SERVE JESUS

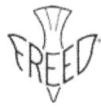

BY ROBIN S.
Jan.19, 1955 – Apr. 7, 2008

I was born on the west side of Long Beach, California, one of nine children. My father, a former Golden Gloves and Navy boxer, was at least a second-generation alcoholic, and a violent one at that. My mother, always hard-working and responsible, also came from a dysfunctional family. Her stepfather was an alcoholic and her mother was a hopeless codependent.

My first recollection of learning about God was in Sunday school, which I attended for only a short time. My grandmother also used to talk about Jesus and spirituality, in between bouts with my alcoholic grandfather. My childhood was filled with an atmosphere of my parents arguing. My father would often physically abuse my mother and/or us. I spent many nights hiding out at the drive-in theater because Dad would come home violently drunk.

The role I played in my family as a boy was fairly insignificant. It seemed like I was starving for love and attention from my parents or from anyone who would give it to me. My older brother and I started playing music when I was around nine or ten. Within a year we were playing in a full band and opening at dances and parties. During this period, I was introduced to glue-sniffing and for the first time became addicted to a mood-altering chemical.

OVERCOMERS OUTREACH

In the late sixties, I began hanging out with an older crowd. This was in the midst of the hippie movement and the Vietnam War protest. I started drinking more, using barbiturates, and getting arrested. Low-riding (cruising around town in our modified cars) and gang-banging became a way of life for me. The homeboys became my family. My use of drugs worsened and I was arrested several times for numerous crimes (possession, under the influence, etc.) I then spent one year in Boy's Republic, a juvenile facility.

When I was sober, I always felt inadequate and unimportant, but when I used drugs, I felt brave and I felt like I fit in. Drugs gave me a sense of worth, so I became more and more dependent upon them.

When I was in the gangs, we were always trying to out-do each other with the different crimes we'd commit. Snatching purses, burglarizing houses, and gang-fighting were just a few of the things we did to get recognition from the world.

I spent a lot of time going in and out of jail. After my stay at Boy's Republic, I made up my mind to stay away from alcohol and drugs and to try and become a responsible person. I decided that it was OK to drink, because after all, everyone drank and it was socially acceptable. I got involved in a relationship that lasted three years but it ended mostly because I drank too much.

During the next ten years, I did a lot of traveling. I went to Colorado to visit my dad, where I decided to be a controlled alcoholic unlike my father. He was the one person I did not want to be like—a violent, raging alcoholic.

After leaving Colorado, I spent some time back in California. In exchange for room and board, I helped my uncle build a fifty-foot trimaran (three–hulled sailboat). Here, I learned the boat-building skills that later played a big part in my life.

My drinking and using progressed. I began "slamming" cocaine (taking the drug by using a needle) with some new so-called friends. I had used the needle only a few times in my life, but now slamming became a romance. I fell in love with this new-found way to use drugs, not knowing that it would nearly kill me someday.

Still making my geographical changes, I ended up in Redding, a small town in northern California. There, I got together with some friends I had known in my teens. I have to be honest; at this point in my life, I was having a lot of fun. I was playing music, going fishing, hunting, and camping, as well as going to a lot of parties. I moved into a large house

DRUG ADDICT SET FREE TO SERVE JESUS

in Redding where I lived with several other people. They all liked to do drugs as much as I did. We would snort or shoot up speed and party for days at a time.

I then met my future bride. On several occasions we would stay up and talk after everyone else had finally gone to bed. We had a lot in common. Both of us came from divorced families and both had alcoholic fathers. I liked her a lot, but she was too young for me, so I never thought about our getting together. She ended up going back to Pennsylvania with her mother and the party house closed down.

I roamed around Redding for a couple of months. Then I found out that the girl and her family were on their way back because it didn't work out with her alcoholic father. We all decided to get a house together. Her mom and I were good friends, but at the time there seemed to be no reason for me to get involved with this family. I was single and I really didn't need anybody. After all, I lived in my motor home van, played my music at parties and bars, and pretty much did everything on my own. But somehow I found myself living with this family and I really didn't know why.

During this time, I fell in love with that young lady. We started out as good friends and we didn't know that God had His hand in it. Her mother (who is, today, a walking miracle herself) found out that her daughter was in love with me and promptly told me to tell her that I didn't really love her. Then she asked me to leave, which I did.

I went back to Long Beach and continued to drink and use as if nothing had ever happened. Time passed and the next thing I knew, I was picking this young lady up at the bus depot. Something kept us together despite all the problems and adversity.

I suffered a serious injury to my hand due to my drinking and using. This gave me the perfect opportunity to get prescription pain pills and to stay loaded all the time. One day, with all the free time I had, my girlfriend and I went driving around looking at different boats in the boatyards of Wilmington. We came across a forty-foot trimaran that was nice, but it needed a lot of work. We decided to buy this boat and rebuild it. We lived on the boat and it was in this place (a junkie-infested, skid-row area of Wilmington) that I finally started to hit my bottom.

Day in and day out, I stayed loaded on one thing or another. I would either sniff carburetor fluid, smoke PCP, drink cheap wine, or shoot up heroin or cocaine. One way or another, I managed to obliterate myself from reality. This went on for about two years and during that time, I broke my leg, had many visits to the county jail, and woke up several times strapped down in a hospital bed, not knowing how I got there.

I put this girl through hell on earth. I physically and mentally abused her while under the influence of drugs and/or alcohol. I would sometimes go to an AA meeting to get the heat off me from my girlfriend, my mom, or anyone who would confront me about my drug problem. But I never really did it for myself. My girlfriend didn't know that I was shooting up heroin. Every time I fixed up, I never knew if I would live through it. I was living a life of complete insanity!

At this point, we ended up staying at my mom's house. My girlfriend and Mom had found out about a traditional 12-step group and decided to get help for themselves. I never felt so alone in my whole life. They had finally gotten off of the codependent merry-go-round and I couldn't manipulate them anymore. They told me that if I wanted to keep drinking and using, it was my decision, but they were going to get on with their lives.

Other things started happening that made me open my eyes. I noticed that my uncle Dean had a totally different life after becoming a Christian. You could see the difference in his eyes. He always seemed to be happy. I wondered what it was that changed him, and I wanted what he had.

Despite those things, my addiction worsened. I began overdosing on heroin. My morning shakes required a drink of some sort just so I could function when I had to go to work. Every day I was faced with the problem of getting money for drugs or alcohol. I had been going in and out of AA for a long time, but I couldn't seem to grasp the idea. Today I realize I had been going there for all the wrong reasons.

One night, after coming down from an overdose of heroin, I remembered my uncle Dean. I asked my mother what had changed him and she said God had changed him. She said that although I had been going to AA, maybe I ought to try God also.

I'll never forget that night. As I laid in my bed, I cried out to God for help and the story of Bill Wilson came to my mind. I decided that if God revealed Himself to Bill W. dramatically, it could also happen to me. I asked God to please help me because I could not go on like that any longer. I asked God to reveal Himself to me, and He did—the very next day!

The next morning, my mother was working delivering magazines as she always did, and as she was driving she turned on the radio. A Christian station just happened to be on. Bob and Pauline Bartosch were

DRUG ADDICT SET FREE TO SERVE JESUS

on the show talking about a Christian 12-step program called Overcomers Outreach. My mom quickly wrote down the phone number. When she returned home, she put the number down on the table in front of me and left.

I called and Bob answered. He told me about Overcomers and he also told me that he himself was a recovering alcoholic. That blew me away. I couldn't believe that he was a minister, a man of God, and he had the same problem that I had. The difference was that he had gotten help and had been sober for thirteen years. I just found it so hard to believe. He told me that the Overcomers met on Tuesday nights, gave me directions, and then we hung up. A little while later, I started feeling sick. I was getting the shakes. I called him back and I told him that I couldn't wait until Tuesday, that I needed to talk to someone that day. He arranged for me to meet him at their house that night. After much persuasion, my girlfriend finally agreed to go with me.

We arrived at the Bartosch home and as they opened the door and welcomed us in, I could feel the warmth and love. I'll never forget the wooden "EASY DOES IT" plaque that hung on the wall. We all sat down and I started telling them my story. My girlfriend didn't know that I had been using the needle and I felt relieved to get that off my chest. As I went on with my confessions, Bob stopped me with tears in his eyes. He told me something that would impact me for the rest of my life.

A couple of years earlier, their oldest son had had a friend named Robin. That friend and I not only had the same name, but he was also a musician and an addict/alcoholic. That Robin had also been using heroin on a regular basis and had come to Bob and Pauline for help. This was on a Thursday night. They arranged for Robin to go to a treatment facility the following Monday since there wouldn't be any beds available until then. But Robin didn't make it until Monday; he died of a heroin overdose the next day, which happened to be Good Friday. This touched me in a way that is hard for me to describe, except to say that I felt like Robin died so I could live. It made me think about Jesus dying on the cross for my sins.

Bob and Pauline felt the similarities between me and the other Robin were too close to be just a coincidence. I had arrived at my moment of clarity. I felt that God had answered my prayers to reveal Himself to me and I became willing to go to any length to get clean and sober. Bob asked me if I would agree to go into treatment immediately if he could find a place. I said yes. After calling several places, Bob found one that would take me that night. Right before we left, we all sat around the kitchen table and prayed. At that moment, I felt a peace I had never felt before. Somehow, I knew that everything was going to be all right.

Today, I have been clean and sober for several years. As a direct result of Overcomers Outreach, my girlfriend and I accepted Jesus Christ as our Lord and Savior. We were also married when I was a year sober and Bob performed the ceremony. My wife Tammy and I now have three beautiful daughters. We are learning what it means to have a personal relationship with Jesus. We know that He loves us and we love Him.

Jesus allowed us to rebuild that broken-down sailboat, which played a big part in keeping me sober. Through Jesus being our "Higher Power," working the 12 Steps, and trying to serve Him on a daily basis, my wife and I are growing spiritually more and more every day. We had the privilege of leading an Overcomers group for several years in Bellflower, California, and we were blessed to see other peoples' lives transformed. We both enrolled in college to study for the ministry, and I was ordained as the pastor of a church in Long Beach, California.

Our congregation consisted of recovering drug addicts, ex-gang members, bikers, and others who have a hard time fitting into a traditional church. One of the many ministries that we offered at our church was Overcomers Outreach. The Lord has blessed our lives so much, and He's given us the opportunity to see miracles happen in many other lives too. We've had a purpose in life and we are excited about God's plans for us.

I have found that if you leave the door of willingness open and seek God with all of your heart (Jer. 29:12), He will meet you wherever you are, and can set you free!

FROM BLACK MAGIC TO THE POWER OF CHRIST

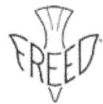

BY BERNARD M.

My mother was only fourteen years old when I was born. My father had walked out on her a few months earlier, claiming that the child she was carrying was not his. However, it was not hard for her to prove that he was the father, since she was white and my dad was black.

I lived with my grandmother until she died when I was four years old. I then went to live with my mother who was now eighteen. For the next three years, I made her life very difficult. For example, I set fire to three apartments and once to myself—I still have the scars to prove it. The strangest thing is I blacked-out all the bad things I did to her. I can't remember anything before I was thirteen or fourteen.

By the tender age of seven, I had to be put in a home for boys and girls. Then I was adopted by a distant relative, an uncle of my mother's cousin; he died two years later. His wife (my new mom) decided that we should move to her home state, which everyone thought was best because of my chronic running way. I had already spent three nights in jail before my tenth birthday.

By the time I reached my teens, I was dabbling in black magic. I had found a place to direct my anger and the hate I felt. I wanted the power to stop people from hurting and rejecting me. If people would not love me, then they would fear me, I would see to that!

OVERCOMERS OUTREACH

Because I was mulatto (biracial), I was never accepted anywhere, not among blacks or whites. What I got from the black arts was acceptance, and I went for it. The only problem? Satan is not a thing to be played with. By the time I was saved, I had been into séances, spells, and worshiping of demons.

During this period, I ran away and went back to my real family. My mother said she could not handle me, so I lived with her brother. I was not mean to them like I was to Mom, but I was not good for them either, because I got them involved with black magic.

At this point I started drinking and stealing alcohol from my uncle. By my second year with them, I got into trouble and the cops said it would be a good idea for me to move back to my adopted parent. I took the hint and left. Within a few months of my return, I noticed the alcoholism really had a hold on my adopted mom and it kept getting worse. Fighting was the norm; drunks would come over to party at our house and I soon learned the fine art of stealing from our inebriated houseguests.

Even at the young age of fifteen, I was already asking the question, "Why am I here?" I came very close to successfully committing suicide. I took an overdose because I wanted attention. My attempt got me into the hospital, where I almost died.

Fortunately that year I started to open up to new ideas. One night while watching TV, I turned on a Christian show and listened. I called in, thinking I would have someone to talk to while the news was on. While I was talking to this guy, something happened that surprised me. He asked me if I was struggling with things no one knew about. Of course I denied everything, but he sure got my attention! If this was from God, then I wanted to know more.

He asked me if I wanted to be set free and invite Jesus into my heart. I said yes but I didn't want anyone to overhear me pray so I took the phone outside, and as I tried to balance the phone and hold the door open, I said the sinner's prayer. An amazing thing happened! I felt a weight lift from my shoulders and a peace in my heart as if Jesus had been waiting to come in. As soon as I opened the door, He rushed in!

My new friend told me to get rid of my black magic stuff. The very next day I tried to. I went into the woods with a bag full of books and spells on how to raise spirits, etc., but when I tried to set the bag on fire, it would not burn. That night I called my friend back and told him what happened. He told me to pray over it as I burned it, asking God to deliver me from its hold. The very next day I did that. This time I went

FROM BLACK MAGIC TO THE POWER OF CHRIST

to the backyard and filled our metal trash can with the junk. I prayed and put two matches into the can, it started to burn, and burn it did! In fact it burned a hole in the bottom of the can. My stepfather blamed the neighbors. I never did tell him what really happened.

My life changed radically. I was no longer the same person. I endured a very difficult process because the enemy did not want to die out of my life without a fight. Fight he did, but the battle was won by God. The next couple of years were up and down, but progressively better. I totally changed in school. My grades improved so much that I graduated six months early and joined the Marines as my father had done.

I survived boot camp and was sent to a new duty station. It was there that I started attending an old-fashioned Pentecostal church and even went out street witnessing. I was reading the Bible and applying it to my life and my knowledge of the Word grew rapidly. After I was transferred to Hawaii, I met other Christians who led me to a Baptist church. I felt compelled to attend even though I preferred the Pentecostal church. I did like one thing they did—they studied the Word. Within a few years, I was witnessing and leading others to Christ, doing visitation, and working on the bus ministry.

Then some brothers dared me to ask a certain girl out on a date. While dating her, I began to make selfish decisions and started to backslide. We became sexually active. So what did I do? Well, like any good Christian boy, I got married, which was not the best thing to do. I now know that I should have repented and asked for help, or at least requested premarital counseling. I had stopped many of my church activities and once the novelty of the marriage wore off, I had too much time to think. I soon found that a six-pack would help me think better.

Once that started, I descended as rapidly as I had risen. I was doing things I had sworn I would never do again—drinking, smoking, drugs, cheating on my wife, etc.

My wife and I moved, and after we relocated, I believed it would be better for us if we did not go to church, because I was not living a godly life. I didn't go to church unless I was really hurting. My drinking progressed to the point where it was the center of my life. I visited nightclubs regularly, and I often stayed out all night, sometimes even days at a time. My spiritual life had dwindled to reading the Bible in emergencies.

During routine drug and alcohol testing in the Marines, I had a positive urine test. Like a dummy, I admitted I was smoking and abusing alcohol. I felt I needed to confess to save myself. Even though I was promised help, I never got it. I fought hard to stay in the military since I had never been in trouble before, but they wanted to make an example of me, so I was discharged eight months later. With a three-month-old daughter, no money, and nowhere to go, I left the Marines hurt, rejected, and ashamed. I was too frightened to be bitter at God, but resentment set in. Within a few months, I also lost my car.

We moved into my adopted mother's home, where alcoholism was king. Drinking was an everyday thing and drugs were the reward for hard work. Before long, my best friend was helping me use the needle for drugs. I never believed I would sink so low, but here I was—needle in arm, drink in hand. I was disgusted with myself.

My wife and kids went back to her mother while I attempted to get my life together. I cried like a baby the day they left, so of course I had to get drunk to deal with my grief. That was the most pain I can ever remember feeling but more was to come. We had to sell everything we had. People took advantage of our vulnerability and my self-esteem was at minus zero.

I started working security jobs and things continued to get worse. Of the places I could get work, the quickest were nightclubs and bars, and of course, wheeling and dealing goes with the turf there. I even started working security for porno shops. It was ironic that a child of God was working to protect the children of darkness. I felt just like the prodigal son working in a pig-pen, but his story had a better ending because he went home; I went for more.

I attempted to clean up my act, but I did nothing to clean up my heart. I started "doing geographics." I circled the country twice in two years. I went north as far as Maine, south to Florida, and then back to Hawaii. During the time I was moving around, my wife went on welfare and moved into low-income housing. My bright thinking told me to go live with her and let her continue collecting welfare while I worked and saved money. Even though dishonest, I thought it was a great idea, except that I used all my money on partying.

My worst move was accepting a job on the merchant ships. I was always gone and I never did save any money. While I was playing on the high seas, my wife had an affair. Worse yet, she was having it with her sister's friend. With the threat of losing my wife and kids, I quit my job and moved back home. But it was too late, because when I came home, she ran off with him. The pain I felt is best described as throwing up

FROM BLACK MAGIC TO THE POWER OF CHRIST

barbed wire. My emotions went from one extreme to another: love to rage, promises to threats. It was the beginning of the end.

My wife got smart. When the family had moved into the low-income housing, I wasn't included on the lease. Since I refused to leave, she and her sister got a restraining order. They had to lie to get one, but it worked. I went back to shipping, which lasted only a few months, just long enough to hit another bottom. I lost thirty pounds and thousands of dollars. In my despair, I cried out to God for help.

God heard my cry. I asked for help and my employer sent me to the East Coast for treatment, but I believed I needed to act like I didn't want to be there, so I sabotaged my treatment. They were smarter than I thought, because in four days they sent me back, saying I needed more help than they could give me.

Before they sent me packing, I went to an Alcoholics Anonymous meeting and that meeting changed my whole life. The name of the meeting was "To Thy Own Self Be True." That has become the foundation of my recovery. After getting rejected for treatment, I got scared, because I believed if I really were crazy, I would be the last to know. I went home to Hawaii and was accepted into a residential program, which was the best thing in my life outside of getting saved. I was able to buy some time and learn what my real problem was—ISM (I-self-me).

As I became clean and sober, and the knots started to untie, I got hungry for spiritual things. Being humbled, I started to seek the Lord and people started coming into my life who knew Jesus. I cannot say that after I got clean everything in my life became perfect; in fact, the opposite was true. My wife divorced me, I lost my family, and I saw my kids put in foster homes because of my ex-wife's bad relationship with her boyfriend. She even charged him with molesting my daughter. Through all this, I didn't drink. Now that's a miracle!

I had started listening to Christian radio while I was fighting for my family. I was not going to church yet, but I was praying, reading, and listening to teaching. While using Alcoholics Anonymous as my main support, I heard a man who taught the Bible in a comprehensible way. In fact, I would tell others he sounds like he's sharing at an AA meeting.

Then I found out that the church he pastored was moving to town and I started to attend slowly at first, because I didn't want to get religious. I just wanted spirituality. I began to see that the Steps and the Bible made a great combination. As I worked the Steps and studied the Bible I got hungry for more. I started applying what I was learning and things started to change. Every time the doors at church were open, I was there. I got into service at both church and AA—I knew I needed both. Unfortunately, both were telling me I didn't need the other. I've seen too many alcoholics relapse in church, thinking God has healed them.

Well, because I'd seen the balance work in my life, I had a vision to start a Christian support group, a place where people in recovery would be supported with the comfort we have from God (2 Cor. 1:3–4). While this was on my heart, I heard a "Focus on the Family" radio show featuring a recovering alcoholic who was a Christian. With that inspiration I was off and running. I had gotten so active at church that I shared my vision with my pastor and soon started a support group.

But all was not complete. I felt compelled to get Christian recovery material that offered the balance of AA and the Scriptures. One day, I heard about a "Christians Reaching the Addicted" Conference in Denver. I could not afford to go, so I decided to pray about it. I shared it with my pastor and he wanted to ask the church to send me. The meeting we had started at church was growing and God was blessing and using it, so they felt the training would be good. I could not believe it, but God worked out all the details for me to attend the conference.

I thought I would be the first to bring the 12-step recovery concept to the church, so you can imagine how blown away I was when I got to the conference. I felt like a kid in a candy store!

One night at dinner, I was sharing all that the Lord was doing in my life, how He used the AA program to bring me back to church and what my vision for recovery was. Imagine my shock when I found out that I was talking to the people I had heard on the radio—Bob and Pauline Bartosch! As Pauline shared, I felt as if my heart was going to explode. The way they had started their ministry was exactly how God was working in Hawaii, even our dove-shaped logo was the same. We bonded instantly.

Through the week, I was privileged to attend some behind-the-scenes meetings. Bob and Pauline made sense when they said, "Why reinvent the wheel?" and so I decided to link my church support group to OO. With that, the Lord told my heart that He would do great things if I didn't care who gets the credit. The conference continued and relationships grew. The last night we realized that everyone was talking about support groups but not one meeting had been held there. So Pauline passed the word that we would have an open AA meeting right there in the hotel lobby!

Words cannot describe the love and togetherness that was felt during that meeting. We laughed and cried and shared God's love with each

FROM BLACK MAGIC TO THE POWER OF CHRIST

other. That one meeting itself was better than the whole week of the conference! The Lord sat in on that meeting. After we shared, they closed the meeting with the reading of "A Vision for You" from *The Big Book* of Alcoholics Anonymous. We finished with hugs and tears, knowing that the Lord had recharged our hearts.

With my heart aflame, I came home to Hawaii. Trials and testing awaited me like never before. My children were in foster homes and my ex-wife had falsely charged me of abusing them. She later admitted she lied, but the damage had been done. I was falsely accused of doing drugs while in the ministry. Things got so bad I thought I was losing my mind.

Yet with all that, it has not stopped the Lord from completing His plan. Today we have two OO meetings going here in Hawaii, and people in the program are coming to the Lord and being discipled. Yes, I have learned that nothing can separate us from the love of God.

Our vision is to establish and develop Overcomers Outreach meetings island-wide and state-wide. With God's help and your prayers, it will happen!

20

JESUS, MY LEANING POST IN RECOVERY

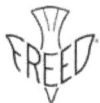

BY PHILIP B.

I was born with a cleft palate that required thirty-five plastic surgeries to repair. The first operation was performed when I was only two days old, the last one when I was sixteen years old. Despite the surgeries, I was left with a speech impediment that profoundly affected my life.

When I started school, my surgeries were scheduled at times when I wouldn't miss any classes, such as summer vacation, spring break, and Christmas. I just couldn't win: holidays meant another trip to the hospital and going to school meant getting chastised for something that wasn't my fault. Blaming God came easy at an early age.

It's not surprising that I started drinking when I was twelve and began using marijuana by the time I was fourteen. It was the only way to deal with pain and rejection. My substance abuse continued to get progressively worse until I was twenty-three, and I took my first step towards recovery by checking myself into a drug and alcohol rehabilitation center for twenty-eight days. There I was first introduced to 12-step programs.

What they had to say sounded fine for those who were too weak to manage their own lives. Staying clean was no problem for me. I just made up my mind to do it and I stayed that way for four years. I didn't need help from anyone. I was my own boss and I could get along just fine by myself.

OVERCOMERS OUTREACH

I had the same attitude about religion. Church was for weaklings. I kept the Ten Commandments; what more could I do? I felt that I was in pretty good standing with the Lord. Why complicate life by going deeper? So I didn't.

I continued to live a drug-free life. It was easy to see the benefits of sobriety. I felt so much better about myself, yet something wasn't quite right. I just couldn't put my finger on what it was.

During this time, my mother was slowly dying of cancer. I lived at home and saw the suffering she went through every day, yet through it all she kept the faith and never stopped praying. One day while we were talking, I got out the family Bible. I handed it to her and she wrote this message, "May you find joy and comfort from this book. Remember your mother's teachings. I know you remember them, please use them. Be good to your father and brother. 'Til we meet again. Love, Mother." I didn't grasp what she was saying at the time, but I was certainly moved. That message was the last thing my mother ever wrote. She died two days later.

My world collapsed that day. My mother, who had been my leaning post for so many years, was gone. I was alone. I knew she had given me the Bible to help me, but I couldn't make heads or tails of it, so I didn't even try.

I began drinking and using drugs again. I got married. I tried everything except the right thing. The following summer I just gave up and attempted suicide. It was then that I realized that I had reached my emotional bottom. I needed help and I couldn't do it by myself.

Three months later, I started attending church again after a fourteen-year absence. I didn't know if it would help, but it sure wouldn't hurt. After about a year in church, talking with friends, I felt like I was getting somewhere, but it was a struggle.

A friend of mine suggested I attend a 12-step program. Although I had attended some years before, I was ready to try again now. The meetings were on Sunday evenings. I thought, *Church in the morning and the 12 Steps at night. Maybe this is what it will take.* When Sunday came, I went to church and I got down on my knees and prayed. It was a simple prayer, but a sincere prayer. I handed my life over to Jesus and asked Him to show me the way.

Fifteen minutes later, my eyes were opened to the Word of God for the very first time. I read Matthew 18:21–35, which is the parable about forgiveness, in which Peter asks Jesus, "Sir, how often should I forgive a

JESUS, MY LEANING POST IN RECOVERY

brother who sins against me? Seven times?" And Jesus says to him, "No! ...Seventy times seven." Jesus then proceeds to share the parable of the master who wants to settle accounts with his servants. One servant, who owed him ten thousand talents, wasn't able to pay. The master forgave him the debt, and yet that same servant shortly thereafter had a fellow servant imprisoned because he could not pay him money he owed him.

After reading that passage, I understood what my mother meant about "joy and comfort from this book." I was saved that morning. I found Jesus. He is the leaning post that I needed and all I had to do was ask.

That very same day I went to a 12-step program, where I told my story. Afterwards someone handed me a typed page with Matthew 18:21–35 on it along with an explanation of the verses about forgiveness. Days just don't get any better than that. I continued to go to the meetings and got a lot out of them. But I was also hungry for Scripture. My church had no Bible study and I was slowly coming to a standstill.

I talked with the person who had given me the paper about my problem. She suggested I attend an Overcomers meeting. It was a 12-step program that also used the Bible. So I went. It was amazing to hear these people talk about the same things that I was going through and using the Bible to get them through it. All this was new to me.

I returned home with my Overcomers handbook and started reading the recommended Bible passages. It was then that I learned that the Bible, and all the wisdom it contained, was at my beck and call. It says it all!

Years ago I used to pick up the Bible and dust it off. Now it doesn't lay flat long enough to gather any dust. I open it up every chance I get. Each day brings a new challenge. Overcomers helps me to meet that challenge with an open mind and an open Bible.

I owe thanks to a lot of people for helping me get where I am today: my mom, who never gave up on me and prayed constantly for me; friends along the way who helped me more than they'll ever know; Overcomers, who made a good thing even better; my friends in the group whom I call on quite often; and most of all, I thank Jesus, because it's through Him that all good things come to pass.

21

SUCH AN ADDICT!

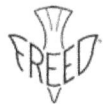

BY JEFF M.

How did this happen? Was I born this way or did I catch this disease along the way? I really don't know and it doesn't matter anyway. What does matter is that it has nothing to do with what a bad person I am, and it helps me to realize that I actually have a disease that cannot be cured, but it can be arrested.

Thanks be to God, today I am in recovery. I have a debt of gratitude to all those who reached out and taught me the way out of my active addiction. I can only try to repay them by sharing my story in the hope that it might help someone else—maybe you!

I am the eldest of three children, and I grew up feeling responsible for the family. My parents divorced when I was nine, and it wasn't long before I had taken over the cooking, babysitting, and cleaning chores to help my mother while she was at work. I began making money at odd jobs and learning to be self-reliant. It was up to me to succeed or fail.

We moved around a lot and I was the "new kid" every year in school until the eighth grade. I always did well in school, as this seemed to please the adults in my life. My childhood wasn't really bad and I didn't go without very much, but I considered myself poor when I compared myself to my friends.

I was forced to attend Sunday school until I was seven, and the actual church service was required attendance on holidays. I came to believe that

God existed but that He was too concerned about important things to have time to care about me. I figured He might be interested in me after I died. I assumed that my time here on earth was entirely in my hands.

By the time I was twelve, I had learned of the pleasant effects of alcohol, as I frequently served as bartender at family gatherings, helping myself to sips of each drink I prepared, just to make sure it was right. I learned to like the taste and particularly enjoyed how it made me feel. It wasn't long before I started showing up at parties or dances with a small container of whiskey so others would realize how cool and grown up I was. I always drank and occasionally shared with others.

Within a year, I had discovered the wonderful world of drugs. Pot, LSD, peyote, mushrooms, and prescription pills were easily acquired and I spent a lot of time finding new blends through experimentation. I became known as a hard partier and graduated from high school as one of the guys who could drink more than anyone else. My identity was established.

Knowing that it was up to me to make it in this world, I kept my grades up through high school so I could get out of town by going to college right after graduation, and so I did. I managed to earn a bachelor's degree in three years by attending a year-round college, graduating as a deck officer in the Merchant Marines at the age of twenty.

I loved going to sea and advanced quickly, but back on shore, I seemed to have a lot of trouble. I got married mainly to establish a life on land, but my heart was at sea. I was most comfortable being a key part of the crew and the operation of the vessel. I was in control and doing something that made me feel very important. Life ashore felt alien, and I sought relief through my good old friends, drugs and alcohol. Cocaine became my very best friend because I found that the combination enabled me to consume more alcohol without showing any effects. Before long, I came to enjoy the effect of cocaine even more than alcohol; however, my wife grew lonely and we divorced within a year. I discovered that the blend of alcohol and cocaine was all I needed in order to feel good. I began to make a lot of money, purchased whatever I pleased, had a great job and lots of friends, and accumulated a nice bank account. I thought I had it made.

Yet one morning, after being up all night as usual, as I watched the garbage collectors coming down the street, I wondered if this was all life was supposed to be. I realized that although I had all the things that were supposed to make me happy, I was not. So I started smoking free base

SUCH AN ADDICT!

cocaine and found a new love. Soon, nothing else mattered and I started cashing in my assets. I went to sea in order to support my habit. As soon as I had enough money saved, I quit the ship and resumed partying. Jobs became scarce, but I didn't care. I still felt in control.

I married again and managed to keep my using a secret from my wife. What a relationship that was. I lost so much weight that she thought I was seriously ill. By the time she discovered that I was using, I had spent over a hundred thousand dollars on drugs. She left me, saying she couldn't handle being with me. So I remarried my first wife who was much more understanding of my ways.

Jobs were hard for me to come by, and it didn't help that I tested positive for cocaine during a pre-employment physical, which ended my seagoing career. Still, as long as I had cocaine, I didn't care. I still felt in control. Good addicts like myself know that when things stop working out, the usual solution is to run away and sell things in order to obtain more drugs. If I ran out of cocaine, there was still alcohol. By that time I had learned how to drink myself into oblivion. That stopped all feelings, but somehow the remorse would not die. It would return full force the very next day.

I divorced again and found a job as a janitor, which paid well enough to keep me in cheap vodka. I had a car and a garage apartment and still felt in control. I started working in a grocery store part time and could soon afford some cocaine again. It was working out for me once again.

Then came that fateful day when I got pulled over in my car just after the cocaine had worn off. I couldn't pass the field sobriety test and was arrested. I found myself in jail, though not for the first time. I spent all the reserve money I had on bail, hired a lawyer, and fought the case, but nevertheless I was found guilty. I managed to lose the job I had as well. I remember thinking that it was such a shame that I'd have to give up driving now, but I could work at a gas station within walking distance, so I still felt in control!

Since I still possessed a vehicle, it wasn't too long before I started driving once in a while without a license. Within a few months I was facing a second DUI charge, along with driving on a suspended license and a few counts of violation of probation. This time, no one would bail me out. I waited a week, detoxing hard and drying out in jail. I lied and arranged bail with the bondsman who had posted bail for my previous arrest. By now I had no family or friends who would even talk to me, and I had lost another job. But I had unemployment benefits and a bicycle, so I still felt in control!

OVERCOMERS OUTREACH

I asked for my sentencing to be postponed so that I could get help and the judge was impressed. I went for a free evaluation at a treatment center where I was told that I might qualify for an outpatient program and that I definitely needed to go to a detox center. I stayed at the center for a little less than forty-eight hours and felt much better, so I left. I drank on the way home and continued to drink non-stop for a week. Toward the end of that week, I was out of money, out of booze, out of cigarettes, and out of friends. I had sold, traded, or pawned everything of value, and my plan to make money recycling bottles wasn't going to work. I had two large garbage cans full of empty bottles, mostly from cheap vodka. I woke up so sick and shaking so much that I could not walk in public, so I spent close to an hour shaking every last drop from each bottle, one at a time, until I had filled two shot glasses. I spilled half of the first one but as the liquor began to steady my hand, I hoisted the second one, saluting the day and toasting my ingenuity. I still felt in control! I managed to get enough money for another day's supply. Life, as it had become, still seemed to be working.

I found myself at the table, telling myself I didn't want to drink anymore, then taking another drink, swearing "no more," then taking yet another drink. Suddenly a thought came crashing in: I'm not in control! I became very scared, more than I ever had been before. I realized that anything would be better than this.

What was I to do? I needed help and right then. So I cried out to a God I didn't know and said, "If You are real, help me, please, God!" Moments later, the phone rang. It was my dad. He said I sounded like I had been drinking and I admitted to it. He told me that he was headed over and would be there soon. He lived hours away, but I was so relieved that my cry for help had been answered that I put the bottle away and went to sleep.

After a rough weekend of detox, Pop took me to the treatment facility and got me into residential treatment. As the alcohol-induced fog began to clear, I started studying the 12 Steps of recovery. It was so apparent that I needed God in my life, but that was not possible with the God whom I thought I understood at that time. The program, as outlined to me, said I must lay aside all my old ideas about God, so when the opportunity to attend church presented itself, I accepted the offer.

I drank real coffee, stole a doughnut, and went to hear some preaching, hoping the church's roof wouldn't fall in on me. The pastor talked of guilt and never stopped looking right at me, or so it seemed. I was sure he saw me steal that doughnut, yet he said I was forgiven for everything I had done through what Jesus had done for me. I left, feeling convicted and

SUCH AN ADDICT!

excited, only to find a Bible had appeared in my room, open to Proverbs. I read all I could and couldn't wait to go back to church.

When that day came I was mortified because I had no decent clothes to wear, so I went in rags. The pastor talked of shame this time and I realized that I was hearing what I most desperately needed. Then he said that if I was ready, all I needed to do was to open my heart and say yes to Jesus! I found myself wanting Him more than I ever wanted anything else in my life, and I said yes right then and there, in the middle of the congregation, among total strangers.

There were no formalities, no special prayers – I just asked Jesus to forgive me and take over my life. Suddenly, a strange but welcome feeling came over me. Somehow, I just knew that everything was going to be all right. God did for me what I could not do for myself. He gave me peace of heart and a sense of security I had always sought but never found until that moment. My journey with Him had begun!

I joined the church and was baptized within two months. I worked the Steps with a sponsor and got into service with both the church and the 12 Step fellowships in my area. Overcomers Outreach served as the bridge between the two for me.

My personal relationship with God continues to grow, and my relationships with others have prospered as well. I have experienced the greatest joy and the deepest hurt in my new life, for it is a new life that God has led me to. I would not change a thing about my path even if I could, for God had me travel that path to become who I am today. I cried out to a God I did not know or understand and He gave me 12 Steps to come to Him.

I'm still such an addict that at times I try to run the show, and that is when life gets hard. My spiritual awakening is simply that God provides everything I need at all times.

During those times in my life when I was using and drinking, I thought I was in control. I could always find an excuse or a way out. Now I have surrendered, He is in control, and I need only to look to Him. I give thanks for what He has given, as well as what He has taken away, but especially for what is left. My time here on earth is now in His hands. When I finally gave up, He took over.

Today I have hope. Today I have faith. Today I have peace. Today I am such a grateful addict!

22

A BIKER FREED FROM BONDAGE

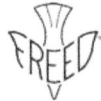

BY JERRY C.

I've been involved with motorcycles most of my life and was a member of a motorcycle club. I'd say that staying loaded all the time and trying to control other people's lives (when I couldn't even run my own) goes pretty much hand-in-hand when living the life of an outlaw on two wheels.

I've spent more time than I care to remember locked up in a prison cell somewhere or another. Since I started doing life on the installment plan at about age thirteen, I've had a lot of time to consider all the wrong and injustice I felt others had done to me and how I was going to get even with the whole world. Yet never once did I think about all the hurt I had caused for everyone I ever loved or cared about. All the suffering I had brought on myself and others might not have happened if I had not been involved in drugs and alcohol.

I don't remember what came first, the drugs or the alcohol. But I'm sure I was hooked from the beginning. Little did I know that I was slowly committing suicide by taking all those substances, but at the time I didn't care. I've been told that most men die of old age before experiencing half of what I've gone through in my thirty-eight years.

I never had much as a kid, so as an adult, when things didn't quite go like I planned while I was trying to work for a living, I'd speed things up a little by taking whatever drug I could get a hold of. Most of the time, I wound up in jail because of this attitude.

I can remember hitchhiking down Pacific Coast Highway in Southern California, while my partner Packy would follow me in his car, looking for someone to sting in a drug or con game. (Packy was later shot and killed by a prison guard during a San Quentin prison incident while we were locked up together in 1976.) After burning someone for several hundred dollars, we would be right back on our regular street corner just twenty minutes later, looking for someone else to con.

I had visions of becoming wealthy by becoming a big drug dealer. It's strange how drugs and alcohol seem to make people like me feel invincible, almost like King Kong! I always thought I was the toughest guy on the face of the earth and I had an irresistible urge to hit people if they dared challenge me. Praise the Lord, He has delivered me from that!

By the time I was twenty-one, I had been jailed too many times to count and had married my first wife. One night after taking Valium all day and closing down the bar near my apartment, a drug deal turned sour. When it was over, I had gunned down two people. A short time later, I was arrested and charged with two counts of first-degree murder. If convicted, I was told I would get the gas chamber. My wife left me.

Once again, God was watching out for me when I couldn't watch out for myself and I didn't even know it. I ended up pleading guilty to a lesser charge a long while later, but was still sent to prison. After being paroled, and with a stronger resentment towards anyone in an authoritative position, my life became more and more consumed with drugs and alcohol. I was in a hole and the only sure way out was death.

In 1982, I found the woman I wanted to spend the rest of my life with. Had this wonderful woman known what was to come about in the next few years, I'm sure she would have run away. Why is it that the ones we love are the ones we always seem to hurt the most? Well, to make a long story short, after all my promises to change and my countless vain attempts to quit drinking, my wife, Donna, decided to take our three children and run for her life.

I slipped further and further into the abyss. For now the reality was all too clear that I had lost everything that was precious to me. I could no longer drink away the pain nor chase it away. I had, as we say, hit my bottom. If God for some reason were to erase all the memories of my past, I would pray He would never let me forget that in the end, no amount of drugs or alcohol would allow me to escape, even for a minute,

A BIKER FREED FROM BONDAGE

the reality at hand. That no longer worked. My friend in the bottle had finally let me down.

I had now become willing to do whatever it took to get sober. For me, however, I knew it would take being in a drug- and alcohol-free environment. My thought was that I needed an easier, softer way out of my addiction. Boy, was I in for a big surprise!

I had searched everywhere and had come up empty. And then after realizing I had no place else to turn, I remembered my sister-in-law had given me a book she had gotten from her church. Searching my car, I found a *FREED* booklet lying on the floorboard in the back seat. On the front was a phone number, so I decided to give it a try. When I dialed the number, a sense of fear came over me. Perhaps I somehow knew that I was finally going to find help, or perhaps the addicted part of my personality knew it would soon lose its crutch and was fearful. The phone rang a couple times and then a man on the other end with a warm friendly voice said, "Overcomers Outreach; this is Bob. Can I help you?"

That phone call was to be the turning point for the rest of my life. Bob listened to all I had to say and then he gave me the number of a local OO group leader, which I called right away. In a short time, two members of OO had me in a car on the way to the local detox. While there, they took my vital signs and made me blow into a breath analyzer. Everyone got very excited when they found out I was .40 (four times the legal limit in most states). I sensed I was about to make a quick trip back to jail, so I made a quick exit instead.

I awoke the next morning in the wet ivy of a neighbor's yard, sick as ever. I wandered home, took up a loaded gun, and promised to use it on myself before I would take another drink. As I sat contemplating shooting myself, a strange thought came over me. If there was truly a God, He must be in a church somewhere and He must certainly have more power than me. So I went looking for a church. I was going to have my war with God and He was either going to change my life forever or strike me dead with lightning.

I had always heard the doors of a church are always kept open. I never stopped to think they had to be locked to protect the church from being robbed by people like me. After trying to get in a church building for a while, I gave up and left, only to return later. Then I was greeted by a man named George.

George was the pastor at the church and he was a couple of years younger than I was. He made me feel quite comfortable and welcome. He allowed me to come into his church, and after not knowing what to say, he began to tell me the story of Jesus and how He had died on the cross for me. It may sound funny, but I think God had taken over George's body and He Himself was sitting there talking directly to me. For the first time in my life, I knew God was real. George got on his knees with me and prayed as I asked Jesus to come into my life. One of the Scriptures George shared with me was 2 Corinthians 5:17 "When someone becomes a Christian he becomes a brand new person inside. He is not the same anymore. A new life has begun." That sure happened to me.

That day, I entered a detox house. It turned out that I entered a thirty-seven-day recovery program. This place was literally the last house at the end of the road for me. As I began to see God's gracious love pouring out of all the people around me, my desire to become sober was overwhelming. Every day became a new experience for me as I learned more and more about myself. As I was taught how to apply the 12-step program to my life, life itself began to take on a whole new perspective.

I was told I only had to change one thing about myself and that one thing was everything. Well, everything as I know it has changed through the fellowship we share at OO. I'm learning to deal with life on God's terms, not always on Jerry's.

Having the 12 Steps of our program broken down into related Bible verses has allowed me to clearly see God's will for me. What a blessing to have fellow Christian addicts all seeking God's guidance together! To this day, the suggested topics in the *FREED* booklet restore my serenity when I begin to slip back into my old self. Most of all, OO has allowed me to know myself as I really am, and to live a sober, productive life one day at a time, by turning to God, instead of to myself, with my problems.

Praise God for the program of Overcomers Outreach and for the miracles it has produced in my life!

23

OUR SON'S ADDICTION LED TO OUR RECOVERY

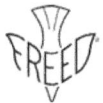

BY PAT M.

Our family seemed to be typical for a Southern California family. We lived in a modest home in the suburbs. We enjoyed our membership in a large, well-established church. We spent weekends together around the house or taking a trip to the desert for camping and off-road vehicle fun. I was active in church helping with outreach ministries, attending weekly Bible studies, and was a Lay Renewal Team member for a number of years. Our son attended a private Christian school and I was very involved with his school activities from preschool years through the ninth grade. We felt assured that he was in a safe place and was receiving the best education possible. Our son's life outside school was balanced out with Little League baseball, Pop Warner football, and Boy Scouts, all of which we participated in as a family. Little did we know that a nightmare was about to begin.

One evening, during a scout awards banquet, our son was to receive special recognition; however, he did not appear. To our surprise, we found him behind the facility, drunk on the wine that the adults were serving for dinner. We were embarrassed, hurt, confused, and angry.

This was one of the first episodes of many that we as parents were split on how to handle. I felt he should be confronted or punished, and my husband felt that the inevitable hangover would be lesson enough. As time went on, this disagreement on how to handle situations became more intense. It wasn't long until our son was caught with liquor in his locker at school. He was immediately suspended for three days. Our first impulse was to go to school and defend him, not realizing at the time that we were losing control of our son and his behavior had extended beyond the experimentation stage. The school did not want him to return. I assured the administration that his assignments would be completed at home. As it turned out, I managed to graduate the ninth grade for the second time, along with my son.

Things on the home front didn't look much better than school. My husband, who had used alcohol and drugs for ten years, assured me that his first-hand experience with such situations would keep them under control. He spent hours lecturing, intellectualizing, and minimizing our son's behavior, both to myself and our son. At the same time, I was yelling, crying, and feeling more desperate on a daily basis.

My husband and I spent hours agonizing and arguing over our son's behavior. We had in-depth, heart-to-heart family discussions about our concerns and fears and within hours we were right back where we started. Our turning point came one night when we returned home unexpectedly and found our son and a friend smoking pot in his bedroom. When we came towards his room, he and his friend jumped out the window and ran away. We were left with the cold hard reality that things were getting progressively worse and nothing we were doing was making the slightest difference. My husband and I stayed up all night trying to come up with some answers and wondered what would happen next.

We finally determined that somehow we had to get some outside help. The next day I made an appointment with our pastor for some guidance and insight, hoping he would have some easy answers for our family situation. Much to my surprise, not only did he not have the answers, but he very clearly stated, "I would like for you, your son, and your problem to leave this church." Needless to say, I was in shock. I felt rejected, confused, and terribly angry.

After discussing this episode with my husband, who was in a state of utter disbelief, we agreed that we must find help somewhere else. He went to the Yellow Pages and found our first link with recovery. We located a counseling center fifteen miles from our home and took our son in for an appointment the very next day. To our surprise, what we found there were other families experiencing similar situations. No one judged or condemned us for not being the perfect family. It was so healing to be

OUR SON'S ADDICTION LED TO OUR RECOVERY

able to discuss our crisis on a day-to-day basis and to share how we were sorrowful and frightened that our son was slipping away.

Each time we met with other families at the center, we found ourselves becoming a little stronger and clearer concerning the destructive power of the disease of addiction. My husband and I were beginning to see some relief in our struggles and arguments over our son's behavior. We began to understand that we truly were powerless over his behavior. Up until this point, we had wrongly assumed that there must be something we could do to fix or change him. It soon became clear that we had plenty of our own personal issues to deal with, besides our son's. Thank God we became willing to do that.

After two months of consistent attendance at individual and family counseling with weekly support groups, our son was admitted to an inpatient chemical dependency treatment center. We were encouraged that he would have ongoing professional help, learn how to work AA's 12 Steps, and gain information on how the family would fit into his recovery.

During this time, my husband and I attended the Palmer Drug Abuse Program as well as meetings at the treatment center in order to maximize our recovery. As we shared with other families, got sponsors, and started working our own 12-step programs, we were beginning to feel less stress and confusion, and we were learning how to set some healthy boundaries for ourselves. We were no longer blaming ourselves or each other; we started working on mending our marriage relationship. For the first time in what seemed like an eternity, we began to be united in dealing with our son. The greatest challenge for me was realizing that the son we had raised hadn't turned out to be the person I thought he was, and this was difficult to accept.

Prior to our son's discharge from the treatment center, we sat down as a family with the counselor and wrote up a contract (a written agreement covering family members' behavior) that we could all live with. As parents we felt better equipped and stronger than ever. Our hope was that we would be a family in recovery and return to some sense of sanity. We were never under the illusion that the inpatient treatment program was a magical cure-all; like all sick families, we had plenty to work on.

The first few days reunited as a family were a bit awkward. Following his three-month absence, it was a major adjustment for us to have our son back home again. He gave us the impression that he was willing to go along with our expectations and guidelines, and we were so relieved.

Yet I was terrified just one week later to find a gun under his mattress! I immediately called one of the counselors at the treatment center who advised me to call the police. Within minutes, they appeared at the house. My husband rushed home from work and we all waited for our son's return. Upon his arrival, the police questioned him about the gun. At first he vehemently denied it, but finally admitted that he had found it in our shed where some belongings were being stored for a friend.

After this encounter, we as a family decided to revise our contract. We felt it was time to set limits like never before, so we told our son that if he could not live by the contract, he would have to find somewhere else to stay. It was at that moment that our strong-willed son decided to pack up and leave! Wow! What a blow that was to me. I was under the illusion that he would have done anything to stay. Without the Serenity Prayer, our 12-step support group, our phone list, and the Lord, we would have lost our sanity in the days that followed.

We just couldn't figure out why our family was going through this nightmare. We still did not have a new place to worship because the pain of being turned away from our church was still too devastatingly fresh in our minds. Even so, we always knew the Lord was there for us. At that time, there was no such thing as Christian 12-step support groups or any Christian recovery that we knew of.

Weeks and months went by and the only thing we received from our son was an occasional nasty phone call. He would blame us and attempt to make us feel guilty for all the things he was experiencing. It was obvious to us when we talked to him that he was doing some kind of drugs, and though this worried me, I didn't want to know too much. It was so very hard not to say, "Come home and everything will be OK." Instead, as advised by other parents who had gone through similar experiences, we told him to call his counselor and the treatment center and go to the meetings at the Palmer Drug Abuse Program. Even though we loved our son as much as we ever had, we could not let him live in our home while he was destroying himself with drugs and alcohol.

We were confident that more prayers were needed so I took a huge risk and told a dear friend about our deep, dark family secret. For the first time, we found unconditional Christian love. She and her husband committed our son to daily prayer and then eventually, with our permission, they had him put on the prayer chain for the entire church. That little church in Roy, Utah, still prays for our son today! It was so healing

OUR SON'S ADDICTION LED TO OUR RECOVERY

to share with fellow Christians about our pain and have no judgment or condemnation.

Our son's drug use escalated to the point where he began to have minor run-ins with the law. It wasn't long before he found himself in juvenile hall, and then on to a county probation camp. Our visits to camp were traumatic. I had a hard time seeing our son in a locked facility. Our discussions seemed to focus on the need for all of us to be in recovery, not just Mom and Dad. There were times when he said all the right things and we felt hopeful and optimistic; on other visits he was so disrespectful that we chose to terminate the visit rather than subject ourselves to the verbal abuse and finger-pointing.

We continued to work on our issues of guilt and shame, beginning to realize that we were not the failures we had once thought. Our marriage relationship was becoming stronger and more unified than ever. When we had to deal with our son's addictive behavior, we were able to set loving boundaries. Our enabling dysfunctional behavior became a thing of the past. At one point, our son referred to us as "black belt Al-Anons." That remark showed us beyond a shadow of a doubt that we were giving out a different message than before—the right one!

It has never been easy, walking this new road of tough love. There have been times when we have doubted and questioned our choices and decisions but held onto each other, always seeking the Lord's guidance. We discovered early on in our recovery that God's Word and the 12 Steps were totally compatible. We had no problem attending secular meetings as Christians. We realized that we were there to share experience, strength, and hope, not attend a church service. No one ever attempted to regulate whom we chose as our "Higher Power." We were always respectful of others, never passing judgment on their relationship with God.

We began praying each night, asking the Lord to show us a way we could help other Christian families like ours. We knew the pain and rejection we experienced from the church was not of the Lord. We were convinced that God was interested in healing and restoration, not condemnation.

By this time, we had sold our house and were ready to move to another area. Our son was in jail and expressed a desire to go once again to a treatment program. We were elated! By the grace of God, it was on the exact day of our escrow closing that all was approved, which meant we had the money to pay for his treatment program. He was now eighteen and it would be the last time we would be in a position to pay for that type of treatment.

After four months at the treatment program, we were overjoyed to see him clean and sober. Soon, he left the program to live with his sponsor. It seemed like we had our son back again. He would come around every weekend, help with projects, and of course he would give me all the hugs and kisses I had missed so much. He even had his sense of humor back. Then, for some unknown reason, our son convinced himself that he could use drugs socially. How saddened we were to immediately see the changes when he got back into the disease.

During this same period we had found a new home church. Our approach was extremely cautious at first, but the warmth and acceptance of the new church family was comforting. We approached the pastor and expressed an interest in starting a 12-step program for Christians in the community. We were still not aware that there were any such groups out there. He was hesitant to embrace the idea and never really gave a reason why. This caused me to want to leave many times, but we never seemed to be released by the Lord to do so.

Finally, about a year later, we had a special speaker come to our evening service. It was not normal for our pastor to bring in someone to share the kind of testimony we were about to hear. A gentleman by the name of Ed C. told his story of cocaine addiction and his recovery through the Lord and a 12-step Christian group called Overcomers Outreach. I almost jumped out of the pew! It appeared to be exactly what we were looking for. My husband nudged me and said, "This is an answer to prayer!"

After the service, we couldn't wait to speak with Ed C. and his wife. They invited us to their meeting so we could see this group in action. Two nights later we attended our first Overcomers meeting seventy-five miles from home. They gave us a handful of literature, a word of encouragement, and told us they would keep us in their prayers. The next week the pastor, who had been so hesitant about starting a group of this kind, resigned. This too seemed to confirm God was in control and we were where He wanted us to be. We took the information to the assistant pastor and he gave us approval to start a group immediately. We contacted the Overcomers Outreach main office and ordered a variety of literature for our first meeting. We knew other Christians who were working a 12-step program, and began to share this new concept with

OUR SON'S ADDICTION LED TO OUR RECOVERY

them. There was no doubt this was the vehicle God wanted us to use to help other hurting Christian families.

Our first meeting was attended by three of our friends. It was very refreshing for the five of us to be working our 12-step program and acknowledging Jesus Christ as our "Higher Power." As the weeks went by, the room began to fill with others. We quickly realized that it was not the people of our own church who would attend, but those from many other churches in our area. I went to several Christian counseling centers to inform them of this new group in our area and how it might help their clients who were in counseling and needed a support group. They were very receptive and our group started growing on a weekly basis.

As time went on, it became more apparent that there were many who wanted this type of support group. God is sending many people through our doors. We have seen real miracles take place in numerous lives. We find that when people have a safe place to share their hurts and pain, God is present and actively healing. Today, we still see God's hand in this ministry.

My burden all along has been to help Christians make connections with resources and agencies to bridge the gap from pain and suffering to healing and wholeness. When we were at our lowest point twenty years ago, there was no Christian network of support that we could find. We eventually gathered together the core of Christian resources from our area and put on a one-day conference that has become an annual event.

Looking back over the past few years, our family has experienced so much. Our son has had his ups and downs with his addiction and has not yet fully embraced the 12-step program. He is currently incarcerated due to the progression of his disease.

God has used all of this in ways that at times we can't understand. We continue on a daily basis to turn our lives and our wills over to the care of God, knowing that He loves us and has a plan for each of our lives. We are grateful to Bob and Pauline for having the vision for this ministry because we are convinced God is using it to help thousands more just like us.

24

NEW LIFE WITHOUT ALCOHOL

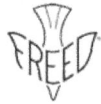

BY VERN A.

I was raised on a farm in North Dakota. I have one younger brother and two older sisters. My mom and dad were strict Christians. They did not believe in drinking, smoking, or swearing. We knew nothing about drugs and did not cheat, lie, or steal. If we did, we got hit either with a hand or a stick. None of my family or relatives drank.

My father wanted nothing to do with any of us kids.

It was very hard work on the farm. We had a thousand or more cattle, about fifteen horses, and also dogs, cats, ducks, pigs, and sheep. We had a very large garden where we worked early in the morning. After we came home from school, my brother, sisters, and I fed and cared for the animals. The farm was not profitable so we never had much money to spend. We farmed more than three thousand acres of non-cash hay crop for feed.

I was introduced to drinking at high school parties, dances, and sports games, and looking back I know that was when alcohol was beginning to be a problem. After high school, I got a classmate pregnant while I was in a blackout. I didn't think the child was mine because the young lady dated other guys, so I denied it until the baby was born. Then I took a blood test, which came out negative, so the case was dropped by the welfare support system. But when Angela was about eight years old, she began writing and calling me her dad and we have continued to correspond for many years like father and daughter.

I married in North Dakota at age twenty-seven and moved to Orange County, California. I finished school and worked in a factory for thirty-five years. My wife could not have children so we adopted a baby girl. I was drinking excessively then. As the years went by my drinking got worse. I was drinking every night when I came home from work and I just couldn't stop. I had many hiding places for my booze so I never ran out. My wife filed for divorce in 1986. My daughter was thirteen when they moved back to North Dakota. It was devastating to lose my family and marriage after twenty years.

Later I met a lady at church. We dated for a year and a half and then married in Las Vegas. This was a horrible mistake because she was also an alcoholic and we were drinking together. She actually dared me to get married. We were so drunk we were barely able to sign our marriage license. When we got to the Little White Chapel, we were dressed in Levi's®, T-shirts, and tennis shoes. We had pizza, beer, and dirt all over ourselves and the other people there avoided us like we were skunks. After the ceremony, the pastor asked if we wanted a video of the occasion and my new wife replied, "Oh, yes!" A marriage not made in heaven, that's for sure. We hung onto each other to keep from falling down drunk. We pretty much came home in a blackout.

Late one night on the way home from dinner, dancing, and drinking, I almost hit a pedestrian. I was covering one eye to see the marks in the road, and the next thing I knew I was home in my recliner. I woke up about five A.M. and remembered almost hitting the pedestrian. I wondered who would take care of my mother if I had hit and killed him and ended up in prison.

By that time I was convinced that I could never stop drinking because I had gone to AA for ten years with no success. I went through the 12 Steps about ten times, and still didn't get it. I finally completely surrendered and asked God to forgive me of all my shortcomings, and if it be His will, to take away the desire to drink. Just like that, I felt a warm tingling feeling go from the top of my head to the bottom of my toes. I said, "Wow! What was that?" God took away the desire to drink that morning, August 15, 1997, and I have not had any desire to drink since. That is a miracle!

I finally retired and got a divorce. Now I have time to work the program by helping others, participating in meetings, and volunteering.

NEW LIFE WITHOUT ALCOHOL

My mother developed Alzheimer's and moved into my home. I helped her until she passed away. It was an honor and pleasure for me to care for her. I was able to sit by her bed and be with her sober when she died and I am so thankful for that.

My life is not that great living alone with no family or relatives, but I have AA for my family. Today, for me to drink is to die! I am forever grateful for AA for sparing my life so I can reach out to others with a message of hope for people like me.

I am also blessed to have Overcomers Outreach for my family. I have been part of a group in Whittier, California. What a joy to know my higher power is Jesus Christ! With the benefit of both AA and OO, I can be happy, joyous, and free both in this life and the next!

ONLY BY HIS GRACE—ONLY FOR HIS GLORY

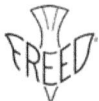

BY ROLF P., GERMANY

If anyone would have said in my best drinking time that one day I would enjoy my life without a drop of excellent beer or delicious wine, that I would regularly go to meetings with "dysfunctional people" and even join a fellowship of Christians praying for others, I would have called that person the greatest fool on earth. Even more amazing, finding myself working for God's purpose and not for my very own personal goals made me see that I was the one who had been a fool.

My alcoholic existence had dominated and nearly destroyed me until I turned my life over to God. Approaching my tenth anniversary of sobriety, I am now allowed to surrender every morning to do His will, fulfill His purpose, and enjoy the tasks He devises especially for me.

I remember well that crucial day when I was sitting shaking and sweating from the last cold withdrawal, receiving the gift of grace over the phone by listening to the message of recovery from Alcoholics Anonymous. I was at the end of my human strength and could surrender for the very first time. I had no power over alcohol and was lost. An AA friend related his story of alcohol abuse and how he found his solution over the darkness of mind and heart. At that moment I discovered the first flash of hope.

When I look back on my life today I know it didn't begin with drinking or other abuse. It's simply a biography of lack of self-esteem (having no God-given self-worth), as well as insufficiency of love for neither myself nor others. I experienced true loneliness because of feeling very special in some different life-pattern, which I did not want to accept at any price. This all caused unfulfilled human relationships and sexual problems, which are a dominant but hidden part of our disease.

My first beer tasted bitter, but later on the beer could not be bitter enough. However, it ended up bringing much bitterness into my life. I felt I didn't really fit into my family or society. They were all cooperative, friendly, and busy people, but I did not have the power to be strong in many situations of life. I seemed to live in another world surrounded by a big wall. My love of movies gave me an escape and refuge for some time. It was difficult for me to speak to people because I felt that they were very superior and I didn't feel good enough.

My brother was six years older than I. He was the big brother I looked up to and admired. I envied his lifestyle: his working, drinking, smoking, joyful partying, sex relations with beautiful girls, etc. When I compared myself to him, I felt unworthy in my own eyes, so I tried to be good in school and in my professional life. I gave it my best shot, but working totally alone is a heavy job when one is facing school or professional challenges. I had an insane and broken relationship with myself; I could not accept or love me! I had no connection with other people and especially with God, although today I know that He protected and saved me from falling into much deeper trouble.

This mental, social, and spiritual disorder consumed me more and more with cravings, turning me into a helpless monster, totally hurt and broken in mind, heart, and soul on the inside, but covered by an outward disguise of dishonesty, denial, arrogance, pride, and selfishness.

As a teenager, I began to discover that all these problems and situations could be coped with and endured with a drink of alcohol. My ability to drink a good portion made me feel grown up. I felt like a real man who could deal with hard life and heavy problems. Drinking made me feel superior to others who could not stand the quantity of stuff I was facing, so I figured I could easily beat those weaklings.

On the other hand, I was trained to really love the alcohol. I could not list all the many fine brands of beer, wine, and liquor I fell in love with. Alcohol became my precious releaser and best companion in daily life. Without knowing it, I was taken over completely. I did not know when I crossed that magic invisible line, losing control over the stuff. I do know that when my father got suddenly ill of cancer and died rapidly, I really

ONLY BY HIS GRACE—ONLY FOR HIS GLORY

lost it completely and began to drown in the alcoholic sea. My life was filled with fear, resentment, anger, hate, bitterness, and, yes, alcohol!

What were the consequences of my love affair with alcohol? I experienced many cold withdrawals in my bed and two urgent surgeries in the hospital because of a bleeding stomach and esophageal varices with 60 percent lethality. Uncountable failures and big problems in all affairs of my life continued for a very long period. My life seemed to have no sense and value anymore and all seemed to be lost. I unconsciously felt the end was near. Worry of losing my life gripped me.

Then I swore to myself, my life's partner, and surely to God, that I would try AA the next time if I failed to stop on my own. I could not imagine that I would have no control about my drinking behavior because I never wanted to drink so much; I just never could stop in time. After some months of self-imagined controlled drinking, I fell in the trap of surrender to it. After falling unwillingly into a six-day binge, I tried with all my forces and knowledge that I had gained over twenty-five years of drinking to overcome the situation, but failed totally. Three days of lonely withdrawal with all the horrible cold and hot roller coasting in total body, mind, soul, and spirit finally brought me to total surrender.

I went to an AA meeting. A friend brought me home, where I had my first open and honest sharing with a member of AA. I was reading the book of AA, crying for joy about the message of hope while still sweating and freezing. The first days on "pink cloud #7" had me living consciously without one drop of alcohol and wandering blissfully through the fresh air.

Amazing grace! Then my AA really began. I was interested in all the people I met and the many books, workshops, and meetings they offered. I had less shame and guilt. My body recovered and the broken relationship in my family and business got better day-by-day. The outward circumstances changed rapidly for good. I received an offer to join a big business project with my brother, fulfilling all the wishes I had my whole life. Security, good income, retirement—all seemed to be realized. Security at last! This was my goal in life, more than I ever dreamed of. And all this was happening to me after just two years of sobriety!

But this was not God's will for me. I knew my brother was ill but the cancer killed him within a few months and all the dreams I had were blowing in the wind. I had to start over and to search again, but this time, I had God working in me. I attended more AA assemblies, more journeys, and more seminars where I was led to the AA Grapevine. I also began corresponding by e-mail with some AA friends from the USA, Australia, and England who had found the "God of their understanding," Jesus Christ. This fervent search for God kept me sober, living, and growing up until today. Then I was led to my special sponsor, friend, and brother in Christ. I was amazed that there was such a total agreement and love within our mutual lives with the same heart beat. On Christmas 1996 he sent me a little Christian booklet that influenced my real spiritual awakening because this resulted in my obsessive hunger for God's healing. I began earnestly to read the Holy Bible the first time in my life, and with His help, I began to understand what it offers for my own life each day.

There are some crucial cornerstones I have to share in my trudging the road of happy destiny. I began to search and attend church services to look for a Christian community to join. I also started attending a special 12-Step/Big Book Group in AA, and began studying the program of Overcomers Outreach, which an English friend passed on to me. I decided one day not to wait for the actions of others but to translate the material by myself, so I started an OO group in our church. Feeling the need and His will for being bound together by Jesus Christ, my partner and I married in His Name in June 1999 and were baptized by our pastor. We began reaching out the OO ministry to other congregations, helping establishing a national 12-Step-network that is now spreading the message of freedom and peace by cyberspace to initiate real Christ-12-Step groups in Germany. We searched earnestly to become members of a real Christian community where we could be placed by God to fulfill His plan and serve His purpose for those broken people who might be marginalized even now in a church society.

My wife and I are both pulling at the same end of the rope; what a blessing. We try to trust, obey, and love our God with all our hearts, minds, and souls, and He promised us the best is yet to come! We take nothing for granted, but pray to be humble and grateful to our Saviour and Lord, Jesus Christ, for all the gifts He bestows to us today.

I have said "good-bye" to my old life, realizing that it was necessary with all its hurts, pain, and damage to bring me to my knees to surrender to God. I now know He has a plan for me, a plan for good and not for evil, to bring a new hope and future when I am searching earnestly, one day at a time.

Today I can accept and love myself, just like God has created me. My alcoholic handicap is a price and pledge for His salvation. He is pottering my different shape of body, mind, and soul, miraculously using my many

ONLY BY HIS GRACE—ONLY FOR HIS GLORY

defects to shape me into what He wants me to be. He and I are working on all this together by His Spirit. The greatest miracle of life is that God loves me just as I am. It took me a great part of my life to understand and trust His amazing grace and divine love with my heart, because my mind will never be able to grasp His abundant gifts.

I am a new creature in Christ!

26

ANTICS OF AN ESCAPE ARTIST

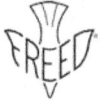

BY PEGGY M.

Once upon a time, on a warm Indian summer evening, a young twenty-year-old maiden undertook a brisk swim in the Pacific Ocean, escaping from Terminal Island Federal Prison in California. In doing so, she acquired a two-year sentence with a five-year special parole. After only a few months of freedom, she violated her parole and had to do another two years. This young maiden was me.

I was not even sentenced yet when I escaped. I had been sent to Terminal Island for a ninety-day observation to see if I was prison material. Well, I guess I showed them!

Running away from my problems always seemed to be my best answer. I ran away from home a few times until I was sent to reform school. That is where I learned about LSD. But it wasn't until I ran away to California that I actually experienced it and marijuana for myself.

The second time I was sent to reform school I walked away for good. I stayed away until I was eighteen years old. During that time I met Jack. The two of us hippies did a lot of partying on hallucinogens and pot.

When I became pregnant and lost the baby to a miscarriage, I started to take life a little more seriously. I went to my parents for help and even tried looking for a job. My relationship with my mother and father had changed for the better. They didn't even report me to the police for being a runaway.

OVERCOMERS OUTREACH

For a short while Jack and I went to live in Denver where his family lived. It was there that I got pregnant with my son. We were still using drugs, but now we were working and mostly using on the weekends.

After our son was four months old we moved back to my parents' home in Tucson. Jack failed to get a job and my parents kicked him out. Even though I kept going out at night to party, I was going through training at the Veteran's Hospital in Tucson to become a medical lab technician.

I met my husband while working as an orderly. He was fresh back from the Vietnam War and introduced me to a heroin habit. Since I had become proficient with needles while working in the lab, it was easy for me to get hooked right along with him.

During my first year of using heroin, we were busted for dealing. My ex went to prison and I got probation, although I had to go to a six-week in-house drug program at a hospital. That is where I was first introduced to 12-step meetings. Although I kept quiet in the meetings and in the group counseling, I managed to leave there with some seeds of hope planted.

Yet later on I was arrested at the US/Mexico border with heroin and was sent to a drug program in Phoenix. Being the rabbit that I am, I decided to take a short break and to go get high with a fellow addict. When we came back to the program, we were sent back to jail again.

However, God had a plan. It was during my second two-year incarceration that I accepted Jesus into my heart. Somehow, I managed to stay clean and sober long enough to earn a furlough home. But it just happened to be the Bicentennial fourth of July in 1976.

Unfortunately, my plans to party had already been set. A friend who picked me up at the prison had a cooler of beer, vodka, and some joints to smoke. We had not even left the parking lot when I started my Fourth of July celebration. He took me to the airport, and when I arrived in Tucson, my other friend met me with some heroin balloons. I fixed one and went home to eat dinner with my family. My face nodded toward the spaghetti on the plate and I woke up in time to excuse myself and go to bed.

The next morning I went to the bathroom to take a shower, but decided to have one more fix. I ended up overdosing and fell against the door. My mother, who was in a wheelchair at the time, could not get the door open so she called the police. I was arrested one more time for possession of heroin. I figured this was surely the end of the line.

ANTICS OF AN ESCAPE ARTIST

While in the county jail, a lawyer told me about a drug program. The one thing different was it was centered on God. Up until that point, I had tried drug programs, hospitals, jail, and prison, and none of those had helped.

I went back to my cell and decided to give God a try. Immersing myself in the Bible for the first time, I actually began to understand portions of it, and the lights came on. I thought, *There might be hope after all!*

Since I was not finished with my federal time, the State of Arizona ran my time concurrent with the feds. The new me arrived back at Terminal Island saying "hello" cheerfully to everyone, even to some of the correctional officers I had displayed an attitude toward before I left. They seemed quite surprised.

But Satan was mad and knew I was vulnerable, being new to the things of God. I found a meeting that was called Addicts for Christ. I went all fired up, to tell everyone that what was being said about God was really the truth. These girls had only known me as a trouble-making drug addict. Little by little Satan kept trying to convince me with thoughts like *They'll never believe you. You'll just make a fool of yourself. Anyway, are you sure this stuff is real?* I ended up not saying a word, and felt so bad about it that I went back to my old ways.

At this point, I vowed not to use heroin anymore and would just stick with marijuana. I promptly got busted on the yard with a joint in my pocket. As I was in the process of being shipped to a maximum security prison in Kentucky, God had me stopped at the federal jail in San Diego. It was there that a friend showed me how to pray in a group with others and asked if I wanted someone in the jail ministry to come visit me. It was with him that I truly learned about salvation and said the sinner's prayer. Now I belonged to God, and Satan was really angry.

I paroled to San Diego and went to Calvary Chapel. Not a lot of people there understood my drug addiction. Unbelievably, I fell back to my old ways once more. After ten years of heroin, I started using cocaine and crystal meth. The next fifteen years were literal hell. I was arrested for residential burglary just around the time when the three-strikes law went into effect. This arrest became my first strike. I went to CRC prison, which was a drug program prison.

I went back a few times on violations, but each time I grew a little stronger in my walk with the Lord and lasted clean a little longer. I was so proud of staying clean for twenty-four hours. The next time I went to

OVERCOMERS OUTREACH

Victory Outreach and lasted three weeks. Later I stayed out a year and a half. I went to church, school, and 12-step meetings.

Even so, I fell again. It was crack cocaine this time, added to my heroin use. Crack took me down faster than any drug ever had. I was arrested for commercial burglary when I was trying to steal four cartons of cigarettes. Strike two. However, this time I knew better.

I had known God and walked away from Him. I didn't deserve to ask for His help. My sentence could have carried six years and would have been double because I didn't show up for my court date. I just told God I would not complain about whatever time He allowed. I only wanted one thing: that God would walk through it with me. I was given two years, and was allowed to go to fire camp instead of prison.

Unbelievably, even this was not my last downfall. When I got out of prison, I had a hard time finding work, a place to stay, and help. I just gave up. Yet a summer spent on the streets, where I was actually homeless, shocked me back to my senses.

I ended up in a Christian rehab for two years, and then I moved out on my own. I was attending church and working, but I had a burning desire to share the news that Jesus is real and He can help drug addicts.

Today, I enjoy a restored relationship with my son who had been adopted by my sister. He has two handsome sons and a beautiful wife. God restores our relationship with Him and with our families if we just let Him.

By God's grace, I have now been clean for nine years! And how blessed I am to facilitate an Overcomers Outreach meeting at my church! I also regularly attend NA (Narcotics Anonymous) and AA.

In spite of my life's many detours, God was working on this escape artist all through those agonizing years. Thankfully, I could never escape Him!

27

FREEDOM FROM FEAR

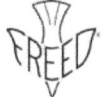

BY AL A.

Fear was my biggest bugaboo in the years before college. I was an extremely bashful, self-conscious, nervous, insecure, and fearful person with strong feelings of inferiority. Change and new experiences bothered me tremendously. I was a compulsive worrier, which led to deep depressions. I had been raised by solid, Christian, church-going parents who loved my two younger sisters and me. My parents raised us the best they knew how.

I didn't drink during high school, believing what my mother had taught me, that it was wrong and sinful. The only extracurricular activities I participated in were band and orchestra. There were other activities that interested me, but because of my fears, I would not get involved.

In college, at the age of nineteen, I had my first drink. I felt like I was doing wrong in having that first glass of wine, but I figured that I would try it just this once. I liked everything about it, the way it tasted, and certainly the way it made me feel. I soon began drinking wine and other alcoholic drinks on a regular basis. Alcohol became very important to me. I still felt that drinking was probably wrong, but because of what it did for me, I didn't care.

College was a completely different experience for me because alcohol enabled me to become a participant in life. I was very active in student affairs. I became very popular, joined a fraternity, and held class and fraternity offices. Drinking seemed to wipe away my worries, fears, and bashfulness. I lived for parties. I had found the answer to living, or so it seemed, and that answer was alcohol. The only problem was that I couldn't always be under the influence, and when I wasn't, all my fears came back.

My dad was the owner of a retail shoe store in Bakersfield, California, and I was invited to join the family business after I graduated from college. My dad did not pressure me, but because of my many fears and my tendency to follow the easy road, I convinced myself to go into the retail shoe business with him. A few years later, I took over the business.

Meanwhile, I married my beautiful wife, Joyce, and we enjoyed a very active social life, all of which centered on alcohol. Even after we had our two daughters, my drinking and alcoholism progressed rapidly.

We pursued an opportunity to open a larger shoe store in Garden Grove, California, closed our Bakersfield business, and moved to Orange County. This was the geographic my wife and I thought would be good for us. We could make a lot more money, I could moderate my drinking, and things would hopefully change. After the move, things did change—they got much worse. My drinking and alcoholism led the way. The shoe business, my relationship with my wife, and life in general were terrible. The only good thing that happened at that time was our son, Joe, was born.

One morning my dad drove from Bakersfield and met me at the Garden Grove shoe store to discuss business matters. He had a lot of money invested in the business. As usual, I had had too much to drink the previous night, so I was hungover and feeling pretty bad at the time of our meeting. After discussing business matters, the subject led to what I knew it would—my drinking. Before getting too far into the topic, I told my dad that I had come to a decision to stop drinking and that I would never have another drink for the rest of my life. I had made many promises concerning my drinking, mainly to my wife; I would say whatever was necessary to get out of trouble with her. I promised her I'd moderate my drinking, quit hiding bottles, and quit sneaking drinks, among other things. Some of those promises I intended to keep, but most of them I didn't. However, that morning I gave my dad my solemn oath and I fully intended to keep it, so I went on the wagon.

As I look back, the blackest part of my life was the period I spent sober after that promise to my dad. I had a wife, a family, a business, and many, many responsibilities. Alcohol had quit working and now I was dry. My past fears, worries, depression, and feelings of inferiority came flooding back. I didn't have God in my life because I had rejected my childhood teachings. I had no answers and nowhere to go.

My wife had begun going to an Al-Anon meeting in Garden Grove. I had heard of Alcoholics Anonymous, but had never heard of Al-Anon Family Groups. She told me a little bit about the program and that she was not attending the meetings for me, but rather to find help for herself. I didn't tell her, but I thought this was a good idea, since she certainly needed help.

During this dry, miserable time in my life, I sought the counsel of a minister of a church in Garden Grove. I told him of the promise I had made to my dad and how I intended to stick with it. He then asked me an interesting question: "How would you drink, if you could drink the way you wanted?" I gave him an answer that I thought he would agree with, having to do with moderate social drinking. He said that if I could drink that way, then I should go ahead and forget the promise I made to my dad, but if I wasn't successful, I should try AA. He told me that there was an Alcoholics Anonymous meeting going on in his church at that very moment and asked me if I would like to check it out. I was so elated that this preacher had given me the OK to drink again that I would have agreed to anything, so he led me to my first AA meeting. I am sure that I hold the record for being the happiest person to ever attend his first AA meeting!

A couple of days after this meeting I thought, *Now is the time to try my luck at drinking again.* I felt sure that since I had been dry for a period of time, I would be successful. However, I realized that I had not been entirely truthful with the minister on how I would like to drink, so I laid out a program for myself.

My first attempt at drinking again was a miserable failure. I got roaring drunk and couldn't stop drinking. I failed in what I had told the preacher and in what I had planned for myself.

After that episode, I took the minister's advice and went back to AA, but I was unable to remain sober over the next couple of years. Things got worse and the disease of alcoholism continued to progress. Because of my drinking, I experienced what it was like to black out and to spend time in jail because of four alcohol-related driving arrests. I experienced what it was like to go on binges, to resort to drinking mouthwash, shaving lotion, and perfume in order to get alcohol into my system. I lost my driver's license, my home, and my shoe business. I went bankrupt and became destitute in every area of my life. Yet I was unable to stop drinking.

We moved back to Bakersfield and I got a job as a shoe salesman in another store. I was working there when I became sober. On December 16, 1970, I had my last drink and returned to AA. At last my recovery had begun. I started attending meetings, reading the *Big Book,* and got into AA's 12 Steps of recovery. Reading chapter 4 in the AA *Big Book* entitled "We Agnostics" and working through the second and third Steps were the beginning of my finding a genuine relationship with God. I believe that God knew I was sincere in my desire to turn my will and my life over to His care, so He revealed Himself to me.

After being sober about four and a half years, I began attending Fruitvale Community Church, where my wife had been taking our children. Here I heard meaningful messages that were instrumental in my conversion. The pastor spoke on the "Sermon on the Mount," and I was amazed at how many places the Bible seemed to be copied from the *Big Book* of AA (instead of the other way around). For the first time I found myself attending church because I wanted to. One morning about this time, I was looking at a pamphlet my daughters had brought home from a Billy Graham movie and it was then that I truly and genuinely accepted Christ into my life.

After a couple of years of sobriety I wanted to change careers, so I sought employment elsewhere and had several job interviews. I was learning that I could work past my fears and successfully confront unpleasant tasks. I learned that it was OK if I became anxious, and that butterflies in my stomach weren't going to kill me. I found that backing away from every unpleasant situation was not living at all, and trying to be constantly comfortable was impractical and impossible.

Instead of accepting any of these job opportunities, I decided once again to go into business for myself. I started a one-man gardening service, thinking I would like strenuous outdoor work. This turned out to be very true and I acquired a landscape contractor's license.

My wife and I still attend the same church, as do our son, daughter, and their families. In our church, Joyce and I have let our continued affiliation with AA and Al-Anon be known, along with the fact that we are both in recovery. We have had many opportunities to help others by sharing our stories and by inviting them to meetings. We found that many people would not attend secular 12-step programs, and also learned that many families in the church were suffering in silence. In January 1984,

FREEDOM FROM FEAR

I started an alcoholic support group for Christians. The group had good results at times but I felt dissatisfied with the format. Finally, Julianna, a young lady from our church, introduced me to the *FREED* booklet of OO. Immediately I knew it was the format I had been seeking. We held our first Overcomers meeting in June 1985. At first it was a struggle to get a new group going. However, we never once doubted that we had the right program.

It became an active, viable group. Our group has definitely been instrumental in leading people to Christ and helping them find sobriety.

God is giving me a second chance. Through our grandkids, I'm experiencing many things I missed out on as a parent. I always loved my children very much, but I couldn't appreciate them the way I'm able to enjoy my two grandchildren! God is number one in our lives, and our lives are filled with the kind of joy that comes from having God at the top of our list. We now celebrate life one day at a time and don't take ourselves too seriously. I pray to be a risk-taker. Can you imagine that from a man who was timid in the extreme?

When I entered AA, I was merely seeking a life of physical sobriety. I thought life would surely be dull and boring without alcohol. Little did I know of the excitement and satisfaction that lay ahead!

Today, I am a totally different person than I once was. I am no longer bogged down by fear. I now know what it is like to venture out and take chances (with God's approval). I am no longer a compulsive worrier, nor do I suffer from depression. God has proven to me that He still performs miracles and that it is probably a bigger miracle for Him to carry us over the mountains than to remove them from our path.

THERE ARE NO COINCIDENCES

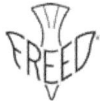

BY CHRISTA B.

In 1987, when my husband Bob and I went to the pool site at a campground near Yosemite National Park, California, we didn't expect to find any other campers. The place had been quiet, almost isolated. But there was a man sitting by the side of the pool watching his wife swim. After introducing ourselves and talking briefly, we discovered they were Christians too. The couple just happened to be Bob and Pauline Bartosch.

We soon learned that this unexpected rendezvous was not a coincidence. We had never heard of an organization called Overcomers Outreach, but Pauline rightly calls it another one of God's incredible miracles. Little did we know the role Overcomers Outreach would play in our lives.

Nor could God's timing have been better. Ironically, at that moment, I was a chemical dependency nurse. I had recently felt compelled to return to Al-Anon because of the challenges in my life, including the fact that my second daughter, age fourteen, was on the poster for missing children.

I was born and raised in Germany as the second oldest daughter in a family of six children. A large family was not fashionable then and I found it totally embarrassing when my mother became pregnant with her sixth child. As World War II refugees, we were poor and considered to be different from the others in the farming community where we lived.

OVERCOMERS OUTREACH

My parents were strict Catholics. Dad was a sincere and hard worker, earning a living at first as a farm hand and later in private business. But somehow we did not fit in. We went to church when others were resting on Sunday mornings from their Saturday night parties and drinking events. Dad had an occasional drink, but would become very ill when others encouraged him to keep up with them. This was also embarrassing. I was uneasy with people outside my family. Even during my career in nursing, I never felt quite comfortable with people. Yet others saw me as a go-getter, pleasant, even entertaining, particularly in places like dance halls where a few drinks helped me loosen up.

My appearance was always carefully staged. I tried my best to look self-assured, yet I remained insecure and desperately needed others to think well of me. I did my best to be pleasing and adaptive so that they would.

My constant aim seemed to be to somehow perfect myself inside and out. I took modeling, singing and piano classes, jazz dancing, and all sorts of schooling while also trying to find Mr. Wonderful and live happily ever after. And, of course, only my successes were worth sharing.

I was more at ease in an environment where I was hardly known. When a romantic relationship in Germany was deteriorating, to protect my pride I pursued a secret desire of mine to emigrate to the United States. My dreams and aspirations were larger than life; above all, I needed to prove to myself and to others that I was on my way towards becoming a success.

My family eventually accepted the fact that I had chosen the USA as my new home. Somehow I enjoyed a new freedom—a freedom from certain rules and traditions that always had seemed to point accusing fingers at me. Yet even the miles could not keep my family and their accusing fingers from following me around; I couldn't escape them totally.

At age thirty I had my first child. The child's father and I experienced a rather rocky courtship, so I chose not to marry him. Nevertheless, I adored my beautiful baby daughter. I remember the pictures and big fuss about President Johnson's first grandchild that same year, but any historical event seemed minor compared to the arrival of my precious daughter. For the first time in my life I was ecstatically happy.

After my baby daughter was born, my husband promised me he would try not to drink anymore. Even as he made that promise, the smell of his beer breath permeated the air. He had just divorced his

THERE ARE NO COINCIDENCES

second wife to marry me, and I, having adjusted to many challenges in the past, was totally certain that I had the ability to somehow fix his past failures. I worked, paid bills, and gradually began to learn that with all my sacrifices and personal efforts, I was unable to prevent my husband's erratic behavior. I felt like I was on a roller coaster ride, which despite some good times, was mostly painful. Soon what disturbed me the most was my own behavior. I became tense and unpredictable and I couldn't even look at my face in the mirror anymore.

Our minister suggested we attend Al-Anon. I'll never forget some of the people I met there, especially Ruth, an elderly seasoned pioneer with pretty, white curly hair. "Do you really believe that God is able to do something about my situation?" I asked her one evening.

Her reply, "Of course He can," seemed so assured. I drove home that evening being aware of a Power greater than myself that could possibly be a reality. But neither my spouse nor I were yet ready to embrace recovery.

We still believed that our lives would change once we moved into our new custom-built chalet-type home on a beautiful canyon site. We were joyous at being able to adopt a beautiful, perfect brand-new baby son just seven months after our three-day-old baby daughter had died. We used these events to put bandages on our pain. We were not yet ready to admit our humanness and failures.

Ultimately, the time came when I had to give up all I had cherished so much to God—my marriage, my material attainments, my sound reputation, and eventually even my image of myself as a parent. Jesus, however, had become real to me and with Him I was ready to rebuild my life. During the years that my daughters were running from life, trying to circumvent their own painful memories by escaping into the world of drugs, I once more was faced with many decisions that demanded prayer, wisdom, and discernment.

With a new and devoted husband at my side, I began attending an Overcomers group started by Bill R. in Riverside. After Bill left, my husband, Bob, and I continued the group, struggling with a temporary drop in attendance, and holding out until a few new faithful supporters arrived. Within a year's time the group began to grow larger, which made it necessary for us to divide into additional groups. We saw God's hand moving in many different lives—and the miracles we witnessed continually encouraged us.

OVERCOMERS OUTREACH

We also began to realize wonderful blessings in our own personal lives. While living away from home, my oldest daughter began to make changes in her life. Since God never does just a partial job, she not only found herself in 12-step support groups, but also at His feet at the same time. Both she and her husband are now recovering from addictions and are wonderful Christians who have started their own Overcomers group, enhancing my life beyond all my wildest dreams.

My beautiful adopted son was elected homecoming king at his Christian high school last year. Unlike with my two wild daughters in years gone by, I never worry whether he is in his bed in the morning.

My ex-husband finally entered a recovery program a few years after our divorce and now lives in Montana.

My husband, Bob, is a miracle. Eight months after we married, he had a near-fatal heart attack and God's grace saved his life. He had triple bypass surgery and today he is physically active and does not rely on any medications. While listening to others in our group, he began to face many of his A.C.A. issues described so well in the Overcomers' *Adult Children of Alcoholics* booklet. He, too, is facing his feelings more openly today, which has helped enrich our marriage. He has accepted that he is a food addict, an addiction he continues to battle every day. At least the foods he is battling are healthy and safe to eat today, and he maintains a perfectly slim figure. When God begins to shower His blessings upon us, He is generous!

Life hasn't been easy, but even so, God has kept giving His blessings. My daughters had good and bad times while growing up, including running away from home and the like. During the time my second daughter was missing, God provided an opportunity for an Overcomers group to begin at our local Juvenile Hall, a new, large, high-security facility. The request had been made to bring more 12-step programs to the inmates. When I listened to the stories of many of the young girls, I could not help thinking of my own daughter and wondering where she was. Was she even alive? A special bond formed between those girls and me. We shared, allowing the Holy Spirit to do the work, and received tremendous blessings.

Then my second daughter came back into our lives. She married at eighteen and satisfied her sentences with the juvenile courts. She is beautiful and without interfering with her life, we enjoy watching her grow through her own challenges. We respect each other's differences and build and encourage them whenever we can.

THERE ARE NO COINCIDENCES

We have four Overcomers groups here in Riverside that no longer need our assistance since they have their own leadership and momentum. We are trusting others to do the tasks we did for more than four years.

Overcomers continues to bear fruit. I experienced a very special blessing Christmas Eve 1991 that I must tell you about. I had recently begun working on an on-call basis in a chemical dependency hospital. Needless to say, I was not too excited when the call came for me to work on Christmas Eve. One of my patients asked for permission to stay up until midnight to celebrate the birth of Jesus Christ! I was in charge of the unit and set up some simple guidelines so others could participate. I had brought a tape with Christmas songs to work that day and I found a New Testament on the unit. After a group of approximately fifteen patients had gathered in the day room, I had a patient read the Christmas story in Luke chapter 2.

The walls were bare. We had some simple seats and a Christmas tree with a few lights. What took place in this humble setting became memorable for the Christians and non-Christians alike who were present. Only the tree lights were lit as we listened to "Silent Night" on our small tape player. With tears flowing, patients said things like, "This is the first sober Christmas that I can remember."

Sobriety is a beautiful thing. After sharing the true heart of the gospel among each other, we agreed to meet again next year. Patients walked up to me and thanked me for the best Christmas they ever had—just a simple setting with the gospel in its midst. The Holy Spirit again had done His work! We are now hoping to add an Overcomers Group to the hospital curriculum.

God continues to give me opportunities to share about recovery. Just recently, I followed up on an offer to lead a 12-step group in a shelter for the homeless. Although the meeting was secular in nature because of outside funding, I am repeatedly blessed as these homeless people share their faith in Jesus Christ, and become receptive to the healing elements as presented in the 12 Steps.

The paper I'm writing on now is splotched with tears, as I have cried a lot while writing this story. These were happy tears, of course, but sometimes it is still painful to look at the past. I imagine if the truth were known, these tears are a mixture of both. It is such a thrill for me to write a small part of this book. It is an honor to share God's handiwork in my life.

29

STUFFED FEELINGS ADDED POUNDS

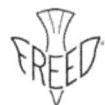

BY LORAINE W.

I grew up in a dysfunctional Christian home. I was the youngest of six children, and soon found out that if I clowned around I could get the attention I so desperately needed. Trying to please everyone would get me attention too. I also found out that being the youngest member of my family gave me no input into the decisions of the family. I felt like a non-person, like I had no identity of my own. I soon learned that I had to role play, according to what my parents wanted, and that meant I was not being quite honest in being myself.

Dad totally dominated the family. Feelings were never allowed to be expressed. His philosophy was, "Do as I say, not as I do." It seemed only two things were acceptable: laughter and over-eating. I was quite good at both. At the time, I did not realize that my overeating was really the way I covered up or stuffed the feelings I was not allowed to express. There were even feelings inside me I was not aware of until I became an adult.

As the youngest, I was often picked on and laughed at for being overweight. I was ridiculed for my stringy, oily hair and at school I was teased and called "Fatty." My self-esteem was very low.

Since, for the most part, a person's concept of God is based directly on that person's perception of his/her earthly father, I grew up not really knowing if God was anyone more than just a grumpy tyrant in the sky.

OVERCOMERS OUTREACH

Fortunately, my parents took us to Sunday school and church every week. I learned many, many Bible verses, which would later prove to be beneficial, although at the time, they were no more than just words in a big, black book.

On December 1, 1963, I accepted Christ as my Savior. I figured that my life would really begin to change because I grew up hearing preachers say that once you gave your life to Christ you would never be the same again. Well, I tried to be different, but life was still the same old thing. I tried to live the Christian life in my own strength, still basically just performing. I would sing the old hymns of the faith, but they were only words with beautiful melodies. I did not really grasp that salvation was a relationship with God through Jesus Christ; I still thought it was a bunch of do's and don'ts.

So I went through life with many bouts of doubt as to whether or not I was even a Christian. I used laughter and overeating to hide the pain of my life. My big smile and continuous laughter won me a few friends. Most who associated with me thought I was happy and easy-going. Looking back, I realize I was basically a robot, never too high and never totally depressed. I was very predictable.

I was active in sports in high school, so I could get away with overeating. Also, sports were a means of getting some of the praise I so craved. I was good at athletics, having played them a lot while growing up. I managed to maintain my weight (145 pounds) in high school after being "Fatty" in grade school and junior high.

In 1973, I got married to a man who was nothing like Dad. Gene was a very loving, kind, considerate man who loved the Lord and loved me dearly. I received much of the love and acceptance from Gene that I had longed for as a child.

Overall, my life seemed quite happy. I found a great deal of security in my marriage, so much so, that I just kept gaining weight. On our wedding day, I weighed 142 pounds; after seventeen years of marriage I had gone as high as 213 pounds! Gene loved me even when I was overweight. He told me there was just more of me to love.

Time after time, I would ask Gene, "Why do I keep eating like this? I can't seem to get control of this problem." Looking back over my life, I finally came to the conclusion that I had lived a life of quiet desperation.

But what was my real problem? Why couldn't I get control of my life, or control my overeating? I thought I was a pretty happy person, at least

STUFFED FEELINGS ADDED POUNDS

I put on a good front. Later I would discover that I was in total denial about my state of happiness.

When I was about forty, I renewed a friendship with a woman I had known since kindergarten. She had become a psychologist. As we shared, I learned a great deal about myself. She explained terms such as "denial," "codependent," "enabler," "boundary-setting," etc. I began to be familiar with these terms. I began to understand myself better, but still there seemed to be something missing in my life. I began to feel like psychology could go only so far in meeting my spiritual needs. Psychology could reveal what was wrong with me, but it could not cure me. It was like a mirror, revealing the dirt on my face, but not enabling me to remove it. Psychology alone left me still a hurting, overweight person.

I was on a diet off and on (mostly off) ever since I was in seventh grade. When I was thirteen years old, I had a thirty-six-inch waist. I took appetite-control pills prescribed by a doctor, but I did not seem to be able to keep the weight off in junior high. I had no discipline, which is the key to losing weight and keeping it off. So the diet route was a yo-yo for me: I would get the weight off and then gain it all back and more. I truly had an eating disorder. I would later learn of my eating problem that it's not what you're eating, it's what's eating you.

All this time I was active in my church. I taught a Sunday school class at various ages in my life, sang in a church choir, and helped in vacation Bible school. I even went on a missionary trip to Mexico when I was in high school. People thought I was a good Christian because I was doing the things a Christian was supposed to do. Yet something was still missing in my life.

I had grown up in the church hearing that a personal relationship with Christ was where it was at, but I did not understand that the power to live that life was a gift from God. All the knowledge I had in my head had not made it those crucial few inches down into my heart. However, this was all going to change soon.

In the early part of 1990, a lady in our church choir asked if there was one person who would be willing to help stuff church bulletins on Friday morning. A few moments passed and when no hands went up, I, being the people-pleaser that I was, raised my hand. Nancy saw it and said, "Oh, bless you!" That made me feel so good!

I had seen Nancy before but did not really know her. She was a tenor and I was an alto, so we did not sit near each other in the choir loft. I thought she was a very beautiful woman; more than that, I had seen something in her life that I wanted. What I saw in her was a real relationship with God, but I didn't know how to get that for myself. I figured if I helped her with the bulletins I could eventually find out her secret. Little did I know what God was about to do in my life through this beautiful woman of God!

I decided I would take on this bulletin stuffing as a weekly project so that I might get to know Nancy. Looking back, I see the hand of God in all my plans concerning Nancy. We hit it off right away and began to share things about ourselves. I told Nancy that my biggest problem was that I was overweight.

As we talked, Nancy asked me if I was familiar with a program at our church called Overcomers Outreach. I said yes, but I thought it was a group designed to help people with drug and alcohol problems, and people who were adult children of alcoholics. Nancy said Overcomers was for anyone with an addictive or obsessive/compulsive behavior in his or her life. I told her that I was certainly a compulsive overeater. Nancy then invited me to Overcomers.

I remember saying at my first meeting that I was a "foodaholic." I also said, "Well, I can't cry." It was impossible for me to cry, nor could I express my feelings of rage, anger, bitterness, or resentment. As I continued to go to meetings, I began to realize that I had used food to stuff down any and all of my feelings. Food, especially sugar, was my high, my fix, my addiction. I looked at Step One: "We admit we were powerless over our [addiction/compulsion]–our lives had become unmanageable." I began to accept the reality of my addiction. I was truly out of control. My life was unmanageable.

As I thought about Step One, I also thought of what Nancy had shared with me: God loves me just the way I am. He loves me unconditionally. Nancy reminded me of that truth very often. I saw in her the unconditional love of Christ. That love was in her eyes, and expressed clearly on her face and in her actions. Nancy consistently walked her talk. I needed to see that.

Step Two says, "Came to believe that a Power greater than ourselves could restore us to sanity." I believe with all my heart that God used Nancy to show me that belief is a choice, but a choice that could be made based on God's Word, which never changes. I knew now that I believed the first two Steps. It just made sense to go on to Step Three. I chose to turn my will and my life over to the care of God on November 5, 1990. That day I completely gave my weight problem over to God. I told Him I would

STUFFED FEELINGS ADDED POUNDS

take it a day at a time—really just a meal at a time. Not only did I give God my weight problem, but by faith I abandoned my entire life to His care. I had come to believe that God was totally trustworthy. I pictured myself climbing into God's lap, believing He is my Abba Father.

On November 5, 1990, I weighed 204 pounds. The weight began to come off without a struggle or great effort. Each day I could hardly wait to meet with God and turn my will and my life over to His loving care for that day. Meeting with God each day for fellowship and a new touch was no longer an obligation as it had been in years past. Now it was a joy! I had truly begun to have a personal, vital, exciting relationship with the God of the universe through His Son, Jesus Christ. What a thrilling adventure God had begun in my life!

Each week I would lose around two pounds–some weeks more, some less. Each week I would also lose the need to stuff my feelings. I found as God had begun to replace my need for excess food with Himself, I was beginning to feel things.

The first gift God gave me was the ability to cry. I remembered Nancy saying months earlier that someday I would be able to cry with her. She was right. I thought it would take years before I would begin to have the ability to cry.

As the weight came off and the feelings came up I had to grieve things I had ignored or just passed over earlier in my life. I had to grieve the loss of growing up without a close relationship with my mom and dad. I had to grieve the fact that I would never have children. I had to work through the loss of a childhood that should have been loving and free from physical, verbal, and emotional abuse.

What transformed my life was the fact that God loved me unconditionally. I chose to believe God that November day, but I did not fully, in my heart, understand it. The tears flowed when that truth seeped into my heart. What a blessing tears have now become!

Now I began to experience my pain from a childhood that I would never have chosen for myself. Through every painful emotion I experienced for the first time, God was there for me. Nancy and the Overcomers were there for me. My husband was there for me. Feeling things was basically all new to me.

During my weight loss, I was able to give God the credit when people asked me about it. There was no room for boasting or bragging on my part. All I could claim that I had done was to give God my will and my life.

I came to realize that a greater joy than the weight coming off was the joy of having a daily walk with the God of the universe. I cry in His presence and know He accepts me and loves me. I feel and believe with all my heart that I am His child. God took from my heart the fear of death and terminal diseases that had always plagued me.

My life is no longer my own. I turn it over to God each day. I know that I am safe in His loving arms. There are days when I have to do this again and again when I've failed to keep my focus on Him. I am learning that God has my very best interest at heart and (as Nancy so faithfully reminds me) that God will orchestrate my life. I need not try to make things work. All I need to do is submit my will to Him and He takes care of the rest. As a result, I've lost more than fifty pounds.

I have noticed that all the verses of Scripture and wonderful hymns of the faith I learned as a child are moving from my head into my heart. I now say in amazement, "Oh, is that what that verse means?" The written Word has become the Living Word for me. Praise God!

Recovery continues to be, as we share in our Overcomers group, the big "P"—process. I will be in process until the Lord calls me home.

I would not trade this last year and a half for anything. I feel like the title of one of John Powell's books, *Fully Human, Fully Alive*. God has been so faithful; I know He will continue to do His will in my life as I continue to submit my will and my life to Him each day. God is my righteousness, my peace, my wisdom, my joy, my strength, my reason for living.

30

A WORKAHOLIC GETS A NEW HEART

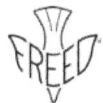

BY KIM G.

The term workaholic for most people is a fairly benign term used to denote a person who is busier than most. Workaholism is not only socially acceptable in our culture, but is also socially encouraged. What most people don't realize is that workaholism is an addiction, and it carries with it the same devastation to the person and the person's family that other addictions have.

Like many addictions, mine had its roots in childhood. I learned at a very tender age that achievements had the effect of making me feel significant, at least for a short while.

I accepted Christ as my personal Lord and Savior at the age of twelve and that made me feel different from the rest of my family. I didn't fit. In high school I became the child whom all the other kids picked on. They called me names and humiliated me on a daily basis. By the time I was sixteen, I felt there was something drastically wrong with me. I thought I was socially unacceptable.

I believed that suicide was wrong, but that God could forgive an accident. So I began walking in front of cars, playing Russian roulette with my life, thinking that I owed it to society to eradicate myself. We lived in a small town and my father used to get phone calls from people who had come close to hitting me and they complained about my behavior. He didn't understand; I'm sure he didn't know what to do.

OVERCOMERS OUTREACH

Sprinkled throughout my early years were my achievements, from positions that I held, to awards won for my poetry and short stories, to my accomplishments in 4–H (including All–'Round 4–H'er of the Year, 1977). Each achievement was my desperate attempt to show the world that I was somebody, that I did have worth.

I was married at the age of nineteen, and my husband and I moved to Tulsa, Oklahoma, to go to Bible school. We spent two years there and moved back to upstate New York several months after my daughter was born. It was there that I began in earnest to find something to fill the empty spot in my life.

When I was growing up, my father was a volunteer E.M.T. (emergency medical technician) and firefighter. I spent a lot of time following him around at the firehouse as he did routine maintenance chores. I had always respected our local E.M.T.s and firefighters, so I began to reason that if I could only become one of them, I would really be somebody. So I became an E.M.T. and I won the respect of my fellow E.M.T.s and my community, but I couldn't respect myself. So I reasoned that if I could become our fire department's second-ever female firefighter, then I would really be somebody. So I completed firefighters' training and became a firefighter. I won the respect of my fellow firefighters and my community, but I still could not respect myself.

During this time, I began to work excessively. In addition to working sixty hours a week at one job, I held two part-time sales positions. Often I would spend all day working and much of the night running the ambulance and fighting fires, trying to rescue mankind. There were times when I left the house and my two girls would cling to my legs and cry because they missed me.

Eventually we moved to a new town and with the move came three important changes. The first change was that my husband became disabled. We had to scrape for every penny merely to survive. Charitable organizations did help somewhat, but they also put incredible pressure on the family unit and treated us as less than desirable people.

The second change was that my husband and I went back to college in an attempt to try to become self-sufficient again. With the challenge of college also came opportunities to achieve. I finished my stint there with two associate degrees (with high honors, of course) and membership in two honor fraternities. My husband and I had been featured in the local paper as being the first husband-wife team to be inducted into one of the fraternities.

A WORKAHOLIC GETS A NEW HEART

The third change was in churches. We began a five-year stint in a spiritually abusive church. By the time we left there the inner pain and turmoil I felt had grown immensely. My perception of God had also been distorted—I viewed Him as holding a whip in one hand and a stick in the other. The whip was because I viewed God as a slave driver, and the stick was used to beat us if we did not perform well enough. Finally, we broke our relationship with that particular church when we moved back to Tulsa to attend Bible school.

By this time we had a family of five and we settled into an apartment in Tulsa. My husband had had a spine fusion a few months previous. We were both students that year, but the entire operation of the household had fallen on my shoulders, including the housework, child-care, and bringing in the income. Even though the inner pain I felt had become unbearable, of course I rose to the occasion.

I spent the year working two and three jobs at a time. I worked eighty to ninety hours per week and spent only two to four hours per night sleeping. Working anesthetized my pain. As long as I was working, I couldn't feel it. I couldn't feel anything. I was numb, and spent several years working like that. I would run on an adrenaline high all day working as fast and as hard as I could. I could not sit still or relax without feeling guilty, and I seemed to need more and more activity to cover the pain.

When I wasn't working for pay I was working at home. It was not uncommon for me to work a sixteen-hour day and come home and bake cookies at night. During that time I suffered periods of burnout. I would back off for a couple of weeks and then plunge forward, full steam ahead.

Eventually, two things occurred that facilitated my hitting bottom. The first happened when I was taken to the emergency room for the third time in as many years, suffering from tachycardia and cardiac arrhythmia—a serious heart condition.

The second happened when my middle child became unruly, almost destroying the family unit. Her behavior became so unruly that we were seriously considering placing her in a foster home. We couldn't do anything with her, so we thought that maybe someone else could.

About that time we entered into family counseling, which saved our family, but at the same time I grew more and more despondent. Financially we were better off than we had ever been. I had a full-time job that I liked, but I was still miserable. All of my work and all of my achievement couldn't make me "somebody." They couldn't fill the emptiness inside.

OVERCOMERS OUTREACH

In January of 1992, I began walking in front of cars again. I worked in downtown Tulsa and I had to cross a four-lane street on my way to and from work. I did so every day without looking to see if anything was coming or not. One day the secretary to the vice-president I worked for almost ran me down. I looked up to see the look of horror on her face as she slammed on the brakes. I thought that I would be in trouble, but no one said a word.

My depression deepened. I could no longer eat or sleep. I lost a lot of weight (I was 5'9" and weighed 118 pounds). I got to the point that I felt there was no hope. One night in February, I fell on my knees and told God that He had three weeks to straighten out my life or I would jump from an overpass that was right down the street from where I worked. I knew that God could answer prayer, but at the same time I didn't think I could sit around and wait for it to fall on me like cherries falling off a cherry tree. So I picked up some books on recovery and began to read.

I picked up a book by Jeff Van Vonderen called *Tired of Trying to Measure Up*. I thought that described me pretty well. True to my obsessive-compulsive nature, I tend to read books from the dedication in the front, to the author's biographical sketch in the back. That book blessed me just by reading the dedication. God began talking to me through that book. There were truths on every page that I had heard before, but for the first time they became real. I realized for the first time that I had been trying to base my self-worth on my achievements and my ability to work. However, my self-worth is not supposed to be based on my behavior, but on who I am in Christ.

Isaiah 9:6 says, "His name shall be called Wonderful, Counsellor..." (KJV). I began to realize that I had the greatest counselor living inside of me in the form of the Holy Spirit. As I turned my will and my life over to the care of God, I began to rely more and more on my resident counselor to orchestrate my recovery. I realized that He knew me better than I did, and He knew what I needed and when.

I was in individual therapy for six months and it was helpful, but I began to feel that I had gone about as far with it as I could go. Recovery doesn't occur in a vacuum; we desperately need the support of other people.

During the first four months of my recovery I read twenty recovery-related books. Many of them carried a list of 12-step groups in the back. It was there that I found the number for Overcomers Outreach.

A WORKAHOLIC GETS A NEW HEART

My husband called and got information on groups in the area, and on August 31, 1992, (my birthday) I attended my first meeting.

To be perfectly honest, I wasn't overly impressed, but I knew that my recovery was a matter of life and death, so I kept going. It took me about six months of regular attendance to be able to open up; I had great difficulty trusting people. During this time I would leave the meetings disappointed because I just couldn't share what was really inside, but at the same time I couldn't wait for the next Monday night for another opportunity to try again. It just goes to show that you've got to keep coming back.

Eventually, I was able to open up and share and allow myself to really be loved. As I listened to some of the more experienced 12-steppers share, I learned a lot about myself, the program, and how the 12 Steps relate to Scripture. I learned how to live one day at a time (something essential for a workaholic). I began applying the 12 Steps to my addiction. Soon I began to see how the 12 Steps could work in other areas of my life. What began as steps, over time became a lifestyle.

My recovery has affected every area of my life. My relationship with my husband is better now than it's ever been. My relationships with my children and family have improved. My relationship with God has improved. No longer do I look at God as the big slave driver. I now see him as the living, caring God that he really is. I am secure in His love. I have the joy of the Lord, and a peace that truly passes all understanding. Even in the midst of tribulation (and we all have tribulation), I don't have to be afraid, because my "Higher Power," Jesus Christ, is with me.

God had truly performed a miracle in my life, working a healing in me both emotionally and spiritually, and yet one thing remained. The stress-filled years of my life took a toll on my heart. I have had a mitral valve prolapse condition since I was a child, but my addiction caused it to worsen to the point where the flaps of the valve didn't close at all. According to my doctors, without surgery I would not have lived to see forty, or anywhere close to it. (I'm thirty-four now).

I had surgery to replace the defective heart valve with an artificial one. During the week before surgery, different Overcomers called me to say they were praying for me. Overcomers showed up at the hospital to sit with my husband while I was in surgery. Two more showed up that night to make my husband leave long enough to get something to eat since he had been without food all day. One group member works at the hospital, and I remember waking up in Coronary I.C.U., finding him standing by my side. I received phone calls, cards, and visits from Overcomers, and daily reminders that I was being upheld in prayer.

Overcomers Outreach has become more to me than just a support group. It has become family. You don't find such unconditional love and caring out in the world, and, sorry to say, you don't find it in a lot of churches either. I am grateful to be alive and to be a part of OO.

I am still a busy person, but I am no longer driven to work. I can relax without feeling guilty. I can actually feel emotions again. Pain is there, yes. There will be pain at times, but I can also feel happiness, joy, and peace. I have learned how to put achievements in their proper perspective. I also know that I will continue to grow. As long as I keep following Christ, life only gets better from here.

31

ADDICT ENCOUNTERS "AMAZING GRACE"

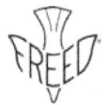

BY DON T.

I was born and raised in a non-Christian home in a small Michigan town, the oldest son of hard-working parents. My father was the shop foreman of an auto parts factory and owner of his own sporting goods store. He was a heavy drinker, father of six kids, fisherman, hunter, and a man who seemingly never slept. My mother brooded over her six kids the best she could, as she was mostly on her own while Dad was busy with his own life.

I was an active kid and was never able to measure up to my own set of standards. By the time I was a teen, I had lost interest in anything that did not involve alcohol or fighting. I was kicked out of school my senior year for fighting. Then I went from job to job, married at eighteen, and enlisted in the Army. While I was stationed in Germany in 1966, I discovered hashish and other drugs to go along with the alcohol that was already a big part of my life. After a few months in Europe, I received orders to go to Vietnam.

Shortly after I arrived in Vietnam, I was introduced to heroin. I spent two tours in Vietnam manipulating the military in order to accommodate my new-found habit. I just didn't care about anything but getting high. I wrote home so seldom that my young wife of less than a year lost patience and filed for divorce. It didn't matter—getting high was the only thing that mattered. During my second tour, I returned to the U.S. just to finalize the divorce, and then managed to remarry before I returned to Southeast Asia.

Upon returning to the U.S. after my tours, I had a great deal of difficulty maintaining my addiction as I had done overseas. The dope was so much more expensive and of lesser potency that I resorted to every means possible to get more money for more dope. Finally, after stabbing a young soldier for just a few dollars, I was arrested by the military police and charged with armed robbery, attempted murder, and possession. After stockade time and a court martial, I was sentenced to nineteen years of hard labor in Leavenworth, Kansas.

Shortly after I settled into prison life—I had accepted my role and was playing the tough guy—God chose to intervene for the first time in my life. For reasons I still don't understand, a military panel selected me as a "victim of the Vietnam war"! They presented me with an offer that I could not turn down. I was told that if I would only subject myself to periodic interviews and updates, the Army was willing to allow me to return to active duty under a special rehabilitation program. I jumped at the chance and left prison after less than one year.

I was then sent to Oklahoma to finish my time in the Army and I managed to live a straight life. I had been reunited with my wife and son, and a daughter was born while we were there. Since I had been cured of my heroin addiction, I never gave it a thought when I drank a little wine or smoked a little dope. Ironically, the Army interviewers never gave it a thought either.

After the Army, I decided to go to college in New Mexico. Everything went along pretty well and I almost felt like a normal person. I tolerated my wife and kids, didn't get drunk that often, and only smoked dope and took acid when it was available. I prided myself for not going out and looking for drugs. Surprisingly, I finished college and found a job in management training with a bank. Except for drinking, drugging, and stealing, I felt the job went well. I was fired because a joint was found in the company truck that I drove. They just didn't understand.

It wasn't long before I divorced my second wife and left my two children. I bounced from job to job and ended up in car sales. It was then that I discovered cocaine. I found that I was a very good car salesman, which was fortunate because I needed a lot more money to accommodate my new cocaine habit. Needless to say, I was never quite able to make enough money for that expensive habit. Within a year, I was arrested and convicted for embezzlement. The Lord stepped in again, because instead

ADDICT ENCOUNTERS "AMAZING GRACE"

of the five to 10 years in prison I deserved, the judge sentenced me to only five years probation. His only stipulation was that I find a treatment center, employment, and a place to live—out of state! I jumped at the chance and returned to Michigan.

I thought, *Surely I must be at the bottom now*. I was divorced for the second time, broke, and owed child support I couldn't afford. I was fresh out of a treatment center (this was before it was the "in" thing to go to treatment) and was, naturally, working a job I didn't like. But even worse, I had returned to my home state not as a hero, but as a loser.

Within just a few months, I was convinced that my world was upright again. I got back in the car business, made some money, made the mistake of hitting the bars, and before I realized it, was back in the saddle again. The next six years were much the same. I married for the third time, but this time I married a born-again Christian. Since I didn't know at that time what that meant, I never gave it a second thought.

During that time, I was asked to go to another treatment center. Since my boss had requested it and was willing to pay for it, I said, "Why not?" I was treatment wise by then and knew that I could easily beat the system again, except something happened that I hadn't counted on. While there, a man witnessed to me about the gospel of Jesus Christ during one of those late-night conversations that often take place in dry-out centers. I politely listened and then went my own way.

The next few months after treatment turned out to be the absolute worst time of my entire life. I was totally out of control. My binges lasted longer than ever before, and each binge included more blackouts and more terrifying stories of my escapades during those binges. On January 16, 1988, after a five-day binge and a two-day black-out, I had really hit bottom. I lost another job. I was broke again, and my family had finally had enough.

I had no one to turn to. My Narcotics Anonymous sponsor walked me around that last night, but I just wanted him away from me. I didn't know what to do.

Then out of nowhere (I know now that it was the Lord's doing), the man who had witnessed to me at the treatment center called. I told him the latest news, and without hesitation, he invited my wife and me to Orlando, Florida, at his expense. He said that he knew someone I needed to meet.

Going along for this ride seemed like any other wild goose chase from my past. I thought the worst that could happen would be a free trip to Disney World. The first morning in Orlando wasn't at all what I had planned. We didn't go to Disney World. We went to visit Amazing Grace. Grace happened to be the elderly widow of one of the pioneers of AA.

Grace greeted us as if we had been close friends all our lives. Then she shared about the spiritual side of Alcoholics Anonymous. Right on the spot she gave her testimony, and then told me, in no uncertain terms, to get on my knees and accept Jesus as my personal Savior. And she did all this within fifteen minutes! Naturally, I fought her at first, but when I realized this lady was not going to give up, I grudgingly followed her instructions.

At first I was a little disappointed. There were no flashing lights, nor could I see or hear the angels in heaven. All I know is, that day was January 21, 1988, and it's been more than five years that I've been sober! Praise God Almighty!

Oh, it has not been easy. In fact, the first few months were bug-crawling tough. But I continued to follow Grace's instructions and became involved in a Spirit-filled church. Those people loved me in spite of myself. Because of that unconditional love and because of God's grace, I have been able to rely upon the strength the Lord has provided. I praise God every morning, all through the day, and every night for His amazing healing in my life.

And His blessings are legion! Incredibly, my family is intact and I am closer to my wife than ever before. I have become a vital part of my step-daughter's life and she means the world to me. Two years ago (against astronomical odds), my wife and I petitioned to adopt a baby. Would you believe that the system allowed this former addict/convict/all-around malcontent to adopt a child? Well, God is in control of everything, and in case anyone should doubt His miracles, we were blessed with a beautiful little five-month-old girl! Praise God! Not even a month later, my seventeen-year-old daughter—whom I had not seen but once in fourteen years—called, and we are working together on a renewed relationship.

After twenty years of job-hopping, would you believe I've had the same job for more than two years? I make less than I ever have, but after all the bills and taxes are paid, sometimes there's even money left over on pay day.

Although God and His love have filled the void in my life, I had realized for some time that there was still something missing. I had no idea what it was until my pastor came to me and said he felt God instructing

ADDICT ENCOUNTERS "AMAZING GRACE"

him to ask me to give my testimony to the church body. I didn't hesitate, and agreed to do this, but I felt that my testimony alone, with giving praise to God for the healing, was just not enough. I knew there had to be others like me who needed ongoing help and support.

AA and NA meetings I had attended seemed to have something missing, so I had stopped attending. Having been led to the Lord by a person who had been intimately involved with the 12-step beginnings (Grace), I knew that God, through Jesus Christ, not just any "Higher Power," was the basis for my continued recovery and happiness.

After many phone calls, I discovered there were no Christian 12-step support groups for addicts and alcoholics in the entire southwestern part of the state of Michigan! After more research, I heard about Overcomers Outreach, and the rest is history. I was asked to give my testimony at my church on Easter Sunday. I had everything outlined, with a few appropriate Scriptures sprinkled here and there, but as often happens, God took over and I never even looked at my prepared speech. I thought I might have said something wrong or had shocked too many people, because hardly a sound could be heard in the church. I closed with the vision of Overcomers Outreach, and to my surprise, after church I was overwhelmed. People I had never met came up to me with tears, hugs, and handshakes—how they thanked me!

I was frightened, yet excited, about our first OO meeting. And when only one person showed up, I was OK because I knew that this was from God, so it must be the right thing to do. For the next two months, I had many a conversation with people in need—phone calls at home and conversations in quiet corners of the church on Sunday—but never more than one or two people made it to the meetings. I switched meeting days and times, looking for the right mix, and then one hot summer day, nobody came. Man, I was heartbroken. I thought, *If this is from God, where are the people? I know the need is there!*

Out of frustration, I called OO and asked to speak to anyone who would listen. The woman who answered took the time to share the story of her group and its struggles. She reminded me to wait on God and to trust in Him and to persevere. If God had not given up, why should I?

She was right. The following week, not one, not two, but four people showed. A week later another showed, then another, and six months later we had a solid core group of nine people. Two people accepted the Lord and two people found sobriety for the first time. We have experienced so much more growth in the Lord and in ourselves that it's hard for me to contain myself when I talk about it. We have even been invited to help another church start its own OO meetings.

    I believe in the 12 Steps, and I believe in the structure of Overcomers Outreach. It has helped the Steps come alive for me and the members of our group. The void in my life was filled by the Spirit of the Lord, and the missing piece I was searching for was found in Overcomers Outreach. The joy that Jesus has brought into my life is so far removed from my old self that it is sometimes difficult for me to comprehend. He has put the pieces of my life back together again, only better than before.

32

RIDING HIGH WITH THE HELL'S ANGELS

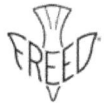

BY JAY S.

I grew up mad at the world, not caring for people a whole lot.
I was born in 1954 in a Navy hospital. For about eight years, my life consisted of moving from one Navy port to another. I never made friends and became a loner at an early age. I never had friends over to play and rarely was allowed to stay over at anyone's house.

Around the seventh grade I started smoking pot and drinking alcohol and I continued to do so for the next twenty years. In fact, I graduated to crank (a dangerous methamphetamine), coke (cocaine), pills, LSD, and Quaaludes–anything that would take me up or bring me down. Usually I tried to go both ways at the same time. I started dealing drugs at age sixteen and moved out of my parents' home into my own apartment. Despite everything, I finished school with honors, which was the best way to prove my father wrong, because he said I couldn't make it on my own.

I got married young, divorced young, and had a daughter who watched her mother and me go through hell. After my drug-filled marriage ended and the courts took away whatever material possessions I had left, I returned to my roots in the South.

There I started dealing crank with the Pagans, a branch of the Hell's Angels motorcycle gang. My anger and pain drove me up the ranks real fast because I was crazy. I would rather fight or shoot you than look at you. Because of the crank, my moods were violent. I became a collector for the Angels, gathering large amounts of money and drugs. I had two people who were the enforcers who rode with me. I was shot twice and cut many times more. And I have done some really bad things that I'm not proud of.

Once I got stopped driving a car with two friends and an ounce of crank was under the seat. I was arrested and sent to jail without a hearing. My reputation in the area got me a ticket to the big house. I stayed in federal prison for eight months, even though I had not been convicted of anything. Society wanted me out of the way. Granted, I deserved every bit of the time I served.

In prison I was confronted by four Confederate Angels, a rival group to the Pagans. They took a shim (knife) and drove it into the muscles under my armpits so I couldn't lift my arms to fight. They said they had a contract to kill me, but that this would be more fun because I couldn't fight with my muscles all torn up. I went to the infirmary for four weeks, and when I got out I hit the first guard I saw, so they put me in solitary confinement. That worked to keep me quiet for a while, but there were some other bad times in prison. I threw a homosexual man over the railing of the second floor and almost killed him for trying to pick me up.

I was released after the eight months when a friend of mine was arrested on drug charges and he told the judge the drugs in the car I had been driving were his.

I got into a lot of jams after that, and a hit was put on me (i.e., a contract for my murder). The Confederate Angels missed killing me, though. They killed two of my best friends who walked out of our clubhouse in front of me. I was going out the door first, when someone pulled me back in and I still don't know who he was. He had no leathers on, so he didn't belong there. Maybe he was an angel of the Lord. The Pagans told me to leave the area, that I was too "hot."

So I left and got married again, which was another disaster. After my experience with this wife, I just went to hell, taking secret flights to foreign countries to pick up large quantities of drugs, and flying back on regular airlines with the contraband in my luggage. I was crazy, but I didn't get caught.

I started to get tired of my lifestyle and started talking to Satan, telling him I wanted out. I knew both sides: I was brought up Catholic and knew about God, I just didn't trust Him. I used to yell at Jesus in my anger because I couldn't understand why He would let me go through so many bad times and still live.

Well, I went on a three-week binge and got a quarter-ounce of coke, a quarter-ounce of crank, some syringes, and beer, and got messed up doing speed balls (combining various drugs). I told Satan at the end of three weeks that I wanted out. Six hours passed by before I woke up from a dream in which Satan was telling me, "I promised you everything and gave it to you, and you want out?" I called him a liar and told him he had used me and taken back whatever he gave me.

Then a hand touched my shoulder and a beautiful light was there and a voice said, "You are coming with me. I have use for you," and I woke up. My room was destroyed. There were syringes stuck in the wall and the furniture was broken. My wrist was deeply cut and I had lost a lot of blood. I should have been dead. Covered with blood, I crawled out of the room and up some stairs looking for help.

The paramedics came and took me to the hospital where they patched me up and wanted to send me home. I caused quite a scene with the hospital's security department because I wanted to be sent to a treatment center but they were reluctant to arrange this. Finally, they agreed. At the treatment center I was locked up and put under observation for a while. I was the first patient this treatment center ever transferred over to a residential drug and alcohol program from the psychiatric unit.

There I met my future wife who worked on the unit and told me about Jesus and His love. While I was there we just talked, and when I was released, she told me if I wanted to see her, it would have to be at her church. I went and it has been a miracle ever since. But that's another story.

While in treatment, I asked this nurse lady why she was always happy. She told me because she had Jesus Christ in her life. The more I saw her, the more she melted my cold heart. Even after reading my charts and records she still saw good in me. She was a beautiful lady inside and out, and not like anyone I would have normally pursued. When I was about to be released from treatment, I asked her out to dinner and she said she couldn't because she worked there and it was against the rules for staff to fraternize with the patients.

A couple of days later I called her and I told her I was having a bad day. Satan was really trying to get me. So she came over, prayed with me, and led me to the Lord. Alleluia! Six weeks later, we got married. She told me that God had told her to leave her job and marry me, which was very

OVERCOMERS OUTREACH

out of character for her. She had been a single mom for several years and it was hard for her to just quit, but she trusted the Lord. We have had a blessed life ever since. We spent our first summer together growing in the Lord. I adopted her two children, and then my daughter from my first marriage who is now fifteen years old, moved in with us.

God directed us to start a 12-step group for people whose lives have been affected by drugs or alcohol and it has grown dramatically.

I was asked to be a deacon in our church, and that amazes me. The first year of our marriage, I had to have a back operation. My liver and pancreas were diagnosed as having borderline cirrhosis and pancreatitis. The Lord healed both of those organs and restored my back. The doctors told my wife that I was a walking miracle; I emphasize that it's God's miracle.

Our Overcomers Outreach group is an answer from the Lord. My wife and I have seen tremendous growth in the twenty to twenty-five people a week who come from all different churches in our area. The group is Christ-centered and run like an AA meeting. The meeting is meaningful for us also, since I am still in recovery and my wife has ACA (Adult Children of Alcoholics) and codependence issues that she is working through. Christ is the center of our home and all three children are active in our church.

The Lord has used us in many ways to help other people and to work as a team for Him. During the past four years, we have started five Overcomers groups in three states. I have been in training to become a pastor and evangelist to work in prisons and drug rehab. I work for an Outreach Ministry in New Hampshire, dedicated to reaching bikers. God is good.

Later, after having served as deacon, I was asked to become an elder in my church. Can you believe it? I am overwhelmed with God's sense of humor. The Lord has pulled our entire family from the murk and mire and placed us on solid ground with Jesus Christ as our cornerstone.

33

GAMBLING AWAY MY DREAMS

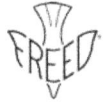

BY WAYNE D.

I was only nineteen years old when I gambled for the very first time. That was thirty-five years ago. By 1990, before I realized what was happening, my wife (my gambling partner for many of those years) and I realized that gambling was beginning to take control of my life.

My wife began to worry constantly about me and we would argue every time we gambled together. Finally, in protest, she gave up gambling.

But that didn't phase me. I just continued to gamble all by myself. I knew in my heart that my gambling addiction was getting worse, so I began to think about all the different ways that I could get the problem under control. However, none of my plans worked and I managed to fail every time I tried to quit, no matter how hard I tried to gamble in a controlled manner.

Finally, in 1991, in desperation I attended a Gamblers Anonymous (GA) meeting which was held upstairs in a church. The doors leading downstairs happened to be open and I realized that some church people were also in the building at the same time. The language at this particular GA meeting was similar to what one might expect to hear in a bar. I left, feeling very out of place, embarrassed because of the rough language, and knowing I wouldn't feel comfortable going back. Yet I knew my gambling was getting worse and I didn't know where else to turn.

OVERCOMERS OUTREACH

Years before, we had purchased a beautiful lot in Truckee, California, on which we planned to build our retirement home. How we celebrated in 1992 as that home went under construction. That home was so special because my wife and I designed it ourselves. I drew up the plans, and the construction was done by friends, family and of course, me. I stayed on the property in a seventeen-foot trailer while my wife stayed with her mother two hundred miles away during the week. She came up on weekends to see the progress of our beautiful new dream house nestled among the pine trees.

Meanwhile, my gambling addiction only got worse. I'm ashamed to say that the money that was supposed to go toward our home went to my gambling instead. Gambling became a twenty-four-hour-a-day obsession for me. I would go gambling and if I won, it merely allowed me to gamble longer. I would not stop to eat, sleep, or even go to the bathroom until I absolutely had to. Even though I knew that eventually all the money would be gone and I had exhausted places that I could cash checks, I could not stop gambling. It was pitiful.

Through desperation and a real desire to stop gambling, I went to a hypnotist who managed to help me for a few hours. Then I went to GA meetings in the Truckee area. I felt uneasy going to the meetings because I still did not feel comfortable saying that I was a compulsive gambler. What I wished I could say was that I used to be a compulsive gambler and that I now deal with an occasional temptation. I didn't want to be one of those compulsive gamblers!

On my way to a GA meeting one night, I stopped by our church to pray about my feelings. That little prayer time became for me a life-changing event. The assistant pastor and I prayed to the Lord, and on the way to the meeting, God made it clear that I was somehow to start a 12-step support group—one believing that Jesus Christ is truly the "Higher Power." With the Lord and the help of the church, we started our group and called it, oddly enough, "Overcomers."

One day I got a call from a nearby town saying that there was an international group called Overcomers Outreach. We got in touch with Bob and Pauline and made our group into a regular OO chapter. Today, through attending church regularly, and most importantly reading the Bible, prayer, and never missing the regular Overcomers meeting, Jesus Christ has truly become my "Higher Power." Dealing with temptation one day at a time, working the Steps, and finding solutions to the gambling problem is beginning to shape me into a man I never thought I could be.

I do not know how much others hurt; I only know how much I used to hurt. My deepest prayer is that if others hurt like I did, that they can find a support group like Overcomers Outreach, believing that Jesus Christ is the "Higher Power"! He will truly set us free if our love for Him is greater than the love that was developed for our addiction.

It's not the problem that is really important, it's finding a solution. Our weakness created the problem; Jesus Christ can be our strength and the solution to every problem, even compulsive gambling!

34

THE RELAPSE ROLLER COASTER

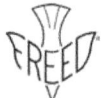

BY MIKE F.

Like so many others, I had my first drink at the early age of fifteen. There was a difference for me, though, because that first drink began a twenty-four-year love affair with alcohol. That first drink was like meeting a best friend for the first time and discovering an instant attraction and affection. From that first experience to the last drink, taken in the bathroom of a treatment center twenty-four years later, alcohol was never far away.

By the age of seventeen, I was married with an infant son and drinking every day. Having dropped out of high school to support my new family, I began to work in a honey factory. Daily drinking at work and parties at night with all my friends, who were still in high school, became my lifestyle.

At nineteen, spurred on by the death of two different friends in alcohol-related accidents, I stopped drinking long enough to get my high school diploma and start college part-time. It wasn't long, though, before I returned to drinking and school went by the wayside. This happened several times as I tried to finish school, but my drinking always got in the way.

By age twenty-three, my employers were complaining, school was forgotten, and my wife was ready to leave. I began to search for some answers. My older brother had come back from the Air Force as a

Christian (a "Jesus freak," I thought), but his life was different and he seemed to have a genuine faith in God. I'd had faith in nothing except my friend, alcohol, which was beginning to turn on me.

On July 25, 1975, I gave my life to Jesus Christ and began my spiritual journey. The conversion was dramatic and the change in my life was instant. The drinking and general insanity abruptly stopped. My wife was converted soon thereafter and together we committed our lives to the Lord. Eventually, seventeen members of my family would become Christians because of the witness of my older brother.

Diving into the Scriptures, church, and anything Christian with the same vigor that I'd had for drinking seemed to promote real growth in my life. My alcoholism was soon nothing more than a bad memory and part of my testimony. I was a new creation in Christ, and the Lord and I together would conquer all problems. Or so I thought.

Less than a year after our conversion, our second son was born. Aaron was a special gift from the Lord following a miscarriage and years of what seemed like a barren womb because of our sick lifestyle. Aaron was a gift in the timing of his arrival and the grace of his personality, which we thought was certainly a sign from God. We would live happily ever after. Following the birth of our third child, a precious daughter, our life was just like many Christian books say a Christian life should be: you accept Christ as your Savior and then sail off into the sunset.

Well, somewhere along the way this nice little Christian family got shipwrecked. Three years after our conversion and still convinced that my alcoholism was behind me, I took a drink. *One drink won't hurt*, I thought. *Just one drink with the boys couldn't hurt*. Working out of state and away from home, one drink seemed innocent enough.

Well, it only took that one drink and I was reunited with that old friend, and friends we were for a while. But soon my friend turned into a dragon. So began a pattern of periodic drinking and periodic sobriety. I kept trying to recapture the fun of my early drinking days, then the high of my spiritual conversion. I was always looking for another high, something to ease the pain I didn't even know I felt.

Several years of this and my weary wife had had enough. Following one more binge, I ransacked the furniture and put my fist through a window. She kicked me out and followed up with a restraining order. She hoped to shock me into doing something about my drinking, but instead my alcoholic mind told me I was free. I figured it was my chance to make up for all I had missed by getting married so young. So I began

THE RELAPSE ROLLER COASTER

a year-long binge of constant drinking and chasing women to ease the pain. We were divorced during that year, and eventually I landed in the Los Angeles County Jail for my second drunk driving offense. I only spent a few days in jail, but to me it seemed like a lifetime, and I began to cry out to God.

Shortly thereafter, I was introduced to Overcomers Outreach. I had been convinced that I was the only Christian to ever fall so far, the only Christian to continue to struggle with an addiction. Walking into my first meeting and finding I was not alone was an overwhelming experience. I wept as I shared my story. At last I had found a group of Christians who seemed to understand the pain of feeling like a failure before God. Through Christian support groups, I began to work on my recovery for the first time. I remained convinced, however, that my relationship with the Lord was the only answer for my addiction.

During this period of new-found sobriety I met Marilyn, a Christian woman who had struggled with alcohol as much as I had. The friendship soon turned to romance and we dated for almost two years. During our courtship we continued to attend Overcomers and our relationship with God and each other continued to grow.

Having some success at sobriety, I began to become somewhat complacent about my recovery. I was certain that the growth I had experienced would keep me from relapsing and I neglected my program. With eleven months and two weeks sobriety, I once again began to drink, setting off another round of periodic binges followed by the intense guilt and remorse that is the nightmare of every alcoholic.

Somehow in the midst of the periodic drinking, Marilyn and I were married, which began a difficult period of adjustment for both of us. Newly wed and both struggling in and out of sobriety made our early married life extremely hard for both of us, as well as for my children. After nearly a year of this struggle, we both came to a point of desperation and became serious about staying sober. I became convinced that God was calling me into counseling. I was certain that working with others was the answer to my problems.

I returned to school with a renewed determination and did quite well for about one semester. However, still believing I could stay sober without working on the inner turmoil and treating my disease, I once again relapsed. This time I was really devastated and I literally gave up and was determined to run away. I had always wanted to go to Hawaii, so one February morning I announced to my wife that we were going to

Hawaii and we would be there by June. With much reluctance, Marilyn decided to accompany me. We arrived in Kona, Hawaii, one month ahead of my schedule.

The first few months were exciting and romantic as we stayed sober and worked on our relationship. We brought my children over for the summer, which made it difficult for us financially. However, we managed to settle into our new life and get established in a church. Once again, I dove into Christian service, becoming an elder and sometimes even filling in for the pastor. I felt ministry would provide the answer and certainly I would never drink if I were serving the Lord in this way.

All seemed to be going well. We established our own business, the church was growing, and God seemed to be working in a miraculous way. The business continued to grow as did my vision for ministry, and I was certain that the Lord would use the business to support our ministry. I had it all planned out, but I was too busy to worry about going to 12-step meetings to work on my own recovery.

Somewhere along the line I took another drink, and before long the periodic binges began again, wearing out my wife, my children, and my pastor. Having to step down from my ministry in the church was a crushing blow and I once again had a feeling of hopelessness. The drinking escalated to the point where I required a drink every thirty minutes just to function.

Finally, with the business suffering tremendously, my second wife ready to leave, and all the other problems brought on by daily drinking crashing in on me, I surrendered. I cried out for help and was admitted for the second time into a treatment center.

Something was different for me this time. I was really beaten and willing to do anything, to go to any lengths, to get better. The years of denial, the years of trying everything to avoid facing the fact that I was an alcoholic began to crumble. For the first time, I was ready to face this dragon that had plagued me for so long. I had the disease of alcoholism and no amount of religiosity was going to cure me.

I conceded that I must work a program of recovery or die of this disease. A daily reprieve was all there was for one as ill as I. For the first time, I began to listen to what others had told me for so long and finally decided to attend Alcoholics Anonymous. As I surrendered to God's will for me, I immersed myself into the program and began working the Steps with my sponsor and dealing with the inner turmoil that had been untouched for so many years. I entered into recovery from alcoholism

THE RELAPSE ROLLER COASTER

and began to accept my daily reprieve, and that daily reprieve has proven to be more than enough.

With about three months of sobriety under my belt, my wife and I traveled back to California to visit family. Unbeknownst to us, we also returned to walk through our greatest trial of all. An early-morning phone call brought the news that is every parent's worst nightmare.

Aaron, my sixteen-year-old son, had been killed in a car accident. The words "Aaron is dead" stung as they rang through my head.

It was as if a huge, heavy, wooden door, like that of a dungeon, had slammed shut behind me with a deafening silence. I could almost smell the dampness. I could feel the dark moisture in the air as the room seemed to close in on me. It took an eternity for my shaking hands to hang up the phone as numbness crept in.

An odd thing had happened just a few days previous. Feeling extremely unsettled, I had taken a long walk. Climbing to the top of a hill to be alone, I had cried out to God, "Why am I here? Why this time?" As clear as any thought can be, the words, "One of your sons is going to die," raced through my mind.

"Lord," I prayed, "even if that is why I am here, I want to be in Your will. Prepare me for whatever You have for me."

I began to sense that somehow in the midst of this nightmare God was involved, even in control. When that door slammed shut with its silent roar, I knew I stood at a crossroads. In one direction was bitterness and despair, in the other was acceptance and peace. Like wild dogs, bitterness and despair pulled me in their direction, but acceptance and peace wooed me with their refreshing coolness.

While walking, only hours after the news of Aaron's death, I passed an open bar. The music played happily, the people laughed, and I could smell the alcohol. I had to make a choice: follow despair, which seemed familiar, or chase acceptance and its balm of comfort. Within the eternity of those few moments, I chose to follow the path towards acceptance. I have had to continually make that choice each time I think of how Aaron was violently ripped away from me at the tender age of sixteen.

In the *Big Book* of Alcoholics Anonymous, one of the writers stresses that acceptance is the answer to all our problems, and without the acceptance found in recovery, I would be unable to go on. First, I had to accept the fact that I was indeed an alcoholic. Then I had to accept that recovery would be a difficult process. So often as Christians, we are looking for the easier, softer way, the quick fix of a miraculous cure. God is certainly capable of miraculous intervention, but more often than not, God utilizes a step-by-step process of recovery to bring healing.

Even the apostle Paul was forced to accept his thorn in the flesh through the grace of God. Now I was being forced to accept the loss of my precious young son. If recovery had not already begun for me, I don't believe I would have survived this loss. The pain is indescribable and recovery does not lessen the pain. Instead, recovery enables me to embrace the pain rather than run from it. The death of my son seemed to unlock the door of denial that surrounded the pain in my life that I had run from for so long.

I am so grateful that the door to my recovery has been unlocked. My life is constantly changing, and usually not according to my plans. Acceptance is the key to trusting that God's plan for my life is best. Recovery began when I no longer denied my pain, but began to work through it with God's help.

My life continues to change and head in unexpected directions, but I am slowly learning to trust God at each new turn. To live a life of acceptance is the greatest of gifts that recovery can bring, allowing us to truly live one day at a time.

35

MY DAILY BREAD ALMOST KILLED ME!

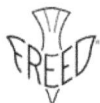

BY LYNN B.

Like many children born in the fifties, I came from a mixed-faith marriage, a volatile union of a Catholic mother and Protestant father. To keep the peace, they decided that my spiritual training would consist of letting me attend various churches and then allowing me pick a faith for myself. Growing up, I often experienced the prayers and principles of God without understanding their purpose or significance.

The only institution with a spiritual foundation that my parents agreed upon was Freemasonry (the Masonic Lodge, related somewhat to the Shriner's Lodge). My first memory of hearing the Lord's Prayer is when it was sung at Masonic installations. When the ceremonies came to the musical interlude, I remember wanting to crawl under my seat with my hands over my ears.

Thus, my initial exposure to the Lord's Prayer was both tedious and torturous. Is it any wonder that I repeated by rote, "Give us this day our daily bread?" It rolled out of my mouth and past my brain without any consideration of the meaning of the words. I learned that prayer was a generic good-luck charm chanted to ward off life's potential harm. I didn't know that the Lord's Prayer wasn't a magic talisman, or that it wasn't something to be invoked in a thoughtless, faithless manner. No one taught me that it was to be a reflective part of my friendship with Christ. No one ever told me that I should be careful of what I ask for when I pray, because I just might get it.

OVERCOMERS OUTREACH

All of my life I had been thin. I could eat anything and never appear to gain weight. Now, at thirty-five years of age, that all changed. I weighed 185 pounds. I was really miserable. My personal life was out of control, and my sick thinking told me that everything would be fine once I was 120 pounds again. Ignoring the true problem, I looked to relieve the symptom by questioning a reed-like friend as to her secret for being slender. Thinness, I believed, was some mysterious talent that I had lost, like forgetting how to ride a bicycle. She replied that I would be slim, too, if I was allergic to as many foods as she was. Oblivious to her pain, I mindlessly prayed aloud, "God, make me allergic too, so I can lose weight."

For most of my adult years, I had lived with a vague malaise that plagued me enough to make my life very uncomfortable, but never enough to seek medical treatment. When I had trouble adjusting to contact lenses, my doctor discovered that the source of my problem was undiagnosed food allergies. Test results showed a reaction to wheat, soy, and almonds.

At first, I was rather numb, and didn't acknowledge to myself how I felt. I kept saying bright, perky things like, "Well, at least it isn't cancer," thereby minimizing and devaluing my pain. In their various forms, soy and wheat are the most common ingredients in foods. Try finding something on a menu in your favorite restaurant or fast-food place that isn't batter-coated, isn't on bread or a bun, or isn't cooked in one of the many forms of soy oil. If I ate out or used canned or frozen meals, it was virtually impossible to avoid the foods to which I was allergic. I still had internal hives no matter how careful I tried to be.

As I began to try to live on my restricted diet, reality sank in. *Give up wheat?* I whined. *That means I have to give up pasta, French rolls, and pizza. An Italian woman, allergic to pizza and pasta?* I complained. This had to be some kind of a cruel joke. I loved my French rolls, my pasta, and my pizza. These weren't just foods, they were my reward when I was good and my solace when I was bad. The truth was that separation from these foods felt as though I was getting a divorce. I was devastated.

The physical discomfort was nothing compared to the emotional deprivation I felt. Eating out anywhere with friends and family, or any kind of social function involving food, left me terribly isolated and depressed. It always seemed to end with my eating a salad and watching my companions enjoy whatever was the delectable specialty of the place. It was difficult to keep from feeling that I was some kind of freak. Life became a living nightmare.

MY DAILY BREAD ALMOST KILLED ME!

After about a year of this misery, my friends and I began to pray for me to be healed. Late one night, I remembered the conversation with my friend, with my flippant prayer about allergies. I couldn't believe it; I had asked for this!

This realization just reinforced my negative views and attitudes toward God. To me, Christ always seemed to be caring, but distant and unavailable. My relationship with God was like that of a helpless child, with Him being my punitive parent. When I prayed, I felt like a little girl who was about to face an unjust father. Fearing his wrath, the child says to his face, "Yes, Daddy," but when she thinks he can't hear, she says softly to herself, "Unfair! You're unfair to me!" Reading the Scriptures often reinforced these feelings of anger and rebellion. The Old Testament story about God punishing the Israelites for murmuring when they had to eat manna every day elicited a similar reaction. Outwardly I said, "God is always right," but inwardly I whispered, "Unfair! God is unfair!"

By this time, the level of insanity in my personal life had brought me into a 12-step codependency group. There I met someone who told me about Overcomers Outreach and I went. OO helped correct my misconceptions of a weak, distant Christ and of God as a punitive father. It was through the OO group's sharing of the Scriptures that I was able to bridge the gap between the head knowledge I had of the Bible and finding a more personal relationship with Christ.

In fact, I first became aware of Overeaters Anonymous and that I had an eating disorder through Overcomers. Prior to Overcomers, I thought everybody ate ten pounds of tangerines for breakfast!

Christ used my allergies to show me that my problem wasn't that I couldn't eat certain foods, it was that they had become idols in my life—substitutes for Christ and the human relationships He wants me to have. When I felt lonely, angry, hurt, or afraid, these emotions changed and were experienced as hunger. I avoided my true feelings through eating or not eating.

Now when I am hungry, I have had to learn to stop and ask myself, *What am I feeling? Am I really hungry? Do I need someone to listen to me, or set a limit on inappropriate behavior, or do I just need a hug?* The allergies forced me to face my lack of relationship with Christ and examine all my other relationships without the numbing protection that eating provided for me.

Christ showed me that I need to be connected with other people, especially women. I have always mistrusted women. He led me to an OA women's group. The old days of eating anything and everything were gone. I let go of the fact that I couldn't eat unless I prepared the food myself. With the support of my OO and OA sisters and my sponsor, I grieved and mourned my losses. Like the Israelites, God requires me to depend on Him daily for manna.

One day at work, I experienced a true miracle. I was extremely frustrated and decided to eat six Hershey bars. Not caring that it would make me very sick, I walked into the break room and began feeding change into the snack machine. It wouldn't dispense the candy. I began to put in more and more money and still no candy. I kicked it in frustration and stood there fuming. Someone walked past me, dropped his money in the machine, and the very candy I had just spent more than five dollars trying to buy came pouring out. I then realized that this was Christ doing for me what I couldn't do for myself, and I softly thanked Him. He is faithful, even when I am not, even when I am a frightened, angry child shaking my fist at Him.

After awhile, my allergy symptoms changed, and I began to have asthma. As a result, I went back to the doctor to have a new series of tests done. The specialist told me that now I had positive reactions only to inhaled allergens. I didn't react to wheat, soy, or almonds after all. People have asked me if I am angry at my doctor, or at the situation of having suffered so much trying to avoid eating foods to which I wasn't allergic. Whether or not I was healed of food allergies, or Christ just made use of a human mistake, I don't know. Either way, it really doesn't matter, as I needed this experience to get my out-of-control eating patterns under Christ's direction.

Now I understand that Christ was never punishing me for complaining about life's unfairness. There is just a natural order that He has laid out. He lets me live out the logical consequences of choosing to have something that isn't good for me. I never knew that until He walked with me as I struggled with food these past years.

Even though I no longer have food allergies, I still can't eat everything I want, whenever I want. Sometimes I am still tempted to eat my emotions, so on a daily basis, I ask Christ to help me.

When the 12-step groups I attend close with the Lord's Prayer, I am mindful of the fact that Overcomers was where Christ brought me together with the people who really taught me to understand the words, "Give us this day our daily bread."

36

WORKAHOLISM IS A LONELY BUSINESS

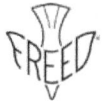

BY DUKE V.

As an only child with no brothers or sisters to play with, I was very lonely most of the time. Even when my parents and I went to visit relatives, I played alone because I had no cousins either. Typically, my parents would sit me in a corner of the parlor by a mirror, give me a set of dominoes and tell me I was to be seen and not heard. I was given all the material things a child could ever want, but it was my father's attention I desired and didn't get. My mother, on the other hand, was always behind me, supporting me in whatever I did.

At about the age of nine, I started to realize I had special abilities. I was a very curious boy and wanted to see how things worked. When I received toys, I would take them apart and put them back together again without any instructions. I would build model cars, airplanes, etc., that way; I never needed the instructions. I was always asking questions, expecting to get answers, which weren't always given. This frustrated me and made me angry.

By the age of twelve, I had already built my first intercom and installed it, complete with wiring, speakers, and switches, in our house. My mom thought this was a fantastic accomplishment. Dad was a very critical person and it seemed that no matter what I accomplished, he made light of it or put me down. This reaction from him made me feel miserable because I didn't think he loved me or approved of me.

OVERCOMERS OUTREACH

Looking back now, I see that I was starting to become a perfectionist in everything I did, from keeping my room neat as a pin, to obsessing on my appearance, to indulging my narcissistic attitude. I did all this in order to gain the approval of my father and others.

When I was a teenager of thirteen or fourteen, my parents were gone from home quite often and I was left to take care of myself. At first I enjoyed the freedom and I learned to be independent. But as time went on, I became lonely and bored. Through my years at high school, I was always seeking approval with the "in" crowd because I wanted to belong. This didn't work out because I was still a loner and wanted control of myself and others. I was also very bored with school. I went through school with only a couple of close friends, both of whom came from alcoholic homes with fathers who were never there for them either.

As a young man, I tried to seek the approval of my father by going to work with him during the summer months. It gave me the opportunity to earn some extra money and to try to get close to him. My father was a machinist and taught me some of the trade. At the same time he told me not to become a machinist myself, which confused me because I enjoyed the challenge of the machine business. I tried to model my father's performance, but I noticed that whatever task I did, my father always seemed critical, no matter how fast or accurate I was. Dad wasn't physically abusive to me, but was verbally abusive by his cutting remarks and by always putting me down.

After graduating from high school I went to work in a machine shop that was owned by one of Dad's friends. I worked there for three years as an apprentice, and after learning all aspects of the machine business, I was put in charge of the shop, including the hiring and firing, making out payroll, having the responsibilities of superintendent, and doing my own machine work. The responsibility of wearing many hats gave me a feeling of power and total control over people, which made me feel more important than my father, because he never achieved the same status.

During this time, I met and fell in love with a naive and innocent young woman named Patty and she and I married. I began working long hours, sometimes as much as sixteen or eighteen hours a day, six days a week. I worked for a small company that had many deadlines to meet, and working overtime was a chance for me to make more money for my family so we could get ahead. I was a perfectionist and was never happy with the job I had done; it was never good enough for me. I constantly strove to learn more so I would have more control over people, places, and things.

WORKAHOLISM IS A LONELY BUSINESS

Because I was so good at what I did, my boss gave me more and more responsibility, which helped me feel important. I thought I was accomplishing a lot at an early age. I didn't know then that I was setting myself up for a lifelong cycle of workaholism. I took on whatever my employer asked me to do and more. I never wanted to fail or turn down anything that might make me feel more important. I never felt that anyone else could do the job as well as I could. When I would go home at night, I never stopped thinking about work. Ideas constantly ran through my head.

In our first seven years of marriage, I never took a real vacation. When I had time off, I would do nothing but work around the house while still thinking about work. We purchased a home, a new car, and many other toys. There certainly wasn't room for God in my life, even though I was a convert to Catholicism and went to church every Sunday. All I could think about was work; I had replaced God with work in my life.

During this time, I noticed my employer began to drink heavily and I soon realized he was an alcoholic. He became verbally abusive towards me, which reminded me of my father. I now realize that I looked to this man as a father figure. I wanted his acceptance and approval, but I only got lip service. I started harboring feelings of anger and resentment and became abusive with my employees. I treated them as I was being treated by my boss. I also began to take some of my anger home. My boss had promised to give me his business someday, but instead was "giving me the business" every day! I started complaining to my wife and was generally unhappy. My boss's drinking got worse and the business began to decline. This put more of a burden on me, having to take care of the business and take care of him. The long hours and dwindling business came to an end as the company neared bankruptcy and I faced unemployment after sixteen years there.

Fortunately, prior to the business collapsing, I received an offer from one of our clients that I couldn't pass up. It was to run an entire company, five times larger than the one I was working for. The position came with many fringe benefits: a gas credit card, a pay increase, a company car, the free use of my employer's home in Lake Tahoe for vacations, etc. I thought I had the world by the tail but there were a few catches.

One requirement was I had to work a minimum of fifty hours a week, which I did for the next fifteen years! Another was the enormous amount of responsibility; I was on call twenty-four hours a day. During these years I enjoyed the work. I had a chance to learn newer technology and expand my education in my field. I was able to spearhead a lot of new projects and do some advanced design work. But once again I found myself working for a workaholic and an alcoholic, similar to my previous situation that had lasted sixteen long years. He worked seven days a week and anywhere from eight to eighteen hours a day. My new boss expected me to work just as hard as he did, keeping the same hours. He turned out to be verbally abusive to me and everyone else in the company.

In my twisted, pre-recovery thinking, I thought I must not be doing the job well enough, so I poured myself into work even more, attempting to win his favor. I became more controlling of other people within the company. The more abusive my boss became, the more controlling I became with my people.

My boss's father had died and left the company to him. He had four daughters and no sons, so I thought that someday, if I worked hard enough, I might own a part of the company. Once again, I fell into the old trap of believing that those who work more, get more.

Meanwhile, my wife and I had three children of our own, but I practically never saw them except for brief moments on weekends. To compensate for my not being home, I tried to buy their love with gifts and amusements. When we would go places, I was there physically, but mentally I was still at work, hashing through what I had to do the following day. I always wanted to give them the kind of love I had never received from my father, but because of my anger and preoccupation about work, I was usually very critical of my children, repeating the pattern of my father. Rarely did I share a dinner meal with them.

Without my realizing it, I had given my wife the sole responsibility of running the household and acting as both mother and father, which was a heavy burden with three small children. When I would arrive home late at night, I only wanted to relax, whereas Patty wanted to talk because she was stressed with the problems of raising the children. This led to a lot of arguing because I didn't want to involve myself with those problems. I found myself coming home later and later, saying only a few words to Patty, eating my dinner (warmed for hours in the oven), falling asleep at the table, getting up to go to bed, and waking up the next morning to start the cycle all over again.

By this time my workaholism had really gone into high gear and I found myself living on an adrenaline high most of the time. As a rule I was edgy and short-tempered. However, on Sundays when we would take our family to church, we looked like the perfect Christian family.

WORKAHOLISM IS A LONELY BUSINESS

The children were dressed immaculately; we put on our fake smiles and interacted with other parishioners as though everything was just fine. (Later, I found out what "fine" really meant: Fouled up, Insecure, Neurotic and Emotionally unstable!) We were good friends with the pastor and my wife sang in the choir. During the services I would usually doze off or be thinking about work, not really getting much from God or the service. God still did not have an important place in my life.

Usually Patty and I had an argument on the way to church and would resume it on the way home. When my argument with Patty was over, I would start in on the children, criticizing them for not behaving or paying attention during the service. I realize now that this erratic behavior was caused by my coming down off the adrenaline high from my hectic work week. Many Sundays I would end up with a terrible migraine headache and would have to stay in bed most of the day. Needless to say, this did not give my family much quality time with me.

This vicious cycle led to an increase in my drinking, which helped me escape the responsibilities and problems I had. My boss invited me to lunch with him on Saturday and we would drink and mull over the problems at work. Soon we began to go out on weekday evenings and have a few drinks, sometimes so many that I drove home in a blackout. This went on for many years. My boss was like Dr. Jekyll and Mr. Hyde. When he was drinking he was my pal, but back at work he was just as abusive as ever. I felt anxious, hurt, and confused by his behavior. I valued myself less and less, which led to low self-esteem and anger, and drove me even more to obsessively become the best at everything I did.

I wanted and needed his approval, which he refused to give. I began to burn out. My self-esteem I was gone, my mental state was shaky, I had headaches every day, and I was constantly angry. I got to the point where I did not want to go to work. I didn't want to go anywhere or see anyone. I just wanted to sleep. I would wake up several times during the night and pace the floor trying to think of a way to get out of this situation. The money had become an obsession to me and, due to my spending habits, I was deep in debt. I contemplated suicide.

One evening I came home so deeply depressed that I broke down and cried. I told my wife that I had to leave the company; I could not take the stress and abuse any longer. Patty was very kind and understanding, but frightened because of the debt we had incurred, but she supported me in my decision to leave the company, which I did.

OVERCOMERS OUTREACH

In this chaotic struggle, God was beginning to work in my life. I found myself seeking the Lord and asking Him for His will in my life and a change in me. I prayed that He would lead me to a decent employer and job. The answer came when I was offered a position with a man who was a kind, decent gentleman—the total opposite of my previous boss. This new job was a salaried, forty-hour-a-week position, which gave me the chance to renew my relationship with my family. Even though the money was much less, by God's grace we were able to make ends meet. I started feeling good about myself again and was even learning how to set boundaries with the help of my new boss. He insisted on a forty-hour week for me and he did the same. His attitude came as a complete shock to me. He would say, "What you don't finish today, you can always do tomorrow." I was floored; my other employers had insisted I work into the wee hours to complete the job.

My new job seemed like heaven. Unfortunately, after three and a half years, the business started to decline and there was not enough work for me. I chose to leave the company, but remained friends with my former employer.

Just prior to leaving that job that summer, I happened to be at a tool show at the Los Angeles Convention Center, where by chance I ran into my previous employer. He was very pleasant to me and we talked at length. He mentioned that his business was doing quite well and said that if I ever wanted to come back, my old position as plant superintendent was available.

This offer sounded like my chance to return to my old job, but with a better working atmosphere, so we agreed to meet the following week, have dinner, and discuss the possibility of my returning. I had mixed feelings about the meeting. On the one hand, I felt fear and anxiety because of the way this man had abused me in the past, but on the other hand, I had many debts and the money would come in handy. I discussed this option with my wife and after long deliberation I decided to return to my old job.

I realized before even starting back that my old boss had not changed but I had. In the three years with my previous employer, God had given me time to learn about myself and He had begun to heal a wounded part of me. I had even learned to set boundaries for myself. In addition, a men's Bible study that I was attending with my brother-in-law served as a monumental step toward my recovery.

WORKAHOLISM IS A LONELY BUSINESS

In September of 1985, I returned to my old job, but this time with new boundaries and goals. My employer agreed to most of my terms, which included a fifty-hour work week with no Saturdays, a substantial raise in pay with other benefits, and no verbal abuse. For the first few years, all went well. I no longer went to drinking lunches or dinners with the boss; instead, I went home to my family at a reasonable hour.

But things took a turn for the worse when a couple of top employees left and instead of replacing them, my boss dumped their responsibilities on me. I felt obligated to take up the slack. I see now that this was a terrible mistake because I was again working more hours and spending time away from my family. With the added pressures and lack of rest, I began drinking more. Both my drinking and workaholism spun out of control again.

In the midst of all this, I was not even aware of the problems at home. My wife was struggling with the children, who were now teenagers, and I was unable to help her. At about that time, she started attending a 12-step recovery group for ACAs, and we became aware that our youngest daughter had a serious problem with substance abuse. I was devastated. My wife was encouraged to attend Al-Anon and through a Christian friend found Overcomers Outreach. I became interested in her recovery because I could see a definite change in her behavior. Despite everything that was going on in the family, she seemed much happier and had more energy than she had had for a long time.

It was around this time that the final turning point came for me as I went on my last alcoholic binge. We were at a wedding and I got so drunk my wife asked me for the car keys. I refused initially. For the first time, she did not react emotionally to my stupor but calmly said she would take a cab home if I would not let her drive me home.

I let her drive. This whole incident was so surprising because she usually called me every name in the book when I would get drunk. This time she reacted to the situation calmly but firmly.

A miracle happened to me the next day. When I awoke, I felt remorseful and asked God to take away the compulsion to drink. No sooner had I asked Him to do this than a warmth had enveloped me and I felt that I would never drink again. That was many years ago. The Lord delivered me. Since I seemed interested in my wife's recovery, she invited me to attend an Overcomers meeting.

At one of the first Overcomers meetings, I met a person who shared his story and it sounded just like mine; he was a workaholic. He eventually became my sponsor and I am truly blessed by our fellowship. I've been able to use many slogans of the program, some of which sounded corny when I first heard them, but which now I really like, such as: "Easy does it," "One day at a time," "What you don't get done today, you can always do tomorrow," etc.

All around my desk at work, I have momentos of the program that remind me constantly to take life on life's terms one day at a time. The Serenity Prayer hangs above my desk. Now when I have a stressful day, I know I have an Overcomers meeting that I can go to, along with my other 12-step programs. I have friends I can talk to without being judged or looked down upon. I can also ask for prayer from my Christian brothers and sisters. Overcomers Outreach is like another family to me. Most importantly, I feel God's presence in these groups. I've also been able to give something back by volunteering at some of the Overcomers conferences.

Today my life has been made richer because of Overcomers Outreach and other 12-step programs. I have found God, and my friendships and family life are improving because I am able to be honest and truthful.

I enjoy the work that I do, and I still work long hours by some people's standards, but it's much better than before. Today I am able to set boundaries and keep my job in perspective by treating other people as I would like to be treated—with kindness and respect.

37

THE PATCHWORK OF MY LIFE

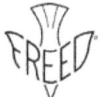

BY FRANCES H.

My passion has always been quilting. I love to see all the colorful pieces come together and form a pattern. I just wish life could be that simple. The pieces of my life were fragmented for a number of years until I stumbled into recovery back in 1983, due to a son who struggled with drug-related problems.

Since I was raised in a conservative Southern Baptist home, such problems as substance abuse were foreign to me. There was never any alcohol in my family and I didn't even know anyone who drank. My family considered such people undesirable.

When I make a quilt, I begin by choosing a pattern, then the fabric (whether bright, dark, muted, or plain) and cut the pieces according to the pattern. Then I sew them together into squares and place them into a master design to form a work of art.

The pattern I chose for my life was to marry a Christian man, have children (more than one, because growing up as an only child was very lonely for me), and to raise those children in a loving Christian home, training them so that they would make the right choices to live productive and happy lives. My ultimate goal was to "train up a child in the way he should go and when he is old he will not depart from it" (Prov. 22.6). I just wish it was as easy as it sounds in the biblical account.

One day I found that my Christian family plan did not seem to be working out. Our eldest child, a son, was exhibiting abnormal behavior and was generally rebellious. Our whole family was affected. Our wonderful Christian home was in turmoil. I spent much time explaining away his behavior (e.g., his friends were influencing him, it wasn't his fault, etc.). I made excuses for him, assuring his high school counselor that he did not smoke because I did not smell cigarettes on him. I waited patiently for him to outgrow this stage, begging him to change, begging God to change him, trying to arrange situations where he would meet someone who could influence him positively, etc. It never occurred to me that he had a disease that I could not treat. These were dark pieces in my life's quilt.

It was during this son's junior high and high school years that I developed physical problems, including depression and panic attacks. My doctor gave me some tranquilizers, which helped for a while but which eventually became a crutch. Later on, I faced the challenge of going off these pills. I even went to a counselor for a while to try and figure out what was causing the panic attacks. Finally, he brought in my husband to discuss our son's constant appeals for money and its effect upon my peace of mind. No solutions were found; my attacks continued.

During this time in my life, my comfort and identity resided in my ability to play the piano. This was my solace, and even though circumstances in our family were out of control and I couldn't seem to do anything about them, I could still function in my job as church pianist.

One Sunday as I was preparing to play the piano for the church service (my husband had gone to northern California to rescue our son from another undesirable situation), I ventured to ask for help from my pastor. He only said, "I'll pray for you, but I can't help you. Just go ahead and play the piano and forget about the situation." So with lots of anxiety and feelings of panic I played, smiled, and pretended that everything was fine.

I concluded that I must keep smiling and keep pretending there was nothing wrong, and that God would eventually provide a solution to the craziness. I believed that my answers should come from within the church and that if they didn't come, I must be doing something wrong. My faith must be lacking. As time went by I became so panic-stricken that I could not continue in my capacity as church pianist. I was devastated. My life was suddenly out of control.

During those years my husband buried himself in his job and hobbies. When he was home, we spent much time arguing, debating, and giving instructions to our son who was not fitting into the ideal family pattern. Mealtimes were the most intense times for all.

THE PATCHWORK OF MY LIFE

It seemed that the entire focus in our family was on this eldest son, just as a spotlight focuses upon a movie star. The other family members were in the background. Our younger son became the family hero, excelling in school and sports, and trying to make up for what his brother was doing. He tried to convince his brother to follow the family standard, but to no avail. Our daughter excelled in school also, and followed the teachings of our family. She stayed busy with her music and detached herself emotionally from us to avoid the family conflict.

I played the role of worrier, interpreter, referee, and policewoman who tried to carry out my husband's orders and report back to him when they were not followed. Our family never really discussed what was going on, but just passively hoped that a solution would come. This problem was literally tearing our family apart. When our son would get in trouble and need money or other help, his dad would help him "just one more time." If my husband was tired of rescuing, I would take over the role. We were on a constant merry-go-round. Each time, we hoped that the immediate crisis might be the last and that our son would turn his life around. Each rescue was like a bandage that helped for a while, but proved to be only temporary. Each time our son ran into trouble using drugs, we brought him back, cleaned him up, believed his promises to change, and hoped that this time he had hit his bottom and would get his life on course. Yet the cycle invariably repeated itself.

I finally came to the realization that I did not even like my son, and was relieved when he was out of the house, even though my thoughts were constantly obsessing about him and his situation. I would spend hours wondering where he was, what he was doing, if he was safe, if he was getting enough food, if he had warm clothing, etc. Another nagging thought was that Christian mothers should not feel this way about their children.

As I tried to accept the fact that our son was chemically addicted, I was devastated. I began to ask myself a thousand questions. What had I done wrong? What could I do to change the situation? I attended Bible studies and looked for answers and even ventured to ask for prayer. The reaction to those requests were anywhere from "Oh, you poor thing" to "If you had done so-and-so, this would not have happened." Then the free advice would flow.

Our son became unkempt, wandered the streets out of work, and expected the family to do his bidding at all times. My biggest questions were, *What will people think of me when they see my son in this condition?*

OVERCOMERS OUTREACH

What do I tell our relatives? Do I say he is just fine (which I don't really know), or should I tell the truth that he is addicted to drugs and alcohol?

The question that nagged me personally was, *How can I possibly be happy when my child is leading such a life?* I was embarrassed, as I felt the whole neighborhood knew about our disastrous problem. As I pondered all these nagging questions and didn't find solutions, I became more and more ill with depression and anxiety. Even though I tried to fool everyone by looking OK, smiling, and pretending, on the inside I was living with the fear of panic attacks. I was always fearful that I would pass out while driving, or at the grocery store, or while playing the piano at church. Still at conflict with my attitude, I felt that those who had addictions or compulsions must be bad people because they obviously made bad choices. The parents of children such as mine must have done something terribly wrong, or their kids would have turned out better. I was haunted by the verse about "training up a child in the way he should go...."

Crisis finally hit our family on August 31, 1983, and God's plan began to immediately unfold right before our eyes. My prayers began to be answered hour by hour, but not in the way I had planned. Because of an automobile accident, we brought our son home and made a phone call to a friend, asking him to come to our house and help us talk to him. Another friend just happened to come by and spent several hours talking and counseling with him. Through the course of the evening, we were encouraged to phone Bob Bartosch, who happened to be a member of our church. He spoke with our son, who agreed to go into treatment! I was numb and incredulous. Our son was getting help, friends had learned about the whole situation, seen him at his worst, and they still loved us. I felt both relief and anxiety, dreading from the start what might happen when he got out in thirty days.

We learned that our son's boss was so concerned about him that she had put his name on a prayer list at her church. Miraculously, his insurance policy paid for his treatment. (He entered the facility thirty minutes before the company's new insurance took over, which would not have paid for it—how's that for a miracle?)

The following Sunday after church, Dave B., who was involved in the Overcomers group, greeted us and said, "I understand you've been through deep waters this week. The Overcomers meeting is at our house tonight. Won't you come?" In just three days I learned that I no longer had to keep a secret and I no longer felt alone.

The first Overcomers meeting was overwhelming. What a relief it was to finally be able to share honestly and see nods of understanding. I

THE PATCHWORK OF MY LIFE

could reveal my true feelings: sadness, frustration, fear, and anger (yes, even anger with God), and no one would give advice or condemn me for those feelings. I still cannot answer the question that Bob Bartosch asked me as he gave me a big bear hug. Why had I waited so long? The encouragement I got there was so wonderful and even though there was still numbness and anxiety, I was given some steps to take to get help for myself.

The first thing I did was attend an Al-Anon meeting. Even though it wasn't a church-sponsored meeting, my new Overcomers friends assured me that I could take what I liked and leave the rest. When I arrived, it was with fear and trembling, but I was at a point of willingness to try just one more time to gather as much information as I possibly could. I needed ideas about what to say and do when the next crisis hit!

What a pleasant surprise awaited me at that meeting. People really listened and didn't give me advice. They just gave a whole lot of hugs. I felt more understanding and acceptance there than at any of my church meetings. And I soon discovered that the program using the 12 Steps was not in conflict with the Bible. In fact, it was the practical way to live those Scriptures that were already part of my Christian walk. I needed to walk through these Steps, giving my son over to God's care.

I continued attending Overcomers. And I continued to attend Al-Anon. One thing that I was made aware of was that I was not responsible for other people anymore; I was only responsible for myself. I was totally overwhelmed one day as I stood at my ironing board and thought about the things I had been learning. I realized that my son had a disease that *he* must take care of, not me. My husband also has a disease called diabetes that he must take care of. I spent most of my time worrying about these two, and wondering what I was going to do. I almost felt invisible. My thoughts and energy had always been on my husband and my children. Who was Frances? I now made it my personal challenge to find out who I was and who God said I was.

As I began attending meetings and practicing the concepts of the 12-step program, my anxiety attacks began to diminish. I was also introduced, through an Al-Anon friend, to a group called Families Anonymous. In that group, I met parents who understood exactly what I was going through, and I continue attending today after almost twenty years. There I know I can find friendship, encouragement, hope, and continual input that is totally relevant to my own situation.

I need to remain focused on my life and allow my son to live his. Now when the phone rings with the next problem or opportunity to rescue,

OVERCOMERS OUTREACH

I am aware that my son must be responsible for himself. I can tell him, "I love you" (and now can really mean it). I can say, "I can't help you," because he has a disease he must take care of himself. I can say, "You know exactly where to get help," because he knows about AA and the available treatment. And I can tell him, "I have confidence in you and know that you will do what is best." You see, when I was solving his problems and rescuing him, I was really saying, "I don't think you are capable of taking care of yourself."

I now have peace in knowing that our son's recovery is not my responsibility. Although he is still struggling, I continue to have hope. I rejoice in the recovery of those his age who I see at Overcomers groups, and am encouraged when I hear them share their victories.

As I review the years since 1983, I can see God's plan and His pieces of my life's quilt fitting together. Perhaps the best part of that quilt is having an opportunity to work in the Overcomers Outreach central office. I love being able to share with others. In addition to sending out literature, I have learned to use the computer. I have pursued other interests for myself, developed my talents, and allowed the rest of my family members to do the same. As these pieces continue to come together in my life, my favorite Scripture has become Jeremiah 29:11, "For I know the plans I have for you, says the Lord. They are plans for good and not for evil, to give you a future and a hope."

God has provided people and resources to help us see and feel His love and grace. My life today is richly filled with new hope, so different than it was a few years ago, even though our son is still not in recovery. I am privileged to attend Overcomers Outreach. I continue to put our son in God's hands and pray that he will someday find recovery. It is important to me to continually keep in mind that I am not in charge of this world, God is!

Today, the pieces of the quilt of my life are turning into an array of technicolor patterns that only God could piece together in His time.

38

NIGHTMARE TO MIRACLE

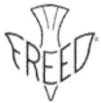

BY MARY JEAN B.

The doorbell rang.

I woke up and looked at the clock. I wondered, *Who would be at the door at two* A.M.*?* (This was the beginning of many two A.M. incidents to follow.) My husband went to the door and I was close behind.

A woman whom we didn't know asked us if we knew where our child was. We thought our fifteen-year-old daughter was spending the night with a girlfriend from school. But, according to this woman, our daughter had attended a party with her daughter where they had gotten drunk, and she had gone to another girl's house to recuperate.

Needless to say, we were stunned and angry. We got dressed and quickly drove to where our daughter was and confronted her. On the way back home, she got the full effect of our anger and frustration for what she had done to herself and to us. Among many other things, we later learned that it usually takes about two years before parents realize their child has a serious addiction problem. Denial is strongly at work for parents in these circumstances and we were a textbook case—a real mess! Thus began the nightmare every parent prays will never happen. For us the nightmare turned into a journey we would never have chosen to take, but God had something very special planned for us down the road.

OVERCOMERS OUTREACH

How could this be happening to us? Our little girl was our pride and joy with her starched pinafores and bobbing blond curls. We had raised her three older brothers with little or no problems. Two had followed in their father's footsteps and chosen military careers upon graduation from high school. Our third son was a year away from graduating college. How could our beautiful fifteen-year-old daughter, who had even more advantages than her brothers, be rebelling and giving us so much trouble and heartache?

We were doing everything right; we regularly attended church, were active in leadership roles, contributed financially, read our Bibles, and faithfully prayed about life's circumstances for ourselves and others. The children too were active in church-related youth group activities. Where had we gone wrong?

We came to dread weekends, since they were party time. The more we tried to control our daughter, the worse the situation became. Tension, anger, loss of sleep, and bizarre and unacceptable behavior became the norm in our home where peace, serenity, and loving relationships had once prevailed. This wasn't living; this was chaos! Suddenly we were dealing with school truancy, a nose-dive in grades, driving under the influence without a driver's license, jails, court appearances, judges, lawyers, wild uncontrolled behavior scenes, leaving home, coming back, and more, all accompanied with an I-don't-give-a-damn attitude. Professional counseling and adolescent treatment programs didn't seem to help either. Our child was on a path of self-destruction and we wondered if it would ever end.

We continued to attend church, smiling on the outside, but dying on the inside, thinking that we were the only ones going through this nightmare. We were afraid to share it with anyone, particularly within the church, for fear they wouldn't understand. Little did we know just how many people sitting in pews around us were experiencing the very same things. God was already at work. He was about to bring some very special people into our lives to help us, and they were right in the church.

About three years after that fateful two A.M. experience, we heard about a Circle of Concern in our church called Overcomers. This was a support group for those who were recovering alcoholics and anyone who was affected by someone who drank. Bob and Pauline Bartosch happened to be the leaders of the group that met on the first Sunday evening of each month.

NIGHTMARE TO MIRACLE

One night, following our daughter's heavy use of substances, we really hit our bottom. We remembered reading in the church bulletin that Overcomers would be meeting that Sunday evening. This could be an avenue of help. What perfect timing for God to perform His first of many miracles. Our daughter, who was so sick, made that meeting and met Bob and Pauline Bartosch and a room full of loving, accepting, recovering Christians. Bob and Pauline recommended a new thirty-day 12-step treatment program at a local community hospital where, as a family, we could begin the healing process.

The next day our daughter was admitted to the recovery program that required the participation of as many family members as possible. That was the beginning of an incredible education for us all. Our youngest son, who was twenty-two years old, was able to join us in family focus week, five days of concentrated sessions learning about the disease of alcoholism. We were introduced to the 12 Steps of Al-Anon and Alcoholics Anonymous.

At the end of the week, each of us had an opportunity to express to our daughter our feelings about how her drinking had affected us. In this same setting, she had the opportunity to express her feelings to each of us also. Our meetings together were especially significant in that we were able to tell each other of our love, support, and appreciation for one another. By this time, sanity was returning to our relationships and underneath the frustration, anger, pain, and craziness, each could feel a lot of love for the other.

It's been a few years since our daughter entered treatment and we've had many opportunities for clear reflection. While the road to recovery has been neither always smooth nor problem-free, we are so grateful for the 12 Steps that show us how to live life one day at a time. The introduction to 12-step daily living was a life-changing experience. It started us on a new road to recovery. We quickly learned that recovery is a life-long journey, not just a short sprint for a person to recapture control of one's own destiny. We firmly believe that control of our lives must be in God's hands at all times, not in our own. During this difficult time, we were provided with tools for living. One of the most valuable principles we learned was that we are not responsible for another person's happiness or actions.

We began attending Overcomers on a regular basis and were surprised to find others there from our church—folks whose lives we thought were trouble–free. What a blessing it was to see other Christians come and receive help and hope and begin their own recovery.

Our story could be the story of countless Christian families who are suffering as we once suffered. Denial, anger, resentments, frustration, blame, bitterness, and even dishonest emotions toward the one we love are some of the overwhelming symptoms that surround families afflicted with the disease of addictive or compulsive behavior. These symptoms were rampant in our home. During those dark days of despair we didn't know if life would ever be normal again. Well, it hasn't been normal (whatever that is), but it has been exciting and rewarding. Our relationship with our daughter is now very special. Today there is an honest expression of openness, respect, and love flowing both ways. Miracles do happen. One happened in our family and it's still in process.

Our biggest surprise was to learn that we didn't have to carry these burdens alone. Our Overcomers family continues to celebrate our miracle with us, and reminds us to keep coming back because it works!

39

SPENDING IT ALL

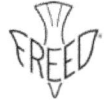

BY JIM S.

It's morning again. I've got to go to work, but there's a sick, sinking feeling in the pit of my stomach. I think I have enough gas to get to work and back. I'd better make a sandwich or I won't get anything for lunch. I'll take the heels of the loaf so that the rest of the family can have regular slices.

Let's see, there are still ten days until payday. I balanced the checkbook last night and we're $150 overdrawn. I wonder how long it will be before my checks start bouncing. It's been getting worse lately. The amount I owe is increasing and it seems like the calls are coming from my bank earlier and earlier in the pay cycle.

It's those phone calls that make me crazy! About 10:30 every morning I start getting the fidgets and actually jump every time the phone rings. I'm afraid to even leave my desk, though sometimes I have to, just to do my job. But I'm always haunted with the thought, *What if I miss a call from the bank and they bounce another one of my checks?* Then my mind races on to the question, *What if I get the call and then I write more rubber checks in order to cover the ones I just bounced?*

I can't go on like this! I'm getting anxiety attacks every morning. My heart pounds, I have cold sweats and those ever-present fidgets. It's so hard to sit still at my desk, but I must try. If my company finds out about all this, I will surely lose my security clearance, along with my job. And without a job, everything else will come unraveled. I just know that my wife will leave me this time if I fail to provide for her. There's another rush of cold sweat and here come the fidgets again!

I just remembered about a support group someone mentioned to me recently. I've been wondering if it could help such a hopeless person like me. But now I'm beginning to be willing to try anything. The group they told me about was called Debtor's Anonymous. I found out there's a meeting at noon today, and another one later in the week. As much as I want to put it off, I realize I can't wait. I need to do something today!

I found the Debtor's Anonymous meeting and all kinds of people were there. Some drove up in Cadillacs and a few rode in on bicycles. I still can't explain how the meeting helped me, but I did feel better somehow. There were people there with huge debts and small incomes who were struggling just to make ends meet every week, I couldn't get over how they could be succeeding in this program and they seemed hopeful. That was the amazing thing. Could there be hope for me?

I've been in the 12-step program for nine months now, and I wish I could say that all my financial problems are solved. Actually, my wife has just left me and is forcing me to give her a divorce. Last night while she was moving her stuff out of the house, I took a long walk. I just don't understand why God is letting this happen, especially now that I'm making progress in recovery. The debts are going down slowly. All my creditors are getting a token payment, even if it's only five dollars per month.

My job transfer five months ago, which cut out all my overtime, really put me in a terrible bind. I started to fret over it until I called my Debtor's Anonymous companions. They held me to the plan, and even helped me formulate an emergency spending plan to get through the first month without working overtime. While I walked last night, I prayed the Serenity Prayer over and over. I finally accepted that I don't have any control over what my wife does. That's when I turned around and headed back to the house. I began to sing hymns and praise songs because I felt like, no matter what, it was all going to work out.

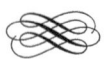

SPENDING IT ALL

Well, it's been one year since the divorce. Without my wife's income, I realized I couldn't afford the six-hundred-dollar-per-month rent. I also didn't need a four-bedroom house all to myself. So now I'm living in a one-bedroom apartment, the cheapest one I could find, but it's OK. It's so close to work I could even walk there if I needed to. It's not far from the university either. And since I've been working my program, God has even given me incentive to go back and finish my bachelor's degree.

I must admit that the clearance investigation gave me a few anxious moments, especially when the government department we work for called me in to discuss my finances. I'm convinced that if I hadn't started Debtor's Anonymous when I did, I would have lost my job for sure. But instead, I was able to show my employer that I was making progress on my debts. In fact, several creditors have been completely paid off! What a miracle! I've even saved enough in my special fund called "Gifts to Me" that I've bought a guitar!

It's been four years now since I joined Debtor's Anonymous. It looks like the group may disband. At one time I would have been devastated, but in the meantime I discovered an Overcomers Outreach group, where I can express my Christian faith along with working my program. Other groups, like CoDA (Codependents Anonymous) and Al-Anon have really been helpful too.

At this point I've found that the money issues don't even bother me anymore, unless the relationships in my life are out of whack. Above all, I must keep my relationship with God straight first. That way, the relationships with my son and fiancée seem to work so much better.

My son is in trouble most of the time. Neither his probation officer nor I can seem to get him to live up to the terms of his probation. I can look back and see how my codependence with his mother contributed to his present condition. But I also realize that I can't let him keep me from doing what is right when he tries to make me feel guilty for his problems.

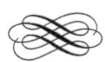

OVERCOMERS OUTREACH

I can't believe it—I finally graduated from college. It only took twenty-one years! I'm almost out of debt. I even took a whole week's vacation this year in New York. Who would have ever dreamed that I would someday fly to Boston, rent a car, and best of all, pay for it all with cash?

God has really taken care of me, even when I didn't understand what was going on. I'm going to be married again in a couple of months. That's real scary, but she is a real practical woman who feels the same way I do about being in debt.

I've been married for two and a half years now. The icing on the cake is that we bought a house a year ago—the first house for either of us. I was so afraid of what the mortgage company would say about my credit history, but I wrote them a letter telling them how I paid off all my creditors, and that I was consistently continuing the practices that got me out of debt. Wasn't I surprised when they offered to loan us a whole lot more money than we were willing to borrow?

God has given us a wonderful son who is just eighteen months old. My oldest son is twenty now and living in another state. My wife's daughter even moved in with us last summer. God is so good.

My failure in my first marriage, as well as with compulsive spending, have taught me a lot about relationships, and have brought me closer to God than ever before. If it hadn't been for all my failings, I would never have gotten desperate enough to turn to a program like Debtor's Anonymous. I could have missed the recovery that God had planned for me. And I may never have found my Overcomers Outreach group that encourages my faith from week to week.

Thank God, I finally hurt badly enough to reach out for help. He was there for me. Today, instead of having a perpetual hole in my pocket, my cup is full and running over, thanks be to God!

CHRISTIAN NURSE NEEDED HER "FIX"

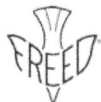

BY PHYLLIS H.

The Scripture verse I could relate to during my roller-coaster years of spiritual successes and failures was Romans 7:15 where the apostle Paul laments, "I don't understand myself at all, for I really want to do what is right, but I can't. I do what I don't want to do—what I hate." That seemed to be the story of my life.

I pled for help and strength from God, but instead I seemed to be left with no energy or desire to continue. Why couldn't I manage to live my life pleasing to God? My husband and I had a nice home and smart children, and were well-known for our community and church involvements. We always managed to portray the mask of looking good in spite of our circumstances. But a gnawing, festering wound within my soul was eating away at my self-esteem. My creativity and joy were gone.

How could this be? I had accepted Christ as my Savior when I was eight years old and had grown to love Jesus as my best friend. However, my spiritual growth came to an abrupt halt when I was fifteen, because I began to date a boy who wasn't a Christian. My Bible reading and prayer were gradually dispensed with until my life totally revolved around this new love. When he broke off the relationship, I was suddenly left without purpose or direction.

How frightened I was! My mind began to question whether God could possibly still love me after I had rejected Him in my disobedience.

Nevertheless, I reasoned that if I was going to hell, I may as well have fun doing it. So it wasn't long before I chose a new group of friends who drank socially. Little did I realize what was ahead.

My first drink of alcohol did something magical to my hurts and pains. I could laugh; I could have fun. And I didn't feel that weight of guilt when I was drunk. I thought perhaps I had found the answer to all my problems.

I continued to attend church as always, and eventually came to the realization after searching the Bible that God did still love me after all. He still wanted me as His child, no matter what I had done. So with humble gratitude, I confessed my sins and recommitted my life to Christ. But instead of celebrating His forgiveness and His great love for me, I began to be filled with a fear of failure and loss and was terrified of losing my salvation again. My doubts began to sabotage all joy, and it wasn't long before I began a pattern of drinking, pleading with God for forgiveness each time, and then promising never to drink again for the rest of my life. I hated myself and seemed to be caught in a vicious trap.

My freshman year at the state university opened up a whole new world of drinking opportunities. By the end of the spring term, I was drinking almost daily just to fight off my depression and guilt. When I returned home for the summer, God gently reminded me of His claim on my life and I once again recommitted my life to the Lord. I realized then that I would need to attend a college where drinking was prohibited if I was just to survive. So I began to attend a Christian college in my area, majoring in Christian ministries the following term, thinking this would solve all my problems. But I was wrong.

The fear of failure continued to nip at my renewed commitment to serve Christ. I was appalled to find that alcohol could be found at this "safe" institution. I gave into the temptation to drink "just one time," and knew that I would need a lot of help if I was going live victoriously.

But then I met my future husband, Ron, and I was hopeful that a life with him would free me from the destructive and demoralizing drinking behaviors to which I was so drawn. We began our married life in the romantic wilds of Alaska. For a while God seemed so close and life was good. But eventually an insidious, deep depression began to haunt me. Then the unthinkable happened: I injured my back. Of course, the doctor prescribed various pills to relieve the pain, decrease anxiety, and help me sleep. My friends encouraged me to use these medications and my husband was happy to see me out of my misery. But I secretly found myself

CHRISTIAN NURSE NEEDED HER "FIX"

thrilled at the way the pills made me feel inside. And so a new cycle of depression, physical ailments, and prescription drug use began.

We soon moved to Oregon and joined a good church, feeling things were beginning to improve again. I tried to believe that finally I would be able to live a fruitful Christian life. Our home became the center for an informal singles ministry, two Bible studies, and much praise music. I joyfully began to write music, lead choirs, and teach Sunday school. The spiritual stirrings of my youth bubbled within and I knew that I would never again fail the Lord!

But then one night, while attending a secular workshop in another town, a new acquaintance began to pour drinks for everyone. I declined a drink, but he kept insisting. For a very brief moment I reasoned that only one drink would be all right. Unfortunately, I was unable to drink only one and almost drowned in the hotel's hot tub that night due to my drunken condition.

I returned home totally devastated, certain that God must despise me. Enthusiasm for ministry evaporated as the long arm of the pit of hell reached into my soul. I found reasons to cancel Bible studies and choir practices. I began working outside the home and enrolled in a rigorous schedule of college classes as I sought to escape my problems and dull the pain.

During that time, our children were born. I became a registered nurse and life looked good on the outside while the torment still raged on the inside. Every time I began to sense God's love and leading, some event would precipitate the use of pills or alcohol and all joy would abruptly cease.

Soaked with the weight of guilt and self-contempt, I continued to portray the looking-good looks as the mask of deception grew heavier. Depression and suicidal thoughts increased in duration and frequency, and it wasn't long before I obtained a prescription for a new, stronger narcotic. I found myself obsessed with maintaining a sufficient supply and resumed drinking. I no longer cared what others thought. I only feared that one of the many doctors I was calling would eventually confront me about drug abuse, so I decided it was time to steal narcotics from work. I was the nursing supervisor, and my coworkers, patients, and physicians trusted me, so there was very little risk. My next opportunity to steal medications would be soon and I was prepared. Fortunately, God intervened before I was able to take this pathetic step of desperation.

OVERCOMERS OUTREACH

The next Sunday I played for worship service and taught Sunday school with a hangover, as usual. Later at home I read a news article about a political figure and her battle with alcohol and prescription drug abuse. I was surprised, because I thought that only street derelicts, drunk drivers, and abusive parents needed treatment for chemical dependency or alcoholism. Then the pastor called to invite me to a special Sunday night meeting. "Phyllis," he said, "I don't know what's wrong, but I really feel you need to come tonight."

A small spark of hope glimmered as I drove to church that night, daring to hope that God hadn't given up on me after all. And what I heard that night propelled me into a new life, free of guilt and full of joy, far beyond my wildest dreams!

I sat there in a dull, drugged haze as the evangelist explained that Christians are God's precious children, and that Satan is determined to destroy us! He went on to say that the day we accept Christ as our Savior, our enemy Satan plots and plans our disarmament, disablement, and demise. In fact, he emphasized, "Those with the greatest potential seem to be the ones hardest hit by Satan's attacks!"

Then the speaker asked if our spiritual growth was repeatedly disrupted by a particular temptation or event. Oh, yes! My heart thrilled. I was filled with both relief and grief as I made my way to the altar. I had been tricked all these years! Satan had planned these attacks to make sure that I would not have an effective ministry or a joyful life. God still loved me and wanted me to be His child after all!

Later that evening I did something I thought I could never do. I discussed the full extent of my alcohol and drug use with my pastor. He facilitated my admission into an inpatient drug treatment facility where I learned that I was absolutely powerless over alcohol or drugs but that God was powerful. Only He could restore me to sanity, renew my spirit, and recreate a new heart within me.

During my first year of recovery I regularly attended Alcoholics Anonymous and continued to grow in the love of the fellowship there. But I longed to share and pray with other Christians in recovery. While on vacation, I visited an Overcomers Outreach group in a local church. I was overjoyed to find others like me who identified Jesus Christ as their "Higher Power." I discovered that I was one of thousands of Christians nationwide who realized their need for recovery and release from various addictions and compulsions.

CHRISTIAN NURSE NEEDED HER "FIX"

One month later I was privileged to share my story of recovery with my church and subsequently began to lead the local Overcomers Outreach group at our church. I am so deeply grateful for the unique fellowship and support I have found in the OO fellowship! My continued recovery has been enriched by a wonderful blend of the Scriptures, prayer, the 12 Steps, a refreshing honesty, and the friendship of other Christians in recovery.

All those years I felt so alone. Satan kept me on a roller coaster of defeat. Yet my Savior was there, waiting for me to put my will and my life into His ever-loving hands. Now that's real power!

41

FROM THE HEART OF AN ACA

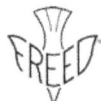

BY BOB NOONAN

Never in my wildest dreams could I have ever imagined that someday God would restore my life from the ravages of being raised in an alcoholic home. But the miracle didn't stop there. He has gone on to use my darkest life experiences to help others to discover the freedom I eventually found in Christ.

I was one of four children raised in a home drenched in alcohol. My father was the alcoholic and my mother was a classic codependent. I learned early in life to practice well the three Don'ts: "Don't talk. Don't trust. Don't feel." I also believed it was hopeless to long for the normalcy I saw in my other friends' families. The anticipatory joy of special holidays was always eclipsed by drunkenness, ranting, never-ending fights, and accusations.

My mother was constantly disappointed that my father chose a relationship with the bottle over her. Several nights a week they would fight until two or three in the morning. That meant that my brothers, sister, and I went to school the next day with very little support.

George Eliot wrote: "If we could hear what goes on in the private lives around us, it would be like hearing the grass grow and the squirrels heart beat, and we would die from that roar that lies on the other side of silence." I was dying on that other side of silence. But I was a good little soldier and pretended that everything was just fine—my contribution to uphold the family image.

In the book *Adult Children of Alcoholics*, Dr. Janet Wotitz wrote about the characteristics of those like me who were raised in such an environment: "We have to guess what normal is...we have difficulty following a project from beginning to end...we judge ourselves without mercy...we have difficulty having fun...and we have difficulty with intimate relationships."[1] No one escapes the alcoholic family unscathed, although I tried.

My grandmother was a great loving influence in my life. To help lighten my mother's overwhelming burdens (i.e., my father's drinking, household chores, the finances, and my siblings and me), she offered to take me to her house. My grandmother, for all intents and purposes, became my mother and her home became my refuge.

Unfortunately, my refuge also became an unsafe place for me to be. When I was five, my step-grandfather—the man who taught me how to ride a bike, swim, and fish—began molesting me. I was overwhelmed with guilt that no five-year-old should have to carry. Yet I still preferred to be at my grandmother's house rather than to endure the pain of loneliness and insanity that engulfed my parents' home.

When I was eight years old my mother finally decided to get help for herself. Since she couldn't fix my father, perhaps she could fix herself. With that, she went to her first Al-Anon meeting, a support group for spouses, family members, and friends of an alcoholic. Not long after that, she piled all of us into the car and took us to our first Alateen meeting, a similar support group for teenagers. It was there that I first became acquainted with the 12 Steps and 12 Traditions of Alcoholics Anonymous. Thanks to my mother's courage to face the truth, she began her journey in recovery and offered her children that same opportunity.

To say the very least, I had a lot of behaviors and thought patterns to unlearn. I can't say that I was even a willing participant when I walked into that first Alateen meeting; however, once there, I experienced unconditional love, acceptance, and understanding that was brand new for me. For the first time in my life I could share my true thoughts and feelings in safety and openness without fear of judgment or criticism. Listening to others share similar pain, hurts, and struggles freed me from feeling desperately alone and gave me great hope.

Because I was raised in a Christian church, the principles of the twelve-step program soon became understandable to me, since I already believed that Jesus was my "higher power." But because of tremendous guilt and shame, it took many years to believe I was eligible for His love and forgiveness.

A year or so later, my father attended his first meeting of Alcoholics Anonymous. He admitted his powerlessness over alcohol, thus beginning the process of recovery as he surrendered his life to God.

Within a few short years our home was literally transformed from the insanity of a war zone to a place of peace were men of all ages came to seek the sobriety and serenity they observed in my father. These men, whose lives were destroyed from the effects of alcohol, were in the midst of facing financial, physical, emotional, spiritual, and marital ruin. They came to my father looking for some answers to relieve their pain.

My father practiced a caring, honest, no-nonsense program. Lives were literally at stake. I often heard him share with others, "Mike, you're still in denial, you're still blaming," or "Larry, you haven't surrendered yet—you're still trying to manage your drinking," or "Jim, you're holding on to resentments and if you don't watch out, you're going to cash them in on a drink. Let go and let God," and "And, John, even though you can't fix your marriage or your financial problems, what are you going to do to stay sober today? All we have is today, take one day at a time."

Because of my father's insistence on a spiritual program and his genuine caring for those who were once like him, many of those people became clean and sober, loving husbands and fathers, and men of good character and integrity. After such a dysfunctional childhood, how blessed I was to eventually witness so many miracles in my own family and in others as well.

From the time I witnessed the power of God in those many lives, I began to feel a strong pull and a consistent calling from God towards ministry myself. I wanted to help ease the burden of others who were held captive. The path God chose for me was a specialized ministry, that of a Christian psychotherapist. Yes, it was true that many other Christian families were being secretly devastated by the disease of alcoholism.

After graduate school, I completed my internship with a Christian counseling group that had a hospital program. I witnessed people suffering from major depression who were often suicidal. Many were diagnosed as Bipolar, or with anxiety disorders, bulimia, anorexia, or substance abuse. All the patients in the program claimed to be believers, but had not yet found any freedom from the bondage that plagued them. About 75 percent of the patients were women, and the majority claimed to come from a home where at least one parent was an alcoholic.

I took this internship with one stipulation, that I wouldn't have to work with any drug addicts or alcoholics. Even though I had the early benefits of a 12-step program and had experienced incredible healing, I had no desire to "return to Egypt." But within several months, I was asked to form and direct a new Christian substance abuse program for this hospital. I wrestled with deep examination of my very soul and dedicated considerable time in heart-wrenching prayer. I had to calm my own great fears of inadequacy and failure.

As I read Romans 8:28, God's truth set me free to do the very thing I was destined to do: "And we know that God causes all things to work together for good to those who love God, to those who were called according to His purpose." God is not the author of sin and I believe He never ordained anyone to be raised in an alcoholic home. However, He did promise that He would use all things to work together for good. First, He drew me to Him because without the great pain I personally experienced, I may have never sought Him. Second, He used my experiences and strengths to help those who were in similar circumstances.

Others may have seen the destructive effects that addiction brought into our lives. They may have witnessed our struggles, powerlessness, self-centeredness, character defects, and resulting dissipation. We had been untrustworthy, confused, and double-minded. But then our lives had been transformed before their very eyes! These people are curious as to what happened to change things so drastically.

I have been rescued by Christ's intervention from the insanity of my past, and have been offered new hope for today and for the future as well. I find myself in a unique position of offering hope to many others. God has called me to carry the message, "Once I was lost, but now I am found!"

All of us who walk the walk of recovery in Overcomers Outreach, are presented golden opportunities to proclaim God's intervention and healing power to our family and friends. We may be surrounded by people who are curious as to what happened to change our lives so drastically. They may be seeking help for themselves or a loved one.

Those of us who have lived through storms of addiction and experienced the healing power of Christ in recovery have the opportunity to be a daily testimony to all those around us who can't help but wonder, "What happened?" Little did I realize that God would eventually redeem my own painful years with huge opportunities to share my experience, strength and hope with literally hundreds of hurting people seeking counseling.

At one time blind to a future, our vision can now become disarming as it pierces through denial and brings truth to the lost. Through the power of God, we can step out of the darkness and into the light. As He takes our hand, He leads us to freedom.

When our broken hearts were put into God's care, we were given hope. Now we can lead others across that bridge to Him, so that He might set more captives free!

42

THOSE OTHER MEETINGS

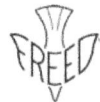

BY BILL D.

From the time I was a small child, I observed that a normally boring older generation seemed to have more fun when they were drinking alcohol. They livened up, and became more entertaining and even a bit scary. My dad, a conservative Lutheran, and my mom, a liberal Catholic, were no exceptions.

While I was in elementary school, I convinced my parents to buy me a guitar so I could copy Elvis, who always seemed to be having a good time. The day came when we had a talent contest in school and I finally had my chance to prove to my parents and my peers that I was someone. Not wanting to be a disappointment, I had never shared about my hearing deficiency. As a result, my rendition of "When the Saints Come Marching In" was horribly out of tune. Needless to say, that was my last guitar performance.

While attending school, the local law enforcement agency held an event with the intention of scaring young people away from drugs. They explained their display case of paraphernalia and substances. For some reason, I was fascinated by this presentation. I remembered seeing Valium in our medicine cabinet at home, and they said if a person took this drug, he would feel rubbery and might even fall down. That sounded good to me, so you know what I did.

OVERCOMERS OUTREACH

When I was thirteen, my parents had a party. I remember being bored and felt that the grown-ups were having all the fun, so I decided to have a beer out in the front yard. The first taste was disgusting. It took a few tastes more to get the effect I was after. Momentarily, life felt OK for the first time, although the next morning I paid the price. Even so, I could hardly wait for my next opportunity to drink.

I spent the next fifteen years chasing that feeling as hard and regularly as I could. In the pursuit, I used any chemicals I could get my hands on with little prejudice, although I managed to avoid needles. When the heat was on, I would switch crowds, poisons, or both.

After high school I settled in with a band, appearing to live the life I once hoped for. (Cocaine was my drug of choice by then, much safer, in my mind, than the PCP I gave up for it.) I found myself building a lighting and special effects show around the band. The band had great potential, but drugs, alcohol, and conflicting egos broke it up. I moved on to different bands and thought I had it made. I could drink, do drugs on the job, have the girls around, and work the hot clubs in Hollywood. This was the good life I'd always longed for!

But at age twenty-four, I was burning out. My body was rejecting the way I was treating it, fear and paranoia were settling in. Needing a change, I packed my camping gear and started my life over in a small farm town on the California coast. Since I was broke and could no longer party, I stuck to cheap beer. In my quest for knowledge, I enrolled in a community college and took a course in psychology. During the second week of classes, the topics were addiction and alcoholism. Thus began my great awakening. I realized my mental, emotional, physical, and spiritual health were all out of whack, and I was potentially heading for more trouble than the police, car accidents, and drug overdoses I had already experienced.

No problem. I decided to stop drinking and drugging. My life improved. I was exercising, sleeping, eating, reading, and enjoying life. Yet something was missing. One night in class I realized *she* was sitting across the room and looking at me. A few nights later, the girl I'd seen showed up at my house for dinner, carrying a very large purse. Out came a bottle of booze and a pipe. We were off and running. It wasn't long before we decided to get married.

About one year into our marriage, we went to counseling, where we were advised to go to AA and NA. That was a good excuse for us to get wasted in the parking lot afterwards. But the day came when my wife told

THOSE OTHER MEETINGS

me I drank too much. Those were fighting words. Soon afterward, she asked me to leave and soon after that, I found myself consuming every pollutant I could get my hands on.

Finally, in a campground near Pismo Beach, I asked God for help. I decided to meet with a Catholic priest. After listening to me rant and rave about all of the people ruining my life, he asked me if I drank alcohol. I replied that I might have a beer or two when I got off work. He pointed out that if my drinking ever got out of control, AA could help me. A few weeks later those words instantly came back to me. I found a phone book and called Alcoholics Anonymous. When asked if I wanted to attend a meeting, I replied, "Maybe." I was then referred to a local AA meeting that was due to start in fifteen minutes. Even though I hadn't had a shower in a few days, I showed up at the meeting. Even so, they welcomed me and told me to keep coming back.

I attended as many meetings as I could, even though the God talk bothered me. I began to take a chance and pray. I got involved in hospital and institution work. I even tried to rekindle my marriage, although it was eventually dissolved. I began to pray that the God who created Alcoholics Anonymous would reveal Himself to me, and He eventually did. In studying the AA literature in depth, I realized that the Bible and Jesus were both there in a very significant way in the beginning of AA. I couldn't wait to get my hands on a Bible.

By this time I was dating a woman I'd met at an AA meeting. She was attending a little Christian church in the neighborhood so I started accompanying her to the services. It wasn't long before I confessed my need for forgiveness and a Savior and committed my life to Jesus. Joyfully, I proceeded to share my great news with my AA friends at the meetings, but this was met with more than a little resistance. I became disillusioned and began to drift away. Sometimes the advice I received at church did more harm than good, so I ended up at an Al-Anon meeting. That's where I met Paul, who told me about an Overcomers Outreach meeting.

At last, in the Overcomers Outreach meeting, I was free to talk about Jesus as my "Higher Power"! I realized that in addition to AA, the Overcomers message needed to be carried into hospitals and institutions. I was elected as the HIM (Hospitals/Institutions/Missions) Ministry chairperson for Overcomers and began to actively take on the challenge. Little did I know that eventually God would use me to rescue and reestablish the ministry of OO during a crisis and then to go on and become its CEO.

OVERCOMERS OUTREACH

It's my dream to carry out the original vision God gave OO's founders, Bob and Pauline Bartosch, to carry the message of hope for people like me who struggle with addictions, and to be a bridge between traditional 12-step groups and churches of every denomination.

Jesus is my "Higher Power." Sometimes I'm not sure what He is doing or where He's taking me, but I know that He is in control. I can absolutely trust Him. Thanks to Him, I have been clean and sober for nineteen years. That is a miracle!

43

LUCKY

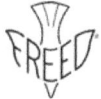

BY JESS MAPLES
(Sept. 10, 1934–Apr. 3, 1989)

Lucky was a pal of mine years ago when I was stationed as a young sailor at an ammunition depot in Nevada. I had been on the Navy base in Hawthorne, Nevada, for eight or nine months when Lucky came aboard. He had one of those disarming personalities that endeared him quickly to everyone who met him, and soon a number of us found ourselves constantly in his company, swimming together, running, and playing ball in our free hours.

Some of us at the depot had developed the unhealthy pastime of going into town for a few beers on Saturday nights. The legal drinking age in Nevada in those days was eighteen, and we rather reveled in our new-found manhood by attempting to down copious quantities of beer. The one who could hold the most, of course, was dubbed the undisputed man-of-the-hour.

One day, several of us were considering whether we should take Lucky along on our next drinking escapade. You see, Lucky posed a bit of a problem for us in that he'd never had a drink in his life. There were moral issues involved here. What would happen with his first drink? What if he got drunk and hurt himself or perhaps got into trouble? With all the inimitable wisdom of eighteen full years of life, we decided to bring him along and let the chips fall where they may.

From his very first drink, Lucky was in trouble. Not only did he enjoy beer, he lapped it up. That first Saturday night out, Lucky got so drunk that he had to be carried back to the base. We decided right then and there that beer was not for Lucky, but he had other ideas. He began going into town with guys who were not in our clique. He got drunk every time he drank, and he drank anytime someone set a beer in front of him.

Pretty soon, Lucky began to change. He started keeping to himself when he wasn't drinking. He slept a lot, didn't eat right, was cranky, and wasn't very nice to be around anymore. To make a long story short, Lucky simply deteriorated rapidly and lost contact with his old friends.

Lucky's story pretty much ends here. One night, while coming back to the base, drunk again and out of control, he staggered into the path of an oncoming car and was killed instantly.

Why have I told you the story of my friend Lucky? Because I want to share with you my belief that alcohol caused Lucky's untimely death. He did not come to us with psychological problems, nor out of a tragic past, nor from a broken home, nor did his ancestry have a bearing on his predisposition to alcoholism. We offered him beer, he didn't seek it out; and we felt guilty for it.

You see, Lucky was a dog. A vigorous, healthy, jet-black, full-blooded Labrador Retriever who drank too much alcohol one day, and it took his life.

Lucky was not unique in his alcoholism. It seems that any species of animal will rapidly become alcoholic if given alcohol to drink. Horses, cats, parrots, mice, dogs—all these have appeared in numerous recountings of stories about animals and booze.

So as much as we try and rationalize that our drinking is due to our particular circumstances, it comes down to the fact that the chemical is the problem. Lucky would have probably lived much longer and continued to be a joy to us if we had not introduced him to booze. At first it was hilarious to see our pal join in the party and get a bit tipsy.

But eventually booze turned on him, bit him like a snake, and destroyed his life.

Thank God, I finally got the message. Eventually, God gave me the power to put the plug in the jug. I've had many years clean and sober that have been a priceless gift to an alcoholic such as myself.

And I've learned that God never makes a mistake. His plans are always the best!

(Editor's note: Jess Maples went to be with Jesus on April 3, 1989. He started one of the first Overcomers groups in the early years. This book is dedicated to him, among others.)

PART IV

OVERCOMERS OUTREACH SUPPORT GROUPS:

A CHRIST - CENTERED PROGRAM OF DISCOVERY

THE HEART OF OVERCOMERS OUTREACH

The purpose of this chapter is to briefly summarize the overall program of Overcomers Outreach and to provide a glimpse into what a typical OO meeting might be like. The following Preamble is the very heart of each Overcomers Group, and is read at every meeting.

OVERCOMERS OUTREACH PREAMBLE

OVERCOMERS is a fellowship of men and women who have been affected either directly or indirectly by the abuse of any mood-altering chemical or compulsive behavior. We believe that as we look to a loving God for help, and put into practice those principles for living which He has given in His Word, we shall find both the strength and freedom we need to live productive and happy lives. We strongly believe that our "Higher Power" is Jesus Christ, our Savior and Lord.

Our five-fold purpose, based directly upon the Word of God is set forth as follows: (1) To provide fellowship in recovery; (2) To be and to live reconciled to God and His family; (3) To gain a better understanding of alcohol and mood-altering chemicals and the disease of addiction/compulsion; (4) To be built up and strengthened in our faith in Christ; (5) To render dedicated service to others who are suffering as we once suffered.

We hold no corporate opinions concerning politics, economics, race, philosophy, science, or any other matter not immediately bearing upon our recovery. While we do believe that Jesus is the Christ, the resurrected and living Son of God, we hold no corporate view concerning denominational preference.

We practice the suggested recovery program of Alcoholics Anonymous, Al-Anon, and other 12-step groups because we believe these to be the practical application of these life-changing principles which are so clearly set forth in the Scriptures.

We welcome anyone who has a desire to stay clean and sober; anyone who has a desire to rise above the pain and turmoil engendered by the addiction of a loved one; anyone wishing to break the bondage of compulsive behavior; anyone who is not opposed to our general method of recovery. We are here to share our experience, strength, and hope with one another. The loving support and genuine caring of fellow members, coupled with daily prayer and the reading of Scripture, prepares us to experience total serenity in Christ, no matter what our outward circumstances might be. Attendance at additional 12-step groups is encouraged. We are dedicated to the principles of anonymity and confidentiality. We guard the anonymity and confidences of other members zealously. Nothing said in these discussions will leave this room in any form. Gossip has no place among us, nor will we share these discussions with outside prayer lists.

Our common welfare must come first. Our leaders are chosen not to govern but to serve. There is only one authority in our group—Jesus Christ, as He expresses His love among us.[1]

WHAT HAPPENS IN AN OO MEETING?

The basic components of an Overcomers meeting are very simple. We meet to praise the Lord; to study the Bible along with the 12 Steps and relevant recovery subjects; to candidly share our experience, strength, and hope in strictest confidence; and to conclude in a circle of mutual

THE HEART OF OVERCOMERS OUTREACH

prayer. Even though Overcomers groups avoid doctrinal issues at all costs, the meeting's focus is specifically based on commonly held tenets of historic orthodox Christianity.

Without a doubt, the incredible power behind the success of those in Overcomers groups is a personal relationship with Jesus Christ. God's Holy Word, linked with the proven tools of the 12 Steps, is the dynamite that helps combat the fear, guilt, anger, loneliness, confusion, and frustration that accompany chemical dependency or compulsive behaviors and their total effects upon the family unit.

Our experience has shown us that healing seems to start with a willingness to be open to God's power through the many sources of help He provides. Our mutual openness provides a channel through which His love can flow and healing can begin. We are a network of people joining together in Christ's Name, learning specific new ways of coping with difficult problems surrounding addictions or compulsions. We find it possible not only to discover survival tools in the face of our addictions, but also to fully experience the abundant life that Jesus promised us in John 10:10, "My purpose is to give life in all its fullness." Yes, He wants what is best for us!

We found that we were the ones who had sabotaged our own recovery through past denial and our unwillingness to let go of our will. Today, we are allowing God to do a new thing within us—something we could never dream up ourselves, no matter how hard we tried!

Those of us in Overcomers have discovered that it works very well to have people with a variety of life's problems present within the same room, where mutual understanding can be achieved. Persons addicted to alcohol, drugs, food, sex, gambling, work, and other crippling compulsions gather to share honestly, and to participate in God's common solution—His miraculous forgiveness and love. Family members of all of the above—known as "codependents," including hurting spouses, worried parents, adult children of alcoholics, and those from dysfunctional backgrounds—are all welcome to participate in this honest meeting of the minds and hearts. Just as the person struggling with an addiction can find recovery, hurting family members can also be FREED from their obsession with their loved one's dilemma and can learn to completely turn them over to the Lord. The family that gets sick together can get well together!

Some of the larger Overcomers meetings divide into different sharing groups, but for the most part the groups are a small, very confidential family of people where safety and anonymity are the rule. Only first names are used to protect the anonymity of each one present. Even though each Overcomers group has a coordinator or facilitator, we believe rotation of leadership is vital to individual growth. There are no gurus in Overcomers. Though the church is not normally accustomed to turning leadership over to untrained lay leaders, we have learned from traditional 12-step groups that trusting the Lord to speak through designated leaders as they share and utilize a simple Overcomers meeting format is the most dynamic, miraculously freeing experience in the world! How exciting to watch these leaders blossom and grow right before our eyes from week to week!

Perhaps the best way to describe what happens in an Overcomers meeting is to quote an intriguing article written by Terry W., a young pastor who visited his first Overcomers meeting in Whittier, California, a few years ago. It's called:

"Honesty"

There I sat, in a setting that I have often sat in before, and yet I felt so out of place. Around me was a group of believers, people who I could tell loved my Jesus. I was both glad to be there, and yet apprehensive. And as the evening progressed, I maintained both of those attitudes.

The evening was filled with all of the normal things done when believers gather. There was singing, a time spent in the Word, sharing of needs, and a time of prayer. There were times when the evening lulled, and then times when it was quite evident that the Spirit of God was mightily at work.

But I guess nothing so impacted me as the first few words that were spoken, for as the leader introduced himself, I knew that this would be an evening far different from others. And all those around introduced themselves, I knew that there was an attitude here that at times is so missing in the church today.

The leader introduced himself by first name only, and right after he stated his name, he also shared the greatest battle and struggle of his life when he stated, "I'm an alcoholic!" And all around the room we went, people admitting their dependence on

THE HEART OF OVERCOMERS OUTREACH

alcohol, drugs, or both. The meeting was the regular fellowship time of Overcomers Outreach, a Christian support group for those dependent and their families.

I felt uncomfortable as the group was going from person to person introducing themselves. I felt as if I should make up an addiction. And yet the real truth is that I too have my vices. I too have those things in my life that leave me helpless and powerless. I too must confess that only when I am honest with myself, God and even others, only then is there hope for strength (2 Cor. 12:10).

Which really leads me to a question for all of us. Do we each possess the same type of honesty that those who attend such a meeting possess? To them, they do not have the option of not facing up. To them, their failure to be honest every day of their lives will lead down a path toward their losing their lives. And the real truth of the matter is that we all are in the same position. We don't have the option of not facing up to truth either, not if we want to experience real life. And if life comes from the life-giver, Jesus Christ, then each of us who allows our attitudes or actions that do not conform to the Word to rule our lives is not living. "For to be carnally minded is death, but to be spiritually minded is life and peace" (Rom. 8:6, KJV).

Honesty is at the same time one of the hardest and yet one of the greatest keys to an effective walk with Christ. It means going to God first with who you really are, and then expressing the desire of who you want to be. People who are willing to stay honest and constantly agree with the Truth in its reality in their lives are people who are used mightily by God.

We don't need pity parties. Nor do we need to feed on each other's mistakes. Instead what we need is a deep commitment to the Truth and a deeper commitment to each other.[2]

Terry's report and reflections, given that he was a newcomer to OO with fresh eyes and impressions, are refreshing and accurate—they truly capture the spirit of an Overcomers meeting.

OVERCOMERS OUTREACH

Meeting Format

One of the main functions of the designated leader is to keep the meeting going on schedule as much as possible. Open the meeting on time.

1. "Hi, everyone, my name is _____. This is the regular meeting of Overcomers Outreach."

2. Opening prayer by leader.

3. Ask for first-time visitors. Welcome them and have them give their first names only. Then everyone responds with "Hi, _____." Go around the group, having everyone in attendance give their first name, along with outside recovery group affiliation if they wish to.

4. If the leader chooses to, he/she may pass out song sheets and have the group warm up with some choruses or hymns of praise.

5. Ask someone to read the Overcomers Preamble.

6. Ask someone to read the 12 Steps, followed by the group reciting the Serenity Prayer in unison.

7. Go around the group giving first names again, and see if there are any sobriety or abstinence birthdays.

8. Topical Study or 12-Step Study. Leader should select enough references to cover a half-hour or less.

9. Sharing Time: Try to make sure that everyone has an opportunity to share within the time allotted.

    Leader Reads the Following Guidelines:

For maximum benefit for the most people: 1) We may ask you to share, but no one should feel pressured to participate and may pass. 2) Please raise your hand to be called upon before speaking, keeping your sharing in the here and now—what you are dealing with this week. 3) Limit your sharing time to about three minutes, allowing everyone in the group to share once before you share a second time. 4) Avoid offering suggestions or methods of fixing another person's problems, allowing individuals to experience their pain without your interference. 5) Please NO CROSS TALK, speak only when it is your turn. 6) Questions can be handled AFTER the meeting so that sharing will not be interrupted. 7) If you have used alcohol or any mood-altering chemical within the past twenty-four hours, we ask you not to share until after the meeting.

10. 7th Tradition

    Leader Reads:

    "We pass the basket to help defray costs of literature and to help support the OO Central Office. In sending a portion of the group's offering to support OO's Central Office, we not only have a chance to give something back for all we've been given, but we also provide the means necessary to carry Christ's recovery message of hope to people around the world."

11. OO Traditions

    "While we finish passing the basket, let's go around the room and read the 12 Traditions of Overcomers Outreach."

12. Leader: ask for a volunteer to lead next week's meeting.

13. Prayer Time. Ask for prayer requests. These should be either regarding ourselves or other group members. Designate someone to begin sentence prayers, and either the leader should close, or designate someone else to close.

14. CLOSE ON TIME. It is very effective to stand, holding hands, and to say The Lord's Prayer in unison, with final exclamation of "keep coming back, it works!"

Note: Once a month the group may want to consider having a "big book study" using either *The 12 Steps Come ALIVE in the Scriptures,* or taking turns reading other chapters from the OO book.

What It Takes to Start an OO Meeting

1. It is important to have the approval of the church's pastoral staff before starting a group so they can be supportive. The pastors usually welcome a group such as OO because it will not take up their time, and gives them a safe place to send families in crisis due to problems of addictions or compulsions.

OVERCOMERS OUTREACH

2. The contact person or group leader should be a Christian who is also in a traditional 12-step recovery program, with continuous sobriety/abstinence for at least one year.

3. It takes a core group of several people who will be committed to meet every week and work on personal recovery issues.

4. It takes a great deal of prayer.

5. Important resources include those items contained in the OO *FREED* booklet, including the outline of the simple but all-important meeting format, a special 12-step study with related Scripture references, guidelines for starting a group, the Leader's Guide, which includes information on group dynamics, "Important Ingredients," and "Helpful Hints for Success." This booklet provides everything needed to start and maintain the group and is available from the OO central office, along with other related materials listed in Appendix A.

View of Our "Higher Power"

Many people ask for an Overcomers Outreach "statement of faith" or doctrinal position. We avoid discussions of specific doctrine in OO groups and instead put our focus upon the person of Christ, our Healer. However, a few basic concepts that describe our position are appropriate and necessary.

Overcomers Outreach maintains that we are all made in God's image but that we are sinners, with an "inner child" that many times needs healing. We inherited our sinful natures from God's first man and woman on earth, and everyone is in need of a Savior. We believe His name is Jesus Christ, God's own Son, who came to give His life that we might live eternally. Because of God's unbounded love for us (we who by rights don't deserve it, as sinners), our "Higher Power" is not one we have created in our own finite minds to suit our fancies, but is the powerful Creator and Lord of the universe. He is not an inanimate object that we can manipulate to our own desires, but is the awesome God who is alive and reaches out His love and presence to each one of us who will accept it.

Jesus of Nazareth was born more than two thousand years ago, walked the earth for thirty-three years, suffered and died upon a cross, shedding His blood for the sins of mankind—and that includes every one of us. The good news is that He rose from the dead and is very

THE HEART OF OVERCOMERS OUTREACH

much alive today! For those of us who accept His gift of love, turning our will and lives over to the care of Jesus Christ means having our sins forgiven—washed totally away—with the promise of eternal life. This message, more than any other, needs to be considered by every person in this world, whether in recovery or not, because it deals with the most important decision we will ever make during our lifetimes, one that will affect us individually for eternity.

OVERCOMERS OUTREACH GROUP TRADITIONS

1. Our common welfare should come first. Personal recovery depends upon God's grace and our willingness to get help.

2. For our group purpose there is but one ultimate authority—a loving God as He expresses Himself through His Son, Jesus Christ, and the Holy Spirit. Our leaders are but trusted servants; they do not govern.

3. The only requirement for Overcomers Outreach membership is a desire to stop addictive or compulsive behavior.

4. Each group should be autonomous except in matters affecting other groups or Overcomers Outreach as a whole.

5. The primary purpose of each group is to serve as a bridge between traditional 12-step groups and the church. We carry the message of Christ's delivering power to individuals and family members who still suffer, both within and outside the church.

6. An Overcomers Outreach group uses The Holy Bible along with the 12 Steps of Alcoholics Anonymous for its tools of recovery. Outside enterprises are prayerfully evaluated lest problems of money, property, and prestige divert us from our primary purpose.

7. Every Overcomers Outreach group ought to be fully self-supporting, declining outside contributions.

8. Overcomers Outreach groups should remain forever non-professional, but our Service Centers may employ special workers.

OVERCOMERS OUTREACH

9. Overcomers Outreach, as such, ought never be organized, but group coordinators network with the Central Service Center, seeing that the group is facilitated through adherence to the *FREED* booklet's "Meeting Format" and rotation of leadership.

10. Overcomers Outreach is, without apology, a Christ-centered recovery group; however, persons of all faiths are welcome. Discussions of religious doctrine should be avoided. Our focus must be upon our mutual recovery.

11. Our public relations policy is based upon attraction rather than promotion. We need to always seek the Holy Spirit's discernment whenever sharing in the media, in order to maintain personal anonymity of all Overcomers Outreach group members.

12. Jesus Christ is the spiritual foundation of all our traditions, ever reminding us to place principles before personalities. We claim God's promise that His power can set us FREE![3]

THE 12 STEPS OF ALCOHOLICS ANONYMOUS *

(Editor's note: These Steps work for any addiction or compulsion. Simply replace the word "alcohol" with your own presenting problem. Study of these steps is essential to progress in this program. The principles they embody are universal and applicable to everyone, whatever his/her personal creed. We strive for an ever-deeper understanding of these Steps and pray for God's wisdom to apply them to our lives. Please note: written permission must be secured from AA World Services, Inc., before reprinting or adapting the Steps.)

1. We admitted we were powerless over alcohol—that our lives had become unmanageable.
2. Came to believe that a Power greater than ourselves could restore us to sanity.
3. Made a decision to turn our will and our lives over to the care of God as we understood Him.
4. Made a searching and fearless moral inventory of ourselves.

THE HEART OF OVERCOMERS OUTREACH

5. Admitted to God, to ourselves, and to another human being the exact nature of our wrongs.
6. Were entirely ready to have God remove all these defects of character.
7. Humbly asked Him to remove our shortcomings.
8. Made a list of all persons we had harmed, and became willing to make amends to them all.
9. Made direct amends to such people wherever possible, except when to do so would injure them or others.
10. Continued to take personal inventory and when we were wrong promptly admitted it.
11. Sought through prayer and meditation to improve our conscious contact with God as we understood Him, praying only for knowledge of His will for us and the power to carry that out.
12. Having had a spiritual awakening as the result of these steps, we tried to carry this message to alcoholics, and to practice these principles in all our affairs.[4]

* The 12 Steps are reprinted with permission of Alcoholics Anonymous World Services, Inc. (See notice on copyright page for additional information.)

OVERVIEW OF THE STEPS

How do we begin this road of recovery? Any one of us who is currently traveling along this pathway will invariably answer: We start at the beginning, at Step One, and with "Number One" (i.e., ourselves). We admit our powerlessness over our addiction or compulsion. We have found that we can simply replace the word "alcohol" in Step One with our own presenting problem—no matter what it is—and it gives us a new beginning, as we place our problem in God's hands. (If we can't think of anything in our life that renders us powerless, we could insert the word "pride" in Step One, and it would fit perfectly.)

The key to these 12 Steps seems to be the ingredient of powerlessness, as noted in Step One. After failing in our own efforts to live with serenity (i.e., clean, sober, and abstinent), we find that we had short-circuited God's power by insisting upon our own will and attempting to retain some of the control ourselves. We find that we no longer need to sabotage the victory He promises to those of us who will simply "let go and let God." When we finally surrendered, it was as if a great load had been lifted from our sagging shoulders. While pondering the first Step, we recognize our own weakness and realize that God has the power to restore us to sanity.

Denial is thrown to the wind with Step Two, as we begin to see our "lostness"—to realistically see the insanity of our lives, and to begin to sense an urgent need for God's power to break our chains and set us free. Whether agnostic, atheist, or disillusioned believer, we can stand together on these Steps. True humility and an open mind can lead us to faith, and every 12-step meeting is an assurance that God will restore us to sanity if we rightly relate ourselves to Him.

With Step Three, we actually made a decision to accept Jesus Christ as our "Higher Power." These first three Steps can be quite similar to a conversion experience and become the basis of a whole new perspective of hope through the Savior that we never dreamed possible. Simply summarized, the first three Steps mean: 1) I can't, 2) God can, 3) I think I'll let Him!

Step Four has us leaping into a "searching and fearless moral inventory." This takes tremendous courage. The opportunity for growth in taking this Step can be excruciating. But as the saying goes, "No pain, no gain!" It prepares us to take the next Step; our life's "spiral" is now headed upward!

Perhaps one of our most difficult assignments in recovery is admitting our shameful past to God, to ourselves, and to another person (Step Five). Our pride is thrown aside, but in so doing, our souls are cleansed by God, and we are given a fresh start. Sharing with another person our most deep-seated guilt and pain seems to take the power out of our bondage and frees us to begin to tackle our relationship with other people.

In Steps Six, Seven, and Eight, we begin to concentrate on cleaning house. Step Six is actually an attitude where we become ready for God to remove our defects of character. During Step Seven, God actually removes our shortcomings when we ask Him. Even though our past may have been sordid and we feel totally unworthy, we are amazed at God's miracles as He actually erases those things that have been holding us back and keeping us from being all that He intended us to be, and He lovingly grants us His forgiveness.

When we come to Step Eight, we begin to work on our relationships. We specifically list the names of all those we have harmed and become willing to make amends to each one. If God has truly "cleaned house" with us in Steps Four through Seven, we will be ready to take this gigantic action step because we have already begun to see the tangible rewards of making things right.

Step Nine has us actively making the amends we need to, not just for the benefit of others, but mainly for our own recovery. In doing so, we are careful not to cause any more damage to ourselves or others by expressing our amends in a thoughtful, appropriate manner. We have found that hidden resentments can sabotage our serenity, so we continually attempt to rid ourselves of resentments as they appear.

By the time we get to Step ten, we are amazed at the progress we have made by taking the first nine, and are surprisingly eager and amazingly willing to continue. We find it important to redo our personal inventories on a regular basis, as more is revealed each time, and our "house" (which we believe is the temple of the Holy Spirit) is kept clean. Promptly admitting our wrongs cleans the slate each time, causing us to be perpetually free.

Without prayer and meditation (Step 11), we will again find ourselves powerless. We begin to take God with us on every step of life's way, praying only for His will (not ours, for a change) and prayerfully seeking His power to continue this recovery road.

The spiritual awakening and relationship with our "Higher Power" that result from taking these Steps cause us to be eager to share this message of hope with others who are still suffering (the essence of Step 12). In fact, we find that unless we give our program of recovery away, we can't keep it very long. The magic ingredient to the ongoing power of these Steps is to continue to practice these principles in all our affairs, relinquishing our control and yielding to God's will for our lives.

As we continue down the Discovery Road, more is revealed with every Step. But we never graduate! It's "progress, rather than perfection," that we seek.

If we really mean business about working our 12-step program, particularly regarding the actual making of amends to others, we will be assured of dramatic results in our own spiritual growth. We surely get the benefits of sobriety, but there are collateral benefits as well.

The following is excerpted from The *Big Book* of Alcoholics Anonymous, as it refers especially to Step Nine. It is rightly referred to as "the promises," held dear by all recovering people:

> If we are painstaking about this phase of our development, we
> will be amazed before we are half way through. We are going to

know a new freedom and a new happiness. We will not regret the past nor wish to shut the door on it. We will comprehend the word serenity and we will know peace. No matter how far down the scale we have gone, we will see how our experience can benefit others. That feeling of uselessness and self-pity will disappear. We will lose interest in selfish things and gain interest in our fellows. Self-seeking will slip away. Our whole attitude and outlook upon life will change. Fear of people and of economic insecurity will leave us. We will intuitively know how to handle situations which used to baffle us. We will suddenly realize that God is doing for us what we could not do for ourselves.

Are these extravagant promises? We think not. They are being fulfilled among us—sometimes quickly, sometimes slowly. They will materialize if we work for them[5]

The rewards of working the 12 Steps are enormous. God provides the faith that had always eluded us in the past, to saturate us with His peace.

Those of us who have been imprisoned by addictions or compulsions value the 12 Steps as priceless tools to use in this business of living. We believe that God has provided them for broken people like ourselves. We found that the basis of our problems was not chemical dependency or compulsive disorders, but just plain living! Merely surviving as a whole person in a sinful world is a tall order! Some of us who are especially fragile have a more difficult time facing life without a chemical or emotional crutch, or escape. The good news is it can be done, with His help—and with a tremendous amount of victory!

We thank God for the tools He has given us just when we had given up hope. The blazing light of His Word shines brightly upon the stepping stones He has provided.

45

THE 12 STEPS COME A-L-I-V-E IN THE SCRIPTURES

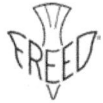

STEP ONE

"We admitted we were powerless over alcohol—that our lives had become unmanageable."

We in Overcomers Outreach have found that this Step translates into the short phrase, "I can't!"

"Hitting bottom" is painful, especially when we have spent a lifetime covering up our problems in order to appear successful and serene, particularly in a church setting. A person who has been using drugs and/or alcohol to "socialize" but eventually "uses" in order to just feel normal has crossed an invisible line into addiction. This can be a lonely, frightening place. Loving someone who is addicted is like loving two people—the drunk one and the sober one (confusing, to say the least). If we are still carrying around the pain of our dysfunctional childhood, we feel stuck in the past and unable to change. It usually takes a painful crisis for any of us to realize our need for help. As long as we think we can handle it (drugs, alcohol, dysfunctional relationships, our loved one's addictions, etc.) we just stay on a roller coaster of denial. We begin to wonder if there is hope for the future.

OVERCOMERS OUTREACH

WHAT THE BIBLE SAYS ABOUT STEP ONE

> *2 Corinthians 1:9 "We felt we were doomed to die and saw how powerless we were to help ourselves; but that was good, for then we put everything into the hands of God, who alone could save us..."*

How can it possibly be good to feel powerless? Then we really feel out of control! After exerting so much willpower into trying to get our addictions and compulsions under control, and then failing miserably, we feel utterly defeated. We are people who have lost hope and have crashed to a painful bottom. How can this possibly be described as "good"? This verse tells us that when we have exhausted all of our own efforts, we are at a point of surrender, and that is good! Giving up hope in our own control measures isn't the end; it's just the beginning of God's divine intervention in our lives. It isn't until we get to a place of admitting our human insufficiency and relinquish our will that God quietly steps in with His own amazing blueprints for our lives. We no longer have to do it alone!

> *Romans 7:18 "I know I am rotten through and through so far as my old sinful nature is concerned. No matter which way I turn I can't make myself do right. I want to but I can't."*

One reason we lost hope was because we have tried, time and time again, to clean up our lives, to no avail. We had blown it so many times that we figured we didn't deserve to be forgiven, even when God offered it. We decided that our destiny is to be a loser, thus we sabotage God's best plans for us. Knowing what we do about our shameful weaknesses and addictions, it's hard to imagine that right in the midst of our very lowest point, God still loves us, accepting us just the way we are, even though we don't deserve it.

> *Psalm 116:10–11 "In my discouragement I thought, 'They are lying when they say I will recover.' But now what can I offer Jehovah for all he has done for me?"*

After years of accumulating bad habits and a list of sins a mile long, it's nearly impossible to believe that we can change! Not only that, we may have done an admirable job of covering up our true condition, or we may have been in total denial about it. Yet deep in our hearts we

THE 12 STEPS COME A-L-I-V-E IN THE SCRIPTURES

know how unmanageable our lives really are. We see the lives of others changing drastically in recovery. Can there really be hope for us too? Enough pain finally brings us to our knees, having to admit our human failures. It may seem like the end, but we find that it is the start of a whole new life—allowing God to manage our lives His way.

> *2 Corinthians 12:9 "...I am with you; that is all you need. My power shows up best in weak people."*

Finally admitting our weaknesses, after avoiding it for so long, makes us realize that our strength is in the Lord, not within ourselves. According to 2 Corinthians 12:7–10, it wasn't until the apostle Paul accepted his "thorn in the flesh" that he experienced any victory! He, of all people, who had even persecuted and murdered early Christians, was transformed into the very person whom God used to proclaim the gospel! Could there be unseen miracles in store for us too?

STEP TWO

"Came to believe that a power greater than ourselves could restore us to sanity."

Following the pattern set in Step One ("I can't!"), in OO this Step means "God can!"

We had lost all hope that things could ever change. Our prayers seemed to stop at the ceiling. Getting to a place of believing that our "Higher Power" (Jesus Christ) can really help us out of the impossible pit of despair of our addiction or obsession with another person is a giant step. This takes the kind of power that only He can provide.

"Restored to sanity" assumes that we've been insane! Most of us resent hearing this, having believed that our problems are due to something or someone else. Rigorous honesty causes us to admit that our lives have become pretty insane, and our addictions or our obsession with another's behavior usually have been involved. Addiction itself is recognized as a form of insanity, because we continue to "use" or drink even though we are destroying our lives. Even when we find some temporary sobriety or abstinence, we may experience a slip back into the same course of destruction. Our Lord has the power necessary to heal us and restore our focus to some peace and serenity we never thought possible, no matter how bad it's been in the past!

What the Bible Says About Step Two

Proverbs 28:26 "A man is a fool to trust himself! But those who use God's wisdom are safe."

We have gone through life gritting our teeth, hanging on tight, and attempting to do things our way. But it seems that leaning upon our human wisdom, or even dictating to God what we think should be done, hasn't worked. In fact, under our own steam we have made a mess of our lives! The Bible tells us to trust God, but it's so hard sometimes when we assume He must have deserted us or that we just don't deserve His intervention. But in order to find victory, we must first be willing to admit our failures and begin to believe that God indeed has the power to make some sense out of our lives.

Romans 5:8–9 "But God showed his great love for us by sending Christ to die for us while we were still sinners. And since by his blood he did all this for us as sinners, how much more will he do for us now that he has declared us not guilty?"

Not guilty? After all we remember about our past, how could God just declare us innocent? The Bible tells us that because our "Higher Power" (Jesus Christ) died for our sins, and rose again to defeat death, we can be washed whiter than snow if we just accept this amazing gift of love. Even though we know that we, of all people, don't deserve God's great sacrifice of His Son upon the cross, salvation can be ours when we proclaim Jesus as our "Higher Power," the living Lord of our lives! Jesus becomes our best friend and offers us hope for the future. The pieces of our sanity seem to come together through connecting with our Maker and allowing Him to rule our lives His way.

Psalm 30:2–3 "O Lord my God, I pleaded with you, and you gave me my health again. You brought me back from the brink of the grave, from death itself, and here I am alive!"

THE 12 STEPS COME A-L-I-V-E IN THE SCRIPTURES

In this passage, the psalmist David had almost given up but kept putting his life into God's care, one day at a time. In order for us to overcome our addictions and compulsions, we must also make that commitment every day. Even though the outlook may seem bleak from a human point of view, we have witnessed other "hopeless" people like ourselves remarkably getting well, so we know that it is possible. God knows our whole story, from beginning to end, and His promises are true!

Mark 9:23 "Anything is possible if you have faith!"

Faith is what's hard. Yet as Jesus was healing people during His pilgrimage here on earth, He said anything is possible to those who believe! The creator of the universe is not restricted to our human standards; His power transcends all of man's puny schemes. His plans are always the best, if we can trust Him!

STEP THREE

"Made a decision to turn our wills and our lives over to the care of God as we understood Him."

Completing the three-part translation of the first three Steps, in OO we sum up Step Three with "I think I'll let Him!"

When we take an honest look at our powerlessness and turn our lives over to God's care (Steps One and Two), that is when He will actually do something about our dilemma—when we are willing to trust Him. "Letting go and letting God" can be tough, quite similar to jumping off a cliff! Trusting our lives to God's care and asking for His will instead of ours may seem foolish. What if we don't like His will for us, and it doesn't fit into our plans? Are we willing to trust Him anyway? Has what we've tried to do before to solve our problems worked? We soon discover that once we surrender, God steps in and does for us what we could not do for ourselves.

WHAT THE BIBLE SAYS ABOUT STEP THREE

Proverbs 3:5–6 "...trust the Lord completely; don't ever trust yourself. In everything you do, put God first, and he will direct you and crown your efforts with success."

OVERCOMERS OUTREACH

Turning our wills and our lives over to the care of God means letting go with complete abandon! Surrendering our wills and our lives to our "Higher Power," Jesus Christ, is to place ourselves under His control, and to be open to His plans for us. Instead of relying upon our self-sufficiency, we become clay in the Master Potter's hand. When we ask Christ to be first in our lives, He leads us into uncharted territory, far beyond our imagination.

Galatians 2:19–20 "...acceptance with God comes by believing in Christ. I have been crucified with Christ; and I myself no longer live, but Christ lives in me. And the real life I now have within this body is a result of my trusting in the Son of God, who loved me and gave himself for me."

In recovery we find that during the years we have been "in control" of our lives we have cheated ourselves out of so much joy! Child-like faith in our "Higher Power," Jesus Christ, causes our lives to have meaning and purpose far beyond anything we ever dreamed possible. His Spirit actually lives within us, and becomes our most cherished Friend, caring about even the smallest matters of our everyday lives.

Romans 12:1 "And so, dear brothers, I plead with you to give your bodies to God. Let them be a living sacrifice, holy—the kind he can accept. When you think of what He has done for you, is this too much to ask?"

As we kneel at Jesus' feet, we realize that we have been bought with a price. We may have abused our bodies—these temporal homes in which we dwell—but are now ready to offer them to God for a good housecleaning. Though we are powerless to be holy or righteous in our own strength, God can use these weak bodies for His glory, if we will only let Him!

Psalm 40:1–2 "I waited patiently for God to help me; then he listened and heard my cry. He lifted me out of the pit of despair, out from the bog and the mire, and set my feet on a hard, firm path and steadied me as I walked along."

THE 12 STEPS COME A-L-I-V-E IN THE SCRIPTURES

The psalmist David testifies of God's deliverance, noting that life is a journey of walking along the new, steady path the Lord provided. As we read through the Psalms, we find that though David experienced total defeat with his face to the ground in hopelessness, he learned that it was OK to be honest with God concerning his true feelings, whether it was anger, fear, or despair. Since God sees to the very bottom of our hearts, it pleases Him when we are honest about what's there.

STEP FOUR

"Made a searching and fearless moral inventory of ourselves."

Digging out a written inventory of our life sounds like a whole lot of hard work. It is, but it pays off! In the past, we may have taken an occasional peek into our past, and it usually just made us feel more guilty! So we may think that we would have to be fearful of any inventory we might do. When a store takes stock of its inventory, it counts every single item, both good and bad. This means that besides all our negatives, we need to consider our positives too, careful not to miss anything!

WHAT THE BIBLE SAYS ABOUT STEP FOUR

Lamentations 3:40–41 "Let us examine ourselves instead, and repent and turn again to the Lord. Let us lift our hearts and our hands to him in heaven. ..."

Taking a close look at the mess we've made of our lives is a tall order for those of us who have been deep in denial. Some of the sordid details can truly be embarrassing. We're hoping that perhaps we can hide these things from God and we would rather pretend that they never happened. We're quite sure that if anyone knew what kind of person we really were, they wouldn't like us. We don't even like ourselves. But God desires for us to turn to Him, sorting out even the most degrading items and putting the whole mess right in His lap. He can handle it—all of it, even though we can't! When we finally get the courage to lift our hearts and hands to Him in submission, we are shocked to see that He accepts us in spite of our blotted record. We begin to discover what freedom is all about!

Psalm 139:23 "Search me, O God, and know my heart; test my thoughts. Point out anything you find in me that makes you sad, and lead me along the path of everlasting life."

What courage it takes to allow God's flashlight to scan every nook and cranny of our being! The psalmist knew that if he was to be freed and cleansed, he must first become honest with himself and God. When we submit to our loving Lord, we seek to please Him and need to be keenly aware of those things that tend to sabotage our relationship with Him. Knowing that life is a one-day-at-a-time proposition, we put our hand into God's, on His path toward life everlasting. Together, we can make it!

Matthew 7:3–5 "...Why worry about a speck in the eye of a brother when you have a board in your own? Should you say, 'Friend, let me help you get that speck out of your eye,' when you can't even see because of the board in your own? Hypocrite! First get rid of the board. Then you can see to help your brother."

We find that we have been so busy focusing upon another person's frailties and problems that we are not in touch with the truth about ourselves. Actually, it has been somewhat of a comfort to compare our condition with someone else whose problems may be worse than ours. We would rather be in the position to help someone else than to have to deal with our own reality. In contrast, the Lord says, "First, get rid of your own sins, addictions, or compulsions." An efficient way to clean house is to catalog every single item—our assets and liabilities—on paper. Then our eyes can take a stark look at our reality. Then we must clean out the cobwebs of our souls in humble prayer to our Savior, Jesus Christ.

STEP FIVE

"Admitted to God, to ourselves, and to another human being the exact nature of our wrongs."

So now it's all out on paper, even our most sordid secrets! It can be overwhelming to consider both the good and bad aspects of our lives all at once! At first it can be difficult to discover any assets, and our liabilities cause us to feel intense shame. We would rather hide most of

THE 12 STEPS COME A-L-I-V-E IN THE SCRIPTURES

it from God, even from ourselves, and especially from another human being! Examining the exact nature of our wrongs and admitting them can be a huge relief! When we can release all of our problems to God, He can handle them! Through Christ's shed blood on the Cross, we are forgiven. When we finally get honest with ourselves, we begin the road to recovery. When we get the courage to "let it go" in the direction of another trusted human being, the chains of bondage are broken.

WHAT THE BIBLE SAYS ABOUT STEP FIVE

James 5:16 "Admit your faults to one another and pray for each other so that you may be healed."

In order for the early Christians to remain close to one another and to be led daily by the Holy Spirit, it was vital that they be honest in all their ways. Sometimes today, due to our denial or shame of our true human condition, we hide—especially from our Christian friends. This is exactly the opposite of what the Bible advocates for our Christian walk. Though it is sometimes difficult to share our truth with another, we can experience a special healing and freedom in the process.

1 John 1:9 "If we claim we have not sinned, we are lying and calling God a liar, for he says we have sinned."

Some people in 12-step programs are spooked by the word "sin" and would much prefer to call it by another name. Yet the Word of God is just too clear that we are all sinners! The good news is that there is a divine remedy for our sinful condition. Jesus Christ has paid the penalty for all of our wrongdoings, if we merely ask Him to. So as much as we might struggle against the term "sin" because it just doesn't fit into our vocabulary, it does fit into God's. It really makes a whole lot more sense to accept our humanness, along with God's gift of love and forgiveness.

Psalm 32:1 "What happiness for those whose guilt has been forgiven! What joys when sins are covered over! What relief for those who have confessed their sins and God has cleared their record."

Once we give up and give ourselves with complete abandon to God, we often wonder what has taken us so long. When peace takes over and

His joy begins to fill us, we realize how long we have sabotaged His power in our lives. To know that our slate is now clean provides incentive to make a fresh start.

> Galatians 6:2–3 "Share each other's troubles and problems, and so obey our Lord's command. If anyone thinks he is too great to stoop to this, he is fooling himself. He is really a nobody."

For those of us who have kept our problems well hidden, trying to solve them by ourselves in an effort to look good, we have totally missed out on some of God's richest blessings. If anyone should be honest about their lives, it should be those who belong to Christ. What better testimony than to live transparent lives, showing how God's power works within His people?

STEP SIX

"Were entirely ready to have God remove all these defects of character."

Giving up some of our pet character defects can be hard when we have hung onto them for so long. Now that we have taken a written inventory and had our souls cleansed by confession to God and another trusted person, we begin to sense a new freedom and growth. We begin to believe that it is worth the risk to take this next step of preparation to allow God to rid us of those things that have held us back from being all He intended us to be. We can't accomplish this on our own—it takes God's power to effectively "clean house," even to the most remote corners of our soul. Removal of all our defects may seem like major surgery!

WHAT THE BIBLE SAYS ABOUT STEP SIX

> James 4:7 and 10 "So give yourselves humbly to God. Then, when you realize your worthlessness before the Lord, he will lift you up, encourage and help you."

It takes a new humility and willingness and a new kind of courage to actually be ready to present ourselves, including all our failings and woundedness, to the Lord. Just when we see no way out of our dilemma,

THE 12 STEPS COME A-L-I-V-E IN THE SCRIPTURES

God steps in and provides divine new hope—hope that in human terms would have been impossible.

Jeremiah 10:23–24 "O Lord, I know it is not within the power of man to map his life and plan his course—so you correct me, Lord; but please be gentle."

Most of us have taken a journey that has included things we are not proud of. We want mercy, not justice, for our past deeds. How awesome that God is merciful to people like us. Our loving heavenly Father does have the power to map a successful plan for our lives, if we will only be honest and allow Him to work in His way.

Hebrews 12:1–2 "...Let us strip off anything that slows us down or holds us back, and especially those sins that wrap themselves tightly around our feet and trip us up; and let us run with patience the particular race that God has set before us. Keep your eyes on Jesus...."

We can be free of the bondage that has kept us ineffective and defeated when we're ready to relinquish control of our lives, along with our defects. God has the power to untangle us from our massive web of failure, and start us on a new path that has a bright future, if our eyes stay focused on Jesus as our "Higher Power."

Hosea 10:12 "Plant the good seeds of righteousness and you will reap a crop of my love; plow the hard ground of your hearts, for now is the time to seek the Lord, that he may come and shower salvation upon you."

Even the prophets of old found that plowing up the hard ground of our hearts can be painful and disconcerting. We become used to the status quo and can't see past it to possible changes or improvement opportunities. If we're willing, God can take the rubble of our past and craft new building blocks that will revolutionize our lives and the lives of those around us.

OVERCOMERS OUTREACH

Micah 7:18–20 "Where is there another God like you, who pardons the sins of the survivors among his people? You cannot stay angry with your people for you love to be merciful. Once again you will have compassion on us. You will tread our sins beneath your feet; you will throw them into the depths of the ocean!"

We are survivors all right! And when God removes our sins and defects, they are gone, no matter how bad they've been. That's why we are in such good hands when we become willing to give them all to Him. We will never understand such love and compassion from an almighty God for such people as ourselves.

STEP SEVEN

"Humbly asked him to remove our shortcomings."

We know if we ask God for anything in Jesus' Name, He will hear and answer us. We may not be accustomed to portraying a humble attitude, so this may seem strange at first. True humility doesn't mean meek surrender to an ugly, destructive way of life; it means surrender to God's will.

We may think that if our shortcomings are removed, we may lose our identity altogether. But having walked through Steps One through Six, we've begun to experience so much peace that we are willing to continue, asking God to unload all those defects from the darkest crevices of our being. We begin to experience a new life, a new spring in our step, a breath of fresh air! We are freed up to be who we really are—made in His image!

WHAT THE BIBLE SAYS ABOUT STEP SEVEN

Isaiah 66:2 "My hand has made both earth and skies, and they are mine. Yet I will look with pity on the man who has a humble and a contrite heart, who trembles at my word."

What a concept! We will never understand how a God who created the universe can have compassion upon finite human beings who fail again and again. Yet all He is looking for is a humble and contrite heart. Jesus

THE 12 STEPS COME A-L-I-V-E IN THE SCRIPTURES

has a special place in His heart for those of us who have been broken, because He has experienced human brokenness Himself while here on Earth. We are very special to Him.

> *1 John 1:9 "But if we confess our sins to him, he can be depended on to forgive us and to cleanse us from every wrong."*

Having walked through a process of routing out our shortcomings and becoming willing to follow through with His plan for us, His power has already started to work. We are ready to humbly seek His cleansing in our lives, trusting our lives into His care with the Bible's assurance that we are indeed forgiven.

> *Isaiah 1:18–19 "...No matter how deep the stain of your sins, I can take it out and make you as clean as freshly fallen snow. Even if you are stained as red as crimson, I can make you white as wool! If you will only let me help you, if you will only obey, then I will make you rich!"*

"Yes, but the sins of my past are just too terrible; there's no way I can be forgiven!" we cry ashamedly. If we hang on to these lies, Satan defeats us. God's Word says we are forgiven, and it's not up to us to decide what God should be thinking or doing. Our role is to merely accept His wonderful gift of love and forgiveness.

STEP EIGHT

"Made a list of all persons we had harmed, and became willing to make amends to them all."

Oh, no—not another writing assignment! Now it's up to us to clear up the wreckage of the past. In order to do this, we need to list every person we have wronged, let go of our resentments (every one), and become willing to make amends to them all, including our worst enemy. How can this help us? By releasing us from the grip of our past, clearing the record, erasing the slate, and allowing us to start over (similar to the way God forgives us in Christ).

OVERCOMERS OUTREACH

What the Bible Says About Step Eight

Matthew 5:23–24 "...If you are standing before the altar...and suddenly remember that a friend has something against you, leave your sacrifice there and go and be reconciled to him, and then come and offer your sacrifice to God."

After spending years blaming other people for our problems, it is difficult to swallow our pride and become willing to make things right with each one, no matter how justified we felt. Making a list of these people is the first step to seeing where we stand in forgiving their trespasses as Christ as forgiven us.

Matthew 6:14–15 "Your heavenly Father will forgive you if you forgive those who sin against you; but if you refuse to forgive them, he will not forgive you."

The Bible really tells it like it is. When I hang on to resentments, I literally sabotage my own recovery and relationship with Christ. It's so hard to let go of situations in which we feel we were wronged. And yet until we're ready to do just that, we cut ourselves off from His power and the joy God has in store for us.

Step Nine

"Made direct amends to such people wherever possible, except when to do so would injure them or others."

Saying "I'm sorry" is difficult enough with people we love; making amends with everyone we have harmed takes courage and God's direction. Sometimes we get a strange reaction from these people. They might not even remember the incident, or they would prefer to keep the relationship hostile. It's important, too, that we're careful about revealing information that might harm someone in our attempt to make things right. The important point is that we will experience a healing in the process of making amends, if we are willing to follow this Step. More often than not, a joyful reunion occurs with the people with whom we build bridges and miraculous healing takes place. This experience is well worth any risk involved.

THE 12 STEPS COME A-L-I-V-E IN THE SCRIPTURES

What the Bible Says About Step Nine

Mark 11:24 "You can pray for anything, and if you believe, you have it; it's yours! But when you are praying, first forgive anyone you are holding a grudge against, so that your Father in heaven will forgive you your sins too."

God sets the perfect example for us because He forgives us our sins and shortcomings. He does this, however, only after we have made an effort to make direct amends to other people in our own lives. This throws a new light into why our lives have been so defeated in the past, as we held on tightly to our grudges. Making things right must begin with us.

2 Corinthians 5:19 "For God was in Christ, restoring the world to himself, no longer counting men's sins against them but blotting them out."

When we learn to forgive others, we must also learn to forgive ourselves. This is the hardest assignment yet! And if He has blotted out our sins, who are we to keep making mention of them? If we insist upon beating ourselves up, we not only snub Christ's great sacrifice for us but we will also stay defeated. This is not God's plan for us.

Colossians 1:20–21 "It was through what his Son did that God cleared a path for everything to come to him...for Christ's death on the cross has made peace with God for all by his blood. This includes you who were once so far away from God. You were his enemies and hated him and were separated from him by your evil thoughts and actions, yet now he has brought you back as his friends."

We, of all people, are now counted as God's friends. Through His Son, we are reconciled to Him. Even though we were total renegades at one time, filled with deceit and hating our brothers, He brings us back to Him if we will only be willing to make amends and sincerely ask with a humble and contrite heart to do so.

OVERCOMERS OUTREACH

Step Ten

"Continued to take personal inventory, and when we were wrong, promptly admitted it."

We've only just begun. We now need to keep repeating the process of taking a candid look at our lives and writing mini-inventories. Now that our record has been cleared by Christ, we need to keep it obstacle-free in order to keep the joy flowing. Our new-found serenity can't afford any more resentments. When we realize we err, the faster we can admit it and ask forgiveness, the freer we will be.

What the Bible Says About Step 10

Psalm 19:12 "But how can I ever know what sins are lurking in my heart? Cleanse me from these hidden faults. And keep me from deliberate wrongs; help me to stop doing them. Only then can I be free of guilt...."

The psalmist knew how hard it was to break a pattern of destruction, but it can be done with His power. Continuing the process of being honest, open, and willing to follow the simple program of life that He designed for us, we stay focused on Him. And the more we chip away, the more that is revealed. He's even promised that we can be free from the guilt that has plagued us for years.

1 Corinthians 10:12 "So be careful. If you are thinking, 'Oh, I would never behave like that!' Let this be a warning to you. For you too may fall into sin. But remember this—the wrong desires that come into your life aren't anything new and different. Many others have faced exactly the same problems before you."

We are admonished that just because we have made the decision to give our wills and lives to Christ, it doesn't mean that life won't eventually have its roadblocks and disappointments. We need to be ready. The very minute we begin to feel powerful again and neglect our 12-step support groups, we may begin to relapse into our old, destructive ways of thinking and behaving. If so, we must take immediate action with the tools God

THE 12 STEPS COME A-L-I-V-E IN THE SCRIPTURES

has given us—they are always there for us! That's why they say in AA, "Keep coming back—it works!"

STEP ELEVEN

"Sought through prayer and meditation to improve our conscious contact with God as we understood Him, praying only for knowledge of His will for us and the power to carry that out."

In order to put God's power to work in our lives, we need to seek the Lord in regular prayer, also listening for His guidance day by day. Taking time to do this may be difficult to fit into our busy schedules, but being on good speaking terms with God can make all the difference in how our day goes. It can determine whether or not we will "use" or drink today; it may decide how we will react to the people we're worried about today. We may have long lists of wants, but seeking His will for us, whatever that might be, is putting our lives in the palm of His almighty hand. Asking for power to carry out His will in our lives keeps us in tune with Him, and on track in this process of recovery.

WHAT THE BIBLE SAYS ABOUT STEP ELEVEN

Proverbs 2:3–5 "...If you want better insight and discernment, and are searching for them as you would for lost money or hidden treasure, then wisdom will be given you, and knowledge of God himself; you will soon learn the importance of reverence for the Lord and of trusting him."

We find that more shall be revealed as we travel along this recovery road. But it depends upon the amount of effort we put into connecting with our "Higher Power," experiencing His presence every day in all of our activities. All He wants from us is a humble and contrite heart; He does the rest.

OVERCOMERS OUTREACH

Psalm 1:2 "But they delight in doing everything God wants them to, and day and night are always meditating on his laws and thinking about ways to follow him more closely."

Spiritual growth doesn't happen overnight. It's a process of working the Steps and meditating upon God's Word, taking as long as it needs to take. Yet we never graduate. We find peace just being on this journey of discovery with Him by our side.

James 5:13 "Is anyone among you suffering? He should keep on praying about it. And those who have reason to be thankful should continually be singing praises to the Lord."

Have we given up on praying because our prayers haven't been answered yet? The Bible says to keep on praying. God does answer prayer, but in His way, in His time. We can have a lot more serenity for ourselves by just having an attitude of gratitude, and lifting our praises to Him who has restored us to a new life.

Romans 8:26 "...By our faith—the Holy Spirit helps us with our daily problems and in our praying. For we don't even know what we should pray for, nor how to pray as we should; but the Holy Spirit prays for us with such feeling that it cannot be expressed in words."

Sometimes we simply don't know how to pray. Not to worry. God understands our stammerings because He looks upon our heart. His Holy Spirit does the work; we just need to rely upon Him and quit trying to be so powerful ourselves.

Colossians 3:16 "Remember what Christ taught and let his words enrich your lives and make you wise; teach them to each other and sing them out in psalms and hymns and spiritual songs, singing to the Lord with thankful hearts."

God seems to love thanksgiving and praise. How can we not praise Him after all He is doing for us? Taking time to do this lifts our spirits and keeps us in contact with His presence.

THE 12 STEPS COME A-L-I-V-E IN THE SCRIPTURES

STEP TWELVE

"Having had a spiritual awakening as the result of these steps, we tried to carry this message to alcoholics and to practice these principles in all our affairs."

Our eyes have been opened. We seem to see things in a different perspective, as God shines His light upon our daily path. The 12 Steps have taken us through some hard places but have released us from bondage and restored our lives! Just when we thought we had no hope, God stepped in when we invited Him and did miracles. We become so excited about the changes in our lives that we are compelled to share this message of hope with others who are still struggling. And we put these principles to work in our lives, over and over again. They work—when we work them.

WHAT THE BIBLE SAYS ABOUT STEP TWELVE

1 Peter 3:15 "Quietly trust yourself to Christ your Lord and if anybody asks why you believe as you do, be ready to tell him, and do it in a gentle and respectful way."

We don't need to hold street meetings and preach about our faith, although sometimes we would like to shout it from the housetops! But we can be ready to share our experience, strength, and hope with others as He brings them into our daily walk. God wants us to do this in a gentle and respectful way. We are free to share, but also to live and let live.

Isaiah 61:1 "The Spirit of the Lord God is upon me, because the Lord has anointed me to bring good news to the suffering and afflicted. He has sent me to comfort the broken-hearted, to announce liberty to captives and to open the eyes of the blind."

How blind we have been in the past! We can hardly wait to tell others that our sight has not only returned, but that we see more clearly than ever before. By sharing ourselves, we may be a source of comfort to those who are hurting desperately.

> *Psalm 96:2–4 "...Each day tell someone that he saves. Publish his glorious acts throughout the earth. Tell everyone about the amazing things he does. For the Lord is great beyond description, and greatly to be praised."*

Not a day goes by that we don't witness some miracle, whether large or small. We can't keep these things to ourselves because it would be selfish. We find that we can't keep it unless we are willing to give it away.

> *Galatians 6:1 "Dear brothers, if a Christian is overcome by some sin, you who are godly should gently and humbly help him back onto the right path, remembering that next time it might be one of you who is in the wrong."*

Even though we think we're completely recovered, we also know how fast we can become "unrecovered"! It may just take one drink or fix to get us going on that downward spiral again. Keeping this in mind, we are in a much better position to share our faith with others.

> *2 Corinthians 1:3–4 "What a wonderful God we have—he is the Father of our Lord Jesus Christ, the source of every mercy, and the one who so wonderfully comforts and strengthens us in our hardships and trials. And why does he do this? So that when others are troubled, needing our sympathy and encouragement, we can pass on to them this same help and comfort God has given us."*

Why have we been through all this? It may have been a difficult road we have traveled with our addictions and compulsions, taking us right down to the bottom. Yet today, in recovery, we are in a position of carrying the message of hope to others who may still be suffering. What a privilege! We dare not be quiet about all that God has done for us!

As we continue to apply the God-given tools of the 12 Steps and Scriptures to our lives on a daily basis, life can become an exciting adventure of discovery and a joyous celebration of victory in Christ.

The Serenity Prayer

God, grant me the
Serenity to accept the things
I cannot change;
Courage to change the things
I can; and
Wisdom to know the difference.
Living one day at a time,
enjoying one moment at a time;
accepting hardship
as the pathway to peace;
Taking as He did, this sinful
world as it is,
not as I would have it;
Trusting that He will make all
things right if I surrender
to His will;
That I may be reasonably happy in this life,
and supremely happy with Him forever in the next. Amen

Reinhold Niebuhr[1]

APPENDIX A : OVERCOMERS OUTREACH PUBLICATIONS

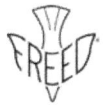

Booklets

    FREED booklet (English, Russian, Spanish, Large Print)
    FREED ACA - Adult Children of Alcoholics
    TNT - Tried N True Teens
    FREED SH - Sex addicts Healed God's way
    OK Kids (ages 5–12)
    HIM Leader Guide
    HIM Step Study Guide
    Steps, Standards, and Traditions Study Guide

Information Pamphlets

    Alcoholism: Sin or Sickness?
    Better Choices for Teens (and Others)
    Chemically Dependent Christian
    Circus of Codependency
    Cocaine/Crack: The Silent Killer
    Disease Chart of Alcoholism
    Does Someone You Love Drink Too Much?
    Dying for a Smoke
    A Personal Letter of Hope from a FREED Homosexual
    Food: Friend or Foe

OVERCOMERS OUTREACH

Group Traditions
Heroin
Higher Power
Hooked on Prescription Pills
Intervention
Letting Go of My Adult Son or Daughter
Marijuana Maze
Methamphetamine Addiction
Practicing Principles
Sexual Addiction in the Church?
Sponsorship
Surrender - Steps 1, 2, 3
Cleaning House - Steps 4, 5, 6
Restoration - Steps 7, 8, 9
Progress - Steps 10, 11, 12
The 5 R's of ACA/DF
12 Steps and Corresponding Scriptures
Which One Is the Alcoholic
Winning Over Gambling Addiction
Working the Steps
Sharing Jesus with My 12-Step Friends
OO introductory brochure

APPENDIX B : INTERNATIONAL MINISTRY

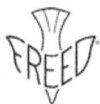

Starting with one small support group in Bob and Pauline's home in California in 1977, Overcomers Outreach became a ministry that encircled the globe. In the United States alone over a thousand Overcomers Outreach Christ-centered support groups were developed in every state. We are also aware that many more groups meet in prisons, treatment centers, sober living houses, rescue missions, and private homes.

Overcomers Outreach Canada, Inc., started in Winnipeg, Manitoba, in 1995 with one group. From that small beginning, it has slowly expanded and matured into eight groups in just the Winnipeg area, as well as twenty or so other groups in other locations across Canada, and their Web site, www.overcomersoutreach.ca, serves the area.

In 1992, Overcomers Outreach was starting in the United Kingdom as well. Thanks to the efforts of a few dedicated individuals, groups started in London and Glasgow and soon spread to Surrey, Essex, Bournemouth, and Belfast. In 2006 the groups began developing OO/UK/EU, and started a Web site, www.overcomersoutreach.co.uk, to serve much of Europe as well as the U.K.

Overcomers Outreach in Germany began in 1997 after God brought Rolf P. in contact with an English friend, Bob T., from Salisbury. Bob sent some Christian booklets and a Bible, and Rolf made his first book translations. In August 1998, Bob sent Rolf the message of OO along with a group starter kit. On June 12, 1999, in Salisbury, England, the first European OO Intergroup meeting was held. Then in 2004, their long-desired dream

OVERCOMERS OUTREACH

of getting online with a German homepage of OO, www.c12undc12.net, became a reality, serving the German speaking nations of Europe. Other European countries that have OO groups include Austria, Italy, Czech Republic, and Spain. Members in Sweden established a Web site, www.overcomersoutreach.se, and have translated some literature to Swedish. OO groups can also be found in China, the Philippines, Russia, Mexico, New Zealand, Malawi, Uganda, Liberia, and South Africa.

Overcomers started in Australia in 2005 as a result of a visit to a group in London earlier that year by Penny W. Groups are meeting regularly in the Sydney and Melbourne areas, and the Web site www.overcomersoutreach.net serves the Australia area.

Requests for group starter kits and information continue to be received at the OO Central Office from all over the world, and the message of Christ's delivering power is spreading through Overcomers around the globe.

APPENDIX C: REFERRALS FOR RECOVERY

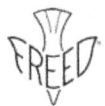

Adult Children of Alcoholics / Central Service Board
P.O. Box 3216 / Torrance, California 90510 / (310)534-1815
adultchildren.org

Al-Anon / Alateen Family Group Headquarters
1600 Corporate Landing Parkway / Virginia Beach, VA 23454-5617
(757)563-1600
al-anon. org

Alcoholics Anonymous
P.O. Box 459 / Grand Central Station / New York, NY 10163
(212)870-3400
aa.org

Cocaine Anonymous
P.O. Box 492000 / Los Angeles, California 90049-8000 / (310)559-5833
www.ca.org

Codependents Anonymous
P.O. Box 33577 / Phoenix, AZ 85087-3577 / (602)277-7991
www.codependents.org

OVERCOMERS OUTREACH

Debtors Anonymous
P.O. Box 920888 / Needham, MA 02492-0009 / (800)421-2383
debtorsanonymous.org

Emotions Anonymous
P.O. Box 4245 / St. Paul, MN 55104 / (651)647-9712
emotionsanonymous.org

Families Anonymous
P.O. Box 3475 / Culver City, California 90231 / (800)736-9805

Gamblers Anonymous
P.O.Box 17173 / Los Angeles, California 90017 / (213)386-8789

Narcotics Anonymous / World Service Office
16155 Wyandotte St. / Van Nuys, California 91406 / (818)787-9706

Overcomers Outreach, USA:
6528 Greenleaf Ave., Ste. 223 / Whittier, California 90601 /
(800)310-3001 info@overcomersoutreach.org
overcomersoutreach.org

Overcomers Outreach, Canada:
844J McLeod Avenue, Winnipeg, MB, Canada, R2G 2T7.
(204)589-3684
(866) 881-2480 (toll-free)
Info@overcomersoutreach.ca
overcomersoutreach.ca

Overcomers Outreach, Germany
c12undc12.net

Overcomers Outreach, Sweden
overcomersoutreach.se

Overcomers Outreach, U.K.
overcomersoutreach.co.uk

APPENDIX C

Overcomers Outreach, Australia
overcomersoutreach.net

Overeaters Anonymous / World Service Office
P.O. Box 44020 / Rio Rancho, NM 87174 / (505)891-2664
oa.org

Sex Addicts Anonymous
P.O. Box 70949 / Houston, TX 77270 / (800)477-8191
saa-recovery.org

Sexaholics Anonymous / Central Service Office
P.O. Box 3565 / Brentwood, TN 37024 / (866)424-8777
sa.org

Sex and Love Addicts Anonymous
1550 NE Loop 410, Ste 118 / San Antonio, TX 78209
slaawfs.org

ENDNOTES

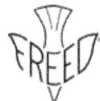

Chapter 1: Beyond Recovery into Discovery

1. *Webster's New Concise Dictionary, Revised Edition* (New York: Modern Publishing, 1987), p. 257.
2. Ibid, p. 90.

Chapter 3: The Founders: Bob's Story

1. *Alcoholics Anonymous, the Story of How Many Thousands of Men and Women Have Recovered from Alcoholism*, 3rd ed. (New York: Alcoholics Anonymous World Services, 1976), pp. 58–59. Reprinted with permission.
2. Ibid, p. 62. Reprinted with permission.
3. Michael Bartosch, "Alcoholism and the Family," monograph while a student at California Lutheran University, 1975, p. 53.

Chapter 5: Bridging the Gap

1. *Twelve Steps and Twelve Traditions* (New York: Alcoholics Anonymous World Services, 1952), pp. 30–31. Reprinted with permission.
2. Ibid, pp. 31–32. Reprinted with permission.

Chapter 6: Birth of a Ministry

1. Jacqueline Weir, "Finding God Through the Twelve Step Programs and the Psalter," *Valyermo Benedictine*, Vol. 2, No. 3, fall 1991, p. 34.
2. *Alcoholics Anonymous*, op. cit., pp. 58–59. Reprinted with permission.
3. Bill W., *Language of the Heart* (New York: AA Grapevine, 1988), pp. 201–202. Copyright (c) by The AA Grapevine, Inc.; reprinted with permission.
4. Bill Pittman, *AA: The Way It Began* (Seattle: Glen Abbey Books, 1988), pp. 184–185.
5. Catherine Marshall, *Beyond Ourselves* (New York: McGraw-Hill, 1961), p. 65.
6. J. Keith Miller, in lecture at Overcomers Outreach conference "Discovery '92."

Chapter 7: From the Pastor: Heart-Mending as the Church's Task

1. Gary Smalley and John Trent, Ph.D., *The Blessing* (Nashville: Thomas Nelson Publishers, 1986), p. 35.

Chapter 8: From the Physician: Healing Body, Mind, and Spirit

1. Stephen Arterburn, *Growing Up Addicted* (New York: Ballantine Books, 1987), p. 65.
2. *Which One Is the Alcoholic?* (Overcomers Outreach, 1992), p. 2.
3. Ibid, p. 5.
4. Anderson Spickard, M.D., *Dying for a Drink* (Waco: Word Books, 1985), p. 41.
5. Ibid, p. 43.
6. *Which One Is the Alcoholic?*, op. cit., p. 3.
7. Ibid, pp. 3, 4.

Chapter 41: From the Heart of an ACA

1. Janet Wotitz, *Adult Children of Alcoholics* (Hollywood, FL, Health Communications, Inc., p.4, 7th printing 1983).

ENDNOTES

Chapter 44: The Heart of Overcomers Outreach

1. Bob and Pauline Bartosch, *FREED* (Overcomers Outreach, Inc., 1992), pp. 7–8.
2. Terry W., "Honesty," Community Informer (Yorba Linda, California,: Community Baptist Church, 1990), p. 4.
3. Bob and Pauline Bartosch, op. cit., pp. 11–12.
4. *Alcoholics Anonymous*, op. cit., pp. 59–60. Reprinted with permission.
5. Ibid, pp. 83–84. Reprinted with permission.

Chapter 45: The 12 Steps Come A-L-I-V-E in the Scriptures

1. Bob and Pauline Bartosch, op. cit., p. 49.

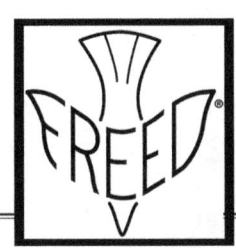

To order additional copies of this book call:
1-800-310-3001
or please visit our Web site at
www.overcomersoutreach.org

Printed in the USA
CPSIA information can be obtained
at www.ICGtesting.com
CBHW021935020424
6252CB00002B/6